Mental Health in the Digital Age

MENTAL HEALTH IN THE DIGITAL AGE
GRAVE DANGERS, GREAT PROMISE

Edited by
Elias Aboujaoude
and
Vladan Starcevic

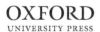

OXFORD
UNIVERSITY PRESS

UNIVERSITY PRESS

Oxford University Press is a department of the University of
Oxford. It furthers the University's objective of excellence in research,
scholarship, and education by publishing worldwide.

Oxford   New York
Auckland   Cape Town   Dar es Salaam   Hong Kong   Karachi
Kuala Lumpur   Madrid   Melbourne   Mexico City   Nairobi
New Delhi   Shanghai   Taipei   Toronto

With offices in
Argentina   Austria   Brazil   Chile   Czech Republic   France   Greece
Guatemala   Hungary   Italy   Japan   Poland   Portugal   Singapore
South Korea   Switzerland   Thailand   Turkey   Ukraine   Vietnam

Oxford is a registered trademark of Oxford University Press
in the UK and certain other countries.

Published in the United States of America by
Oxford University Press
198 Madison Avenue, New York, NY 10016

Library of Congress Cataloging-in-Publication Data
Mental health in the digital age : grave dangers, great promise / edited by Elias Aboujaoude &
Vladan Starcevic.
    p. ; cm.
Includes bibliographical references.
ISBN 978–0–19–938018–3
I. Aboujaoude, Elias, 1971, editor.   II. Starcevic, Vladan, editor.
[DNLM: 1. Impulsive Behavior.   2. Internet.   3. Behavioral Symptoms.
4. Psychotherapy—methods.   5. Telemedicine—methods.   6. Video Games—adverse effects.
WM 176]
RC569.5.I54
616.85′84—dc23
2014033993

9 8 7 6 5 4 3 2 1
Printed in the United States of America
on acid-free paper

Dr. Aboujaoude is cofounder of eTherapi, a telemental health platform. Dr. Starcevic discloses no relationships with commercial entities and professional activities that may bias his views.

Contents

Contributors

Elias Aboujaoude, MD, MA
Clinical Professor
Stanford University School of Medicine
Department of Psychiatry and
Behavioral Sciences
Stanford, California
United States

Craig A. Anderson, PhD
Distinguished Professor
Iowa State University
Department of Psychology
Ames, Iowa
United States

Gerhard Andersson, PhD
Professor
Linköping University
Department of Behavioral Sciences
and Learning
Linköping
Sweden
and
Karolinska Institute
Department of Clinical Neuroscience
Stockholm
Sweden

**David Berle, BA(Hons),
MPsychol(Clin), PhD**
Senior Clinical Psychologist
Nepean Blue Mountains Local
Health District
Nepean Anxiety Disorders Clinic
Penrith, New South Wales
Australia

Zsolt Demetrovics, PhD
Professor
Eötvös Loránd University
Institute of Psychology
Department of Clinical Psychology
and Addiction
Budapest
Hungary

**Lina Gega, PhD, BA(Hons),
BN(Hons), RMN, ENB(650)**
Reader in Mental Health
Northumbria University
Faculty of Health and Life Sciences
Newcastle upon Tyne
United Kingdom

**Simon Gilbody, DPhil, FRCPsych,
FRSA**
Professor of Psychological Medicine
and Health Services Research
University of York
Department of Health Sciences
and HYMS
Mental Health and Addiction
Research Group
York
United Kingdom

Mark D. Griffiths, PhD
Professor
Nottingham Trent University
Psychology Division
International Gaming Research Unit
Nottingham
United Kingdom

Christopher L. Groves, MS
Graduate Student
Iowa State University
Department of Psychology
Ames, Iowa
United States

Doug Hyun Han, MD, PhD
Associate Professor
Chung Ang University
School of Medicine
Department of Psychiatry
Seoul
South Korea

Keith M. Harris, PhD
Adjunct Senior Fellow
School of Psychology
The University of Queensland
St Lucia, Qld
Australia

Sarah E. Jones, MA
Doctoral Student
Arizona State University
Hugh Downs School of Human
Communication
Tempe, Kentucky
United States

Anthony F. Jorm, PhD, DSc
Professorial Fellow
University of Melbourne
Centre for Mental Health, Melbourne
School of Population and
Global Health
Parkville, Victoria
Australia

Sylvia Kauer, PhD
Post Doctoral Research Fellow
University of Melbourne
General Practice and Primary Health
Care Academic Centre
Carlton, Victoria
Australia

Sun Mi Kim, MD, PhD
Clinical Assistant Professor
Chung Ang University
School of Medicine
Department of Psychiatry
Seoul
South Korea

Orsolya Király, MA
Doctoral Student
Eötvös Loránd University
Institute of Psychology
Department of Clinical Psychology and
Addiction and
Doctoral School of Psychology
Budapest
Hungary

Beatrix Koronczai, PhD
Assistant Lecturer
Eötvös Loránd University
Institute of Psychology
Department of Developmental and
Clinical Child Psychology
Budapest
Hungary

Eric Malbos, MD, PhD
Physician and Virtual Reality Exposure
Therapy Specialist
University Hospital of Sainte
Marguerite
Department of Medical Psychology
Marseille
France

Jeffrey G. Miller, DNP, ACRN, APNP
Assistant Professor
Medical College of Wisconsin
Department of Psychiatry and
Behavioral Medicine
Milwaukee, Wisconsin
United States

Katalin Nagygyörgy, MA
Doctoral Student
Eötvös Loránd University
Institute of Psychology
Department of Clinical Psychology
and Addiction
Budapest
Hungary

David J. Peterson, MBA, FACMPE
Administrator
Medical College of Wisconsin
Department of Psychiatry and
Behavioral Medicine
Milwaukee, Wisconsin
United States

Halley M. Pontes, BSc (Psychology),
MSc (Clinical Psychology)
Doctoral Student
Nottingham Trent University
Psychology Division
International Gaming Research Unit
Nottingham
United Kingdom

Nicola J. Reavley, PhD
Senior Research Fellow
University of Melbourne
Centre for Mental Health
Melbourne School of Population and
Global Health
Parkville, Victoria
Australia

Sophie C. Reid, MPsych (Clinical), PhD
Honorary Research Fellow and Clinical
Psychologist
Murdoch Children's Research Institute
Parkville, Victoria
Australia

Matthew W. Savage, PhD
Assistant Professor
University of Kentucky
Department of Communication
Lexington, Kentucky
United States

Vladan Starcevic, MD, PhD,
FRANZCP
Associate Professor of Psychiatry
University of Sydney
Sydney Medical School—Nepean
Discipline of Psychiatry
Sydney
Australia

Robert S. Tokunaga, PhD
Assistant Professor
University of Hawaii at Manoa
Department of Communicology
Honolulu, Hawaii
United States

Aviv Weinstein, PhD
Senior Lecturer
University of Ariel
Israel
and
Senior Research Fellow
Department of Nuclear Medicine
Tel Aviv Sourasky Medical Center
Tel Aviv
Israel

Introduction: www (dot) Mental Health

Elias Aboujaoude and Vladan Starcevic

The Internet and related technologies have reconfigured every aspect of life, and mental health has not been immune to these changes. Although much has been written about electronic challenges to psychological well-being (e.g., violent video games) and seeming digital wonders (e.g., online therapy), a balanced look at the field—one that celebrates the "good" and acknowledges the "bad"—has been elusive, with most scholars firmly planting themselves in one camp or the other. With the lack of cross-talk between the two sides nearly as old as the Internet itself, the time is ripe for an objective, comprehensive assessment of the intersection between mental health and digital technology. It is very much in this spirit that we conceived of *Mental Health in the Digital Age: Grave Dangers, Great Promise* and assembled its expert contributors. A result of reading the book, we hope, will be a nuanced appreciation of the opportunity, risk, and all-round complex richness brought about by this unique collision.

RISKS AND CHALLENGES

The first section of the book focuses on the menace to psychological well-being from the growing reliance on, and misuse of, digital technology, and on the ways in which some old forms of problematic or deviant behavior have been shaped by this technology and some new psychopathologies have been introduced. Since the first reports of "Internet addiction" emerged in the mid-1990s, much research has accumulated into the phenomenology, course, and pathophysiology of this condition. In Chapter 1, Aviv Weinstein and Elias Aboujaoude review that research, offering an up-to-date picture of the conceptualization; etiological factors; epidemiology; course; coexisting psychopathology and health problems; associated personality, social, family and cognitive factors; and psychotherapeutic and psychopharmacological treatment of problematic Internet use. The authors also address the controversies and shifting diagnostic definitions that have plagued the field since its inception and conclude that although knowledge has increased exponentially, there are many unresolved issues that call for further research.

Although problematic video game use shares some similarities with problematic Internet use, it would be too simplistic to treat them interchangeably as many studies and publications too often have. The Internet is typically a medium for obtaining information, enhancing communication and fostering a wide variety of pursuits (e.g., social, sexual, consumerist). Video games, on the other hand, are approached primarily for diversion purposes, and the potentially time-consuming activity that the player engages in tends to be more repetitive and circumscribed in scope than the activities of those who are excessive Internet users. By dedicating a separate chapter by Mark Griffiths and colleagues to an in-depth overview of problematic video game use (Chapter 2), we highlight the importance of differentiating among the various digital activities that occupy online life, because their effects on the person's psyche and their habit-forming potential may differ.

Whether it is a person's Internet or video game use that is of concern, the changing diagnostic definitions, lack of guidance from the diagnostic and classification systems, plethora of online self-diagnosis tools, and dearth of psychometrically sound scales can hinder the clinician's work and confound the data. Chapter 3 by Orsolya Király and colleagues discusses the best tools available to navigate the process of making diagnoses and help draw a clearer line between pathological and adaptive technology use in a technology-dominated world, where some degree of "overuse" seems inescapable. Adhering to those tools will empower clinicians in the art of proper diagnosis and allow for more consistency and better comparisons among research studies.

Neuroimaging is an increasingly popular technique used to shed more light on psychopathology. In Chapter 4, on the neurobiology of problematic Internet and video game use, Sun Mi Kim and Doug Hyun Han provide a thorough review of research in this advanced modality and discuss neurophysiological and genetic aspects. Despite the considerable controversy that still accompanies psychopathology related to excessive Internet use and online gaming, there now exists difficult-to-ignore evidence of biological changes happening in the brain as a result of this new type of human-screen interaction. Rather than dismiss it, it behooves us to try to understand the behaviors behind it and mitigate their negative effects—in other words, to take an approach similar to substance use disorders and impulse control disorders, where similar neurobiological findings have been documented.

Many of us use various technological gadgets to also engage in angry interactions on anonymous blogs, watch gory videos on YouTube, or play violent video games. Violence, especially as depicted and sometimes celebrated and rewarded in video games, has raised particular concerns. Due to the interactive nature of new technologies, the aggression we "practice" virtually might have more offline repercussions than "new" exposure to violence that accompanied every other new media platform from radio to movies to television. In Chapter 5, Christopher Groves and Craig Anderson make an impassioned, data-driven argument that video game violence does lead to increased offline aggression and that energy spent disputing that causality would be better spent mitigating the well-documented and disturbing effects of that link.

Chapters 6, 7, and 8 discuss the effects of the modern technology on certain aberrant behaviors and psychiatric conditions. Thus, the clinical presentation of hypochondriasis—a disorder well described several centuries ago—has been transformed by the information revolution. Instead of consulting books and various printed media, people with health anxiety are now more likely to go to "Dr. Google" and exhibit a behavioral pattern known as cyberchondria. In a chapter devoted to this phenomenon, Vladan Starcevic and David Berle present cyberchondria as an excessive or repeated search for health-related information on the Internet and conceptualize it as a failed reassurance-seeking behavior. In other words, instead of decreasing anxiety or distress about health, cyberchondria only exacerbates it. The chapter also discusses conceptual and theoretical issues related to cyberchondria and ways of preventing and alleviating it.

Cyberbullying is an aggressive behavior born out of the new interaction between humans and technology, and one that has been described as an epidemic among young individuals. Bullying is a well-known problem, but cyberbullying differs in important ways, as Matthew Savage and colleagues explain in their chapter. One distinguishing feature is a new dynamic between victim and perpetrator that allows for a "revenge of the nerds," where technological savviness can replace physical strength as a determinant of power or control. Another characteristic of cyberbullying is the difficulty to protect oneself given how the Internet's penetrance makes potential targets much more reachable and at practically all times. New awareness, public health tools, and specific interventions are therefore proposed to prevent cyberbullying and help the casualties of this problem, both among victims and perpetrators.

The first section of the book ends with a chapter by Keith Harris that analyzes the suicide landscape as reconfigured by the Internet. Although online suicide pacts, webcam suicides, and step-by-step "how-to" prosuicide sites may hog the media's attention, this chapter provides a thorough review of the research behind the sensationalism. The author delves in a data-driven manner into what he calls the "suicidal mind, online" to explicate the high stakes, vulnerabilities, and thought processes behind Googling "suicide." His conclusion is an optimistic one, fortunately. As he compares, with numbers, statistics, and personal observations, the state of "cybersuicide" today to a decade ago, he is hopeful that online-based treatments, sophisticated outreach efforts and increased awareness will prevail, eventually making the Internet and related technologies more a deterrent than an enabler when it comes to suicide.

OPPORTUNITIES AND PROMISES

The optimistic note that the cybersuicide discussion ends on is a good transition to the second section of the book, devoted to the brighter side of the digital revolution and its pro–mental health effects. This section begins with Chapter 9 on psychoeducation and the Internet, written by Nicola Reavley and Anthony Jorm. Obtaining adequate information is a starting point for most interventions in mental health. This chapter shows how difficult it has been to provide high-quality information on psychiatric disorders online and, even more so, how the attempts to categorize mental health websites on the basis of their quality have encountered numerous obstacles. Nevertheless, there has been progress in terms of improving the content of these websites and recognizing the more reliable sources of online information, which makes it easier to access adequate information on the Internet. Encouragingly, there is also emerging evidence that use of mental health websites may lead to better outcomes by promoting knowledge, changing unhelpful attitudes, and abandoning maladaptive behaviors.

Chapter 10 by Gerhard Andersson reviews the booming field of online psychotherapy. The Internet dissolves distances, including those between patient and care provider; this increases access to crucial mental health care, especially for rural patients, those with mobility difficulties, or individuals whose work and life circumstances do not allow them to get to a therapist's office within the workday. Also, the Internet may help confront issues such as stigma and social anxiety that often prevent patients from seeking care. These potential advantages of online therapy may be familiar, but the number of positive controlled efficacy trials reviewed in this chapter may surprise some readers. These pertain primarily to online therapy with minimal therapist involvement but, also, to online therapy conducted in real time with full therapist participation (with or without webcam). Together, the data across several psychiatric diagnoses point to a revolution that is well underway in the provision of psychotherapy.

Although online psychotherapy, including cognitive-behavioral therapy, incorporates some degree of live therapist involvement, computerized cognitive-behavioral therapy refers to a technology-enabled psychotherapy that essentially bypasses the therapist altogether beyond involvement in the initial stages of designing a computer program. An advantage of some therapies is that they can be "manualized" (i.e., described in a step-by-step fashion) to ensure consistent application across a broad range of symptoms and situations, as Lina Gega and Simon Gilbody explain in Chapter 11. Computerized cognitive-behavioral therapy further standardizes therapy delivery, which can greatly democratize access to treatment; in a world where demand for psychotherapy services outstrips supply, that can be a true gift. The chapter also takes a much-needed critical look at the advantages and disadvantages of computerized cognitive-behavioral therapy, including its cost-effectiveness.

At the intersection of advanced technology capabilities and mental health needs lies the new field of virtual reality exposure therapy. In Chapter 12, Eric Malbos introduces us to the dramatic new tools available to the 21st-century therapist: head-mounted displays, motion trackers, and data gloves, which are all meant to allow patients to interact efficiently and realistically with three-dimensional representations of their worst fears or with disorder-specific stimuli. The theory of habituation and extinction by which exposure therapy is thought to achieve its goals in "real life" is shown to work in virtual environments as well. The chapter reviews trials of virtual reality exposure therapy in various anxiety and other disorders and points to advantages of this therapy in terms of decreased time and cost and improved access. With technology becoming more affordable, the assumption that the equipment for virtual reality exposure therapy is too expensive no longer holds, and its "mainstreaming" can be expected in the coming years.

If Internet-based therapy or virtual reality exposure therapy feels revolutionary, consider therapy by means of the cell phone. In Chapter 13 on mobile therapy, Sylvia Kauer and Sophie Reid explain how mental health apps have become the latest manifestation of a digital revolution gone mobile. Apps that track mood, sleep, energy level, and various symptoms in real time are gaining in popularity, and early research suggests that they can increase awareness of the symptom being tracked and lead to measurable symptom improvements. In addition, mobile therapy can include text messages with appointment and medication reminders, self-motivating content and soothing narratives that help reduce anxiety during offline exposure homework. As such, mobile therapy can be useful across a range of psychiatric disorders and presents rich opportunities for research, including the ability to assess wellness as a function of location and better contextualize symptoms and treatment response. With further studies, highly personalized interventions can result.

Whether or not they are based on the latest technology, the therapeutic encounters and interventions have to be documented confidentially and accurately by the clinician or researcher. Radical change is afoot there, too, as the patient chart, that cornerstone of medical practice, gets rewritten in pixels. Chapter 14, the last chapter of the book, written by David Peterson and Jeffrey Miller, is devoted to electronic medical records. The authors explain the pressures motivating the move away from paper records and the many advantages and disadvantages of such a move to the mental health field in particular, where privacy and security concerns may loom even larger and where seemingly inevitable network breeches may be even more ominous. There are also uncertain effects of using electronic mental health records on the quality of the patient-therapist relationship—will the laptop lead the patient to withhold crucial information or cause the therapist to seem aloof or disinterested due to diminished eye contact? Clinicians need to understand how these concerns and issues can be addressed effectively before feeling comfortable with the modern technology encroaching on this aspect of their practice.

PUTTING IT ALL TOGETHER

This description of the book provides a glimpse of an emerging field that has a certain future. Although we do not know exactly how that future will unfold, the trends presented here are clear. Also, the book is written by authors from eight countries and four continents, which demonstrates that in a globalized world many issues are surprisingly similar.

One common denominator to the "negative" aspects of an encounter between digital technology and mental health presented in the first part of the book is that they have been emphasized and sometimes promoted by the popular media. This is not surprising, because the media has an insatiable appetite for everything that is novel and makes for a "good story," especially if the consequences are melodramatic. However, mental health professionals and researchers need to be careful not to fall for hype and, for example, espouse a view that the Internet and related technology are the root of so much evil. Likewise, mass media should not "lead the way" and fill the vacuum by setting their own agenda for action. In fact, much of the controversy stems from the discrepancy between sometimes desperate calls for action by the media and the less strident stance of clinicians and researchers. Authors of the chapters in the first part of the book take this into account and focus on the evidence whenever it is available, while acknowledging the importance of the phenomena that they address. No wonder their approach is cautious; they point to the conceptual and methodological obstacles to research, as driving their measured and somewhat tentative conclusions. Also, they all call for more studies instead of sensational reporting and unproductive, quarrelsome debates.

Popular media are much less interested in psychological therapies and in the way that they have been modified by the modern technologies. The source of the controversy surrounding the "positive" side of the encounter between digital technology and mental health lies elsewhere. The notion that computers, the Internet, virtual reality environments, and even smartphones can decrease the need for traditional therapists or perhaps make them obsolete has been met with significant resistance. Although such ideas have been embraced by public health figures and administrators, especially in view of the promise of improved access to care and decreased cost of mental health services, many mental health professionals have remained suspicious, probably due to a sense that the foundation of their professional identity is being jeopardized by these modern technologies. However, as the second part of the book shows, no one needs to feel triumphant or threatened. Evidence suggests that within a stepped care or an alternative health model, everyone could potentially gain from embracing aspects of modern technology in psychotherapy delivery. For that to happen, further research needs to establish more clearly what type of therapy is most suitable for which individuals, which disorders, and under what circumstances.

In summary, it would be misleading to describe the Internet and related technologies as inherently "good" or "bad" for mental health. As we hope the book will demonstrate, a plethora of data support the argument that, rather than having a unidirectional effect of the modern technologies, much positive and negative can happen, and is indeed happening, at the intersection of mental health and digital life. Continued fragmentation of Internet mental health research reinforces a rift between the "pro" and "con" camps. It does a disservice to the field and slows down the pace of research progress when the pace of technology development is showing no signs of slowing down. This much is clear—the digital revolution is here to stay, and so are its mental health consequences, both positive and negative. The coming together within this book of experts with pointedly divergent interests and points of view to take stock of where we are and where we may be headed is an effort we are proud of. We hope it will start a much-needed dialogue among scholars, clinicians, students and policy makers across the wired globe.

DISCLOSURE STATEMENT

Dr. Aboujaoude is cofounder of eTherapi, a telemental health platform. Dr. Starcevic discloses no relationships with commercial entities and professional activities that may bias his views.

SECTION I
CHALLENGES

1 Problematic Internet Use

An Overview

Aviv Weinstein and Elias Aboujaoude

INTRODUCTION

As the Internet increasingly permeates home, school, and work lives, overuse or misuse of this technology can be expected to lead to marital, academic, and job-related problems (Young, 2004, 2007; Yellowlees and Marks, 2007). Indeed, with expansion of the Internet over the past 15 years, a potentially pathological side to online life has gradually become more apparent, attracting the attention of researchers, clinicians, and the popular media (Young, 1998; Griffiths, 1998, 2000; Shaw and Black, 2008; Aboujaoude, 2010). Many designations have been given to this problem, including "Internet addiction disorder," "compulsive Internet use," "pathological Internet use," and "problematic Internet use." This last term will be adopted in this review, although it has to be acknowledged that with increased connectivity and with the advent of smartphones, it is almost impossible to separate Internet use from other online activities, such as video game playing and texting. This is why some scholars have advocated for another designation that is more inclusive and may be more relevant—"pathological use of electronic media" (Aboujaoude, 2010).

This chapter will cover the evolution, controversies, and advances in the concept of problematic Internet use (PIU). It will describe its prevalence and phenomenology, including demographic, psychosocial, and cognitive features, and will review its coexistence with other psychiatric disorders and personality dimensions. Finally, it will address psychotherapeutic and psychopharmacological interventions as they have been studied to date. To the extent allowed by the literature, the focus will be on PIU, with problematic video game use addressed elsewhere (see Chapter 2), even if most studies have not made a clear distinction among the various time-consuming activities individuals can pursue online.

DIAGNOSTIC DEFINITIONS

At least three different models have been proposed for PIU (Grant et al., 2010; Weinstein and Lejoyeux, 2010, 2013). Some have considered it part of the obsessive-compulsive spectrum of disorders, in that there is a similarity between obsessive-compulsive disorder (OCD) and the intrusive, anxious urge to repetitively check one's e-mail or Facebook page or repetitively play an online video game. This model is supported by some preliminary pharmacological treatment studies with selective serotonin reuptake inhibitors (SSRIs) (Dell'Osso et al., 2006, 2007). PIU has also been conceptualized as an impulse control disorder, characterized by the urge to repeatedly engage in a behavior—going online—that is pleasurable in the moment but can lead to negative downstream effects (Aboujaoude, 2010). A third conceptualization for PIU is as a "behavioral addiction" similar to a substance use disorder (Han et al., 2009). That is suggested by the presence of withdrawal-like and tolerance-like features in PIU as well as by the individual's continued use of the Internet despite adverse consequences—all of which are often seen in substance addiction.

Another matter of debate is whether PIU is a truly discrete psychopathological entity or a manifestation of an underlying disorder. The frequent appearance alongside PIU of numerous other conditions can certainly raise complex questions of causality. Indeed, it has been argued (Pies, 2009) that based on the limited available data regarding course, prognosis, temporal stability, and response to treatment, it might be premature to consider PIU as an independent diagnosis and as such it should not be included in classifications of mental disorders. That, ultimately, was the decision of the *Diagnostic and Statistical Manual of Mental Disorders*, fifth edition (DSM-5) work group, which concluded that current research evidence did not support establishing a new diagnostic category for PIU. The work group moved from a broad conceptualization (along the lines of PIU) to a more narrow one, focusing primarily on pathological online gaming and avoiding use of the term "addiction." That is how Internet gaming disorder, which in many studies is subsumed under PIU (see Chapter 2), was mentioned in the DSM-5 (American Psychiatric Association, 2013), but only as a condition for further study, not an official DSM-5 diagnosis. Thus, the DSM-5 still does not offer sufficient guidance on how to approach individuals with suspected Internet-related psychopathology or how to design or interpret research studies into this topic. Instead, clinicians and researchers have to rely on proposed definitions, along with several screening and assessment instruments developed for PIU and problematic video game use (see Chapter 3).

As the name has caused debate, so have the various diagnostic definitions developed by researchers who believe that PIU is a real and potentially serious psychopathology. Most definitions, however, point to excessive, poorly controlled Internet-related preoccupations, urges, or behaviors that ultimately result in impairment or distress. Among the proposed criteria, four in particular were considered highly relevant to any DSM-5 definition (Block, 2008): (1) excessive Internet use, often associated with a loss of sense of time or a neglect of basic functions; (2) withdrawal, including feelings of anger, tension, and/or depression when the computer is inaccessible; (3) tolerance, including the need for better computer equipment, more software, or more hours of use; and (4) adverse consequences, including arguments, lying, poor school or vocational achievement, social isolation, and fatigue.

Tao et al. (2010) focused on eight criteria (including all four stated above) that they drew from clinical experience. They tested the accuracy of each to arrive at a diagnostic definition that they then validated in a group of 405 subjects. Their definition, shown in Table 1.1, emphasizes the presence of both preoccupation with the Internet and withdrawal (the two criteria with the highest diagnostic accuracy), along with one or more of five other criteria (tolerance, unsuccessful attempts to cut back, continued use despite negative consequences, loss of other interests, and use as a means to escape). When these symptom criteria were combined with three additional criteria (exclusion of other etiologies, clinically significant impairment, and a course of $\geq$ 3 months of $\geq$ 6 hours daily nonessential Internet use), the definition's diagnostic accuracy reached 99.26%, with a sensitivity and specificity of 89.66% and 100%, respectively, and very high interrater reliability.

Table 1.1 Proposed Diagnostic Criteria for Problematic Internet Use

(a) Symptom criteria

Both criteria present:

- Preoccupation with the Internet when offline (thinks about previous sessions or anticipates future sessions)
- Withdrawal, as manifested by dysphoric mood, anxiety, irritability, or boredom after being offline for several days

Also, at least one of the following:

- Tolerance, defined as increased Internet use required to achieve the same satisfaction level
- Persistent desire and/or unsuccessful attempts to control, cut back, or discontinue Internet use
- Continued excessive use despite physical or psychological problems likely to have been caused or exacerbated by Internet use
- Loss of previous interests, hobbies, and other pleasurable pursuits
- Use of the Internet to escape or relieve a dysphoric mood

(b) Exclusion criterion

Excessive Internet use is not better accounted for by another disorder

(c) Clinically significant impairment criterion

Excessive Internet use results in functional impairment, such as academically, professionally, or in personal relationships

(d) Course criterion

Duration of heavy Internet use exceeds 3 months, with at least 6 hours of Internet usage (non-business/non-academic) daily

From Tao R, Huang X, Wang J, Zhang H, Zhang Y, Li M (2010). Proposed diagnostic criteria for Internet addiction. Addiction 105: 556–564.

Most diagnostic definitions and diagnostic scales, however, approach PIU as a rather homogenous activity, focusing on total time spent online and on overall dysfunction, without assessing the nature of the time-consuming pursuit. Yet online activities may differ in associated risks, habit-forming potential, and treatment approaches when such activities are detrimental. Therefore, the user's specific online pursuits should be covered in any comprehensive diagnostic interview, not the least because psychotherapeutic interventions need to be tailored accordingly. As such, it is essential to ask about gaming/gambling, shopping/bidding, sexual preoccupations, and social networking, all the while assessing the amount of online presence expected for the person's work; school activities; and normal social, entertainment, and information needs. Establishing an accurate diagnosis necessitates keeping in mind that a "healthy" level of online life is likely a requirement and that a totally offline existence is no longer realistic or, in most cases, even possible and can itself be a sign of pathology.

CAUSES OF PROBLEMATIC INTERNET USE

The causes of PIU are unknown. Neurobiological theories have been proposed based on neuroimaging evidence and are discussed in Chapter 4. Also, very preliminary data exist on possible genetic contributions, including increased frequency of the homozygous short allelic variant of the serotonin transporter gene (SS-5HTTLPR) (Lee et al., 2008) and the rs1044396 polymorphism on the CHRNA4 gene (Montag et al., 2012). More research is required to explore these findings.

Psychological explanations have also been suggested (Table 1.2). One conceptualizes PIU as an inadequate strategy or self-relaxation tool for coping with stress (Grusser et al., 2005). Alternatively, PIU may result from a need to expand social networks to establish or enhance relationships and improve self-confidence, social abilities, and social support (Campbell et al., 2006; Kittinger et al., 2012; Smahel et al., 2012).

Other individuals, particularly those with heightened social anxiety, may perceive online communication as a safer means of interacting, due to the greater degree of control over one's image and the lower risk of negative evaluation. This, according to some theories, can lead to PIU (Lee and Stapinski, 2012). In addition, the Internet can appeal to individuals who struggle with identity (Ko et al., 2006) and self-concept issues (Israelashvili et al., 2012), in part through giving

Table 1.2 Proposed Psychological Causes of Problematic Internet Use

Inadequate coping with stress
Means of improving social abilities and social support
Attempt to alleviate social anxiety
Means of improving coping with identity and problems with self-concept
Accessibility, affordability, and anonymity of online sexual behaviors
Body image avoidance and preoccupation with being overweight
Need to escape or create a virtual "ideal self"

them the opportunity to improve or change personas. Excessive use of the Internet toward that goal may represent another pathway to PIU. Furthermore, PIU can result from a pattern of compulsive online pornography watching or other online sexual behaviors. This has been seen as a consequence of the accessibility, affordability, and anonymity of online sexual experiences (Southern, 2008). Yet another pathway to PIU may be body image problems and avoidance of real-life interactions because of embarrassment relating to one's appearance; that seems to be the conclusion from research conducted in young French adult females (Rodgers et al., 2013) and overweight American males (Hetzel-Riggin and Pritchard, 2011). Finally, PIU can be a symptom of radical escapism or the need to flee from an unpleasant reality (e.g., in the context of depression) or to create a virtual "ideal self" that is liberated of real-life stressors and limitations. This has been observed among players of certain video games, such as massively multiplayer online role-playing games (Achab et al., 2011; Billieux et al., 2011; Li et al., 2011; Zanetta et al., 2011; Leménager et al., 2013). More research is needed to understand the psychological basis of PIU and to explore neurobiological and genetic susceptibilities that may underlie its pathophysiology.

PREVALENCE

Prevalence data on PIU are limited by methodological difficulties and the heterogeneity of study samples and assessment tools (Kuss et al., 2014). This makes the task of comparing prevalence rates across studies, age groups, and countries difficult. Also, the use of the inherently flawed online recruitment tools in some prevalence studies can further complicate comparisons and inflate figures (Greenfield, 1999; Aboujaoude, 2010). A systematic analysis of assessment instruments by Byun et al. (2009) revealed several research limitations, including inconsistent definitions for PIU or Internet addiction disorder, recruitment methods that may cause serious sampling biases, use of exploratory rather than confirmatory data analysis techniques, and a focus on association rather than causal relationships among variables.

On the most fundamental level, it is easy to see how the lack of consensus on what constitutes PIU can yield substantially divergent point prevalence rates (Table 1.3). According to a worldwide review carried on behalf of the German health ministry, international prevalence rates for PIU range from 1.5% to 8.2% (Petersen et al., 2009). The vast majority of the evaluated studies used questionnaires such as the Internet Addiction Test (see Chapter 3) to arrive at prevalence, rather than the gold standard of the comprehensive clinical interview, in a random general population sample. In the United States, rates have varied from 0.7%, based on a random telephone survey of 2513 adults (Aboujaoude et al., 2006), to a range of 0% to 26.3% of adolescents and college students, based on a review of eight prevalence studies conducted in that age group (Moreno et al., 2011). In Europe, rates of PIU show a broad range as well, varying between 1% in a random survey of 8132 Germans (Rumpf et al., 2014) and another random survey of 3399 Norwegians (Bakken et al., 2009) to 18.3% in

Table 1.3 Prevalence of Problematic Internet Use

Study	Country and Study Population	N	Condition Studied	Prevalence Rates
Greeenfield, 1999	United States, online adult population	17,251	CIU	6%
Whang et al., 2003	South Korea, online adolescents	13,588	IAD	3.5%
Niemz et al., 2005	United Kingdom, online college students	371	PIU	18.3%
Aboujaoude et al., 2006	United States, general adult survey	2513	PIU	0.7%
Pallanti et al., 2006	Italy, school adolescents	275	IAD	5.4%
Kim et al., 2006	South Korea, school adolescents	1573	IAD	1.6%
Deng et al., 2007	China, Hunan province, middle school students	5760	IAD	2.4%
Cao et al., 2007	China, Changsha City, school adolescents	2620	IAD	5.52%
Fortson et al., 2007	United States, college students	411	PIU	25%
Ha et al., 2007	South Korea, school adolescents	452	IAD	20.3%
Jang et al., 2008	South Korea, school adolescents	912	IAD	4.3%
Park et al., 2008	South Korea, school adolescents	903	IAD	10.7%
Bakken et al., 2009	Norway, general population survey	3399	IAD	1%
Ni et al., 2009	China, Shaanxi province, college students	3557	IAD	6.44%
Tsai et al., 2009	Taiwan, college students	1360	IAD	17.9%
Seo et al., 2009	South Korea, school adolescents	676	IAD	3.1%
Lam et al., 2009	China, school adolescents	1618	IAD	10.2% "moderately addicted"; 0.6% "severely addicted"
Tsitsika et al., 2009	Greece, school adolescents	411	IAD	10.4%
Fu et al., 2010	Hong Kong, random household survey of adolescents	208	IAD	6.7%
Christakis et al., 2011	United States, online college students	307	PIU	4%
Poli and Agrimi, 2012	Italy, college students	2533	IAD	5%

(continued)

Table 1.3 Continued

9

Problematic Internet Use

Study	Country and Study Population	N	Condition Studied	Prevalence Rates
Durkee et al., 2012	11 European countries, high school adolescents	11,956	PIU	4.4%
Xu et al., 2012	China, Shanghai, school adolescents	5122	IAD	8.8%
Yoo et al., 2013	South Korea, adolescents	795	PIU	3%
Goel et al., 2013	India, Mumbai, college students	987	IAD	0.7%
Yadav et al., 2013	India, Ahmedabad, adolescents	621	IAD	0.7%
Rumpf et al., 2014	Germany, general population	8132	IAD	1% (entire population); 2.4% (14–24-year olds); 4% (14–16-year olds)
Stavropoulos et al., 2013	Greece, school adolescents	2086	IAD	3.1%
Siomos et al., 2013	Greece, adolescents	2017	IAD	15.3%
Ricquebourg et al., 2013	France, Reunion Island, college students	1,119	PIU	6%
Lai et al., 2013	Hong Kong, high school adolescents	844	IAD	3%
Wu et al., 2013	China, Wuhan province, high school adolescents	1101	IAD	13.5%
Bener and Bhugra, 2013	Qatar, schools and colleges, adolescents and young adults	2298	IAD	17.3%
Li et al., 2014b	China, 31 provinces, elementary and middle school students	24,013	IAD	6.3%
Tang et al., 2014	China, Wuhan province, high school adolescents	755	IAD	6%

Abbreviations: CIU, compulsive-impulsive Internet use; IAD, Internet addiction disorder; PIU, problematic Internet use.

a United Kingdom study of 371 college students (Niemz et al., 2005). A major cross-sectional survey of high school students conducted in 11 European countries investigated the prevalence of PIU in relation to demographic and social factors and Internet accessibility (Durkee et al., 2012). A total of 11,956 adolescents were recruited from randomly selected schools in 11 sites. The overall prevalence of PIU was 4.4%. It differed among countries, correlated significantly with mean hours spent online, and was higher among males than females (5.2% versus 3.8%). Other studies have also shown higher male prevalence (Carli et al., 2013).

PIU has received the most research attention in East Asia, but prevalence rates from East Asian studies can be even more challenging to interpret, in part because many studies use vague terms to describe levels of Internet usage, often without clearly defining or validating them (e.g., "borderline," "excessive," "at risk," and "addictive"). In general, reported East Asian PIU rates have varied from 2.4% (Deng et al., 2007) to 13.5% (Wu et al., 2013) in Chinese middle schools and high schools, respectively, and from 1.6% (Kim et al., 2006) to 20.3% (Ha et al., 2007) in South Korean adolescents.

Not surprisingly, PIU prevalence rates from studies in other countries also show wide variation—from 0.7% in a study of Indian college students (Goel et al., 2013) to 17.3% in a study of Qatari adolescents and young adults (Bener and Bhugra, 2013). Clear and consistent diagnostic criteria, representative samples recruited offline, and validated questionnaires are needed to determine more accurate PIU rates in the future.

COMORBIDITY WITH PSYCHIATRIC DISORDERS

Cross-sectional studies report high rates of comorbidity between PIU and other psychiatric symptoms and disorders. The data, however, are severely limited by the frequent use of self-report questionnaires rather than validated tools or a structured psychiatric interview to diagnose comorbid conditions. Still, the picture that emerges is one where the presence of comorbidities is the rule rather than the exception.

A recent review (Carli et al., 2013) of comorbidity studies that met preset inclusion criteria for the review (adequate size, ascertained diagnostic criteria for PIU, accepted measures to assess comorbid psychopathology) analyzed 20 studies conducted in adults, adolescents, or children. The review found that 75% of the studies reported significant correlations with depression; 57% with anxiety; 100% with symptoms of attention deficit hyperactivity disorder (ADHD); 60% with obsessive-compulsive symptoms; and 66% with hostility/aggression. Of note, no study in the review reported a significant association with social phobia or substance use disorders. Also, the majority reported a higher rate of PIU among males than females.

In the large Norwegian population prevalence study (N = 3399) reported by Bakken et al. (2009), 41.4% of "Internet addicts" reported feelings of depression in the 12 months prior to the study, compared to 15.8% of "nonaddicts." Sleep disturbance symptoms, anxiety symptoms, and alcohol and other substance abuse were also more common (38.6% versus 26.4%, 36.4% versus 5%, and 13.6% versus 1.1%, respectively). Similar to most PIU comorbidity studies, the questions used to assess symptoms were not based on established diagnostic criteria. Table 1.4 lists other studies that have explored the coexistence of PIU and other psychiatric symptoms or disorders; the vast majority are based on self-report questionnaires and symptom checklists, not a face-to-face structured interview.

Three small studies did involve face-to-face interviews of adult patients with PIU. Black et al. (1999) assessed 21 subjects with the Diagnostic Interview Schedule

Table 1.4 Coexistence of Problematic Internet Use and Psychiatric Symptoms and Disorders

Study	Country	N	Condition Studied	Coexisting Disorders/Symptoms and Rates of Association with Psychopathology
Kim et al., 2006	South Korea	1573 adolescents	IAD	Depression and association with suicidal ideation
te Wildt et al., 2007	Germany	23	IAD	Depression, 77.8%
Ha et al., 2007	South Korea	452 adolescents	IAD	Depression
Yen et al., 2008	Taiwan	3662 adolescents	IAD	Higher levels of somatization, obsessive-compulsive symptoms, interpersonal sensitivity, depression, anxiety, phobia, paranoia, and psychoticism
Kratzer and Hegerl, 2008	Germany	30	PIU	Anxiety disorders, 50%
Ko et al., 2008b	Taiwan	2114 high school students	IAD	Alcohol use
Yen et al., 2009a	Taiwan	2793 college students	IAD	ADHD and impulsivity
Yen et al., 2009b	Taiwan	2453 college students	IAD	Alcohol use
Bernardi and Pallanti, 2009	Italy	50 adults from outpatient neuroscience clinic	IAD	High dissociation scores. Also, 4% ADHD, 7% hypomania, 7% binge-eating disorder, 15% generalized anxiety disorder, 15% social anxiety disorder, 7% dysthymia, 7% obsessive compulsive personality disorder, 14% borderline personality disorder, and 7% avoidant personality disorder.
De Berardis et al., 2009	Italy	312 college students	IAD	Alexithymia, dissociative experiences, lower self-esteem, and higher obsessive-compulsive symptoms
Morrison and Gore, 2010	United Kingdom	1319	IAD	Depression
Xiuqin et al., 2010	China	204 adolescents	IAD	Higher levels of obsessive-compulsive symptoms, interpersonal sensitivity, depression, anxiety, hostility, paranoia and psychoticism

(continued)

Table 1.4 Continued

Study	Country	N	Condition Studied	Coexisting Disorders/Symptoms and Rates of Association with Psychopathology
Alavi et al., 2010	Iran	250 college students	IAD	Higher levels of somatization, obsessive-compulsive symptoms, interpersonal sensitivity, depression, anxiety, hostility, phobia, paranoia, and psychoticism
Tsitsika et al., 2011	Greece	129 adolescents	IAD	Depression
Liberatore et al., 2011	Puerto Rico	71 adolescents	IAD	Depression
Kormas et al., 2011	Greece	866 adolescents	IAD	Conduct disorders, hyperactivity
Yen et al., 2011	Taiwan	2348 college students	IAD	Hostility
Cheung and Wong 2011	Hong Kong	719 adolescents	IAD	Depression and insomnia
Guo et al., 2012	Hong Kong	3524 adolescents	IAD	Depression
Wei et al., 2012	Taiwan	722	IAD	Social anxiety and depression
Canan et al., 2012	Turkey	1034 college students	IAD	Dissociative symptoms
Fischer et al., 2012	Germany	1435 adolescents	IAD	Depression, deliberate self-harm, suicidal behavior
Mazhari, 2012	Iran	950 college students	PIU	Impulse control disorders
Yates et al., 2012	United States	1470 college students	PIU	Alexithymia, inferior self-concept
Cho et al., 2013	South Korea	524 male adolescents	IAD	Depression, anxiety

Abbreviations: ADHD. attention deficit hyperactivity disorder; CIU, compulsive-impulsive Internet use; IAD, Internet addiction disorder; PIU, problematic Internet use.

and found the lifetime prevalence of mood disorders and major depression to be 33% and 15%, respectively. Furthermore, 38% had a lifetime substance use disorder and 19% had a lifetime diagnosis of anxiety disorder. Also, in a case series of 20 patients with PIU (Shapira et al., 2000), 70% carried a lifetime diagnosis of bipolar affective disorder (type I or II), 15% had major depressive disorder, 55% had substance abuse, 50% had an impulse control disorder, and 45% had social anxiety disorder. Finally, an Italian study (Bernardi and Pallanti, 2009) used a structured clinical interview to assess psychiatric conditions in 50 adults with "Internet addiction." The study showed that dissociative symptoms were prominent and strongly correlated with severity of "Internet addiction." Also, 4% had ADHD, 7% hypomania, 7% binge-eating disorder, 15% generalized anxiety disorder, 15%

social anxiety disorder, 7% dysthymia, 7% obsessive-compulsive personality disorder, 14% borderline personality disorder, and 7% avoidant personality disorder.

Taken together, surveys conducted among high school and college students show similarly high comorbidity rates with mood and anxiety disorders, but ADHD may be more frequent than among older individuals with PIU (Weinstein and Weizman, 2012). In a study of 752 South Korean elementary students, 33% of those with ADHD also met criteria for PIU (Yoo et al., 2004). Another study in 216 Taiwanese college students showed that 32% of subjects with PIU met criteria for ADHD compared to 8% of regular Internet users (Ko et al., 2008a). This does not establish causality, however, and it remains unclear whether the Internet may appeal to individuals with ADHD or whether excessive Internet use may lead to inattention and ADHD.

Finally, significant attention is being focused on the possible association between problematic video game use and violence or sociopathy. Online video games are discussed in detail elsewhere (see Chapter 2), but studies have often diagnosed individuals who are primarily excessive online gamers as having PIU. A Taiwanese study in 2348 college students assessed hostility in PIU as a function of subjects' specific online activities. It found that those with PIU had significantly higher levels of hostility both in the real world and online (Yen et al., 2011). However, subjects using the Internet for online gaming had higher expressive hostility than those spending most of their online time chatting. Aggression was also associated with excessive Internet use in another study of 2336 South Korean high school students (Kim, 2013).

In summary, a strong association can be seen in both adults and adolescents between PIU and a number of psychiatric conditions. However, these results should be regarded with caution as most studies relied on self-assessment to diagnose PIU. Moreover, although PIU does not have established diagnostic criteria, the comorbid conditions explored in the studies often do. Those formal criteria and diagnostic definitions, however, are often completely ignored in favor of descriptive terms that are open to interpretation and unscientific (e.g., vague "anxiety" instead of generalized anxiety disorder, vague "depression" instead of major depressive disorder). It is also crucial to remember that an association does not mean causation, and it remains unknown whether the various psychiatric problems found to coexist with PIU preceded or followed it. Indeed, the only study to assess psychiatric symptoms that may precede PIU was conducted by Cho et al. (2013) in 524 first-grade male South Korean students. Subjects were assessed at baseline and in middle school 7 or 8 years later. Results showed that baseline anxiety and depression were associated with future PIU. Still, there is no established predictor of PIU.

PHYSICAL AND OTHER HEALTH HAZARDS ASSOCIATED WITH PROBLEMATIC INTERNET USE

Other known health hazards associated with PIU appear related to sleep deprivation or disturbance. A South Korean study of high school students with PIU found that 37.7% had excessive daytime sleepiness (Choi et al., 2009). Insomnia, witnessed snoring, apnea, teeth grinding, and nightmares were more common in individuals with PIU compared to healthy controls (Choi et al., 2009). Also, a relationship between body mass index and obesity rates on the one hand and PIU on the other was seen in two studies (Canan et al., 2014; Li et al., 2014a), suggesting that PIU may be associated with unhealthy eating habits and decreased physical activity.

FACTORS ASSOCIATED WITH PROBLEMATIC INTERNET USE
Personality Factors

Beyond comorbid conditions that might precede or accompany PIU, several studies have examined associated personality dimensions. The list of character traits that have been linked with PIU is long and sometimes inconsistent. It includes lack of perseverance (Mottram and Fleming, 2009); psychoticism (Tosun and Lajunen, 2009); and neuroticism, sensation seeking, trait and state anxiety, and aggression (Mehroof and Griffiths, 2010). In addition, high harm avoidance, high novelty seeking, high reward dependence, low self-directedness, and low cooperativeness were positively correlated with PIU in two South Korean studies (Ha et al., 2007; June et al., 2007), and low novelty seeking was seen in a third South Korean study (Cho et al., 2008). Yet another study, conducted in Taiwanese adolescents, showed a correlation with high novelty seeking, high harm avoidance, and low reward dependence (Ko et al., 2006). Finally, low self-esteem, along with alexithymia, dissociative experiences, and impulse dysregulation were seen as risk factors in a sample of Italian adolescents with PIU (De Berardis et al., 2009). Judging the strength and quality of the studies and the size of the evidence, the best supported association appears to be between adolescents with PIU and the personality dimensions of high novelty seeking and high harm avoidance (with the latter finding seeming to contrast with substance use disorders) (Mehroof and Griffiths, 2010).

It has also been hypothesized that the Internet can influence users' offline personalities, encouraging the narcissistic, grandiose, regressive, and impulsive behaviors that easily manifest in the anonymous, lawless online space in the "real world" (Aboujaoude, 2011). Research into this phenomenon, however, remains very preliminary (Aboujaoude, 2011).

Social and Family Factors

Several small studies have looked at social or family risk factors for PIU. Loneliness, low self-esteem, and low life satisfaction were associated with PIU among Turkish students (Bozoglan et al., 2013), whereas two Chinese studies blamed PIU on recent stressful events (Lam et al., 2009), school stress, poor relations with teachers and other students, loneliness, and family conflict (Wang et al., 2011). Another study, conducted in Taiwan, highlighted the role of substance use, perceived positive parental attitude toward substance use, and living in rural areas (Yen et al., 2007, 2009c).

On the family front, there is evidence that individuals with PIU manifest disrupted family functioning (Senormanci et al., 2014), and PIU has been associated with inadequate family communication, poor family cohesion, family violence exposure (Park et al., 2008), unhealthy family attachment patterns (Shin et al., 2011), and parental rejection or overprotection (Yao et al., 2013).

In general, despite limitations that include small size, nonrepresentative samples and failure to rule out psychiatric comorbidities that may be the root cause (e.g., clinical depression that might be triggering the school or family problem), these studies suggest that certain social characteristics and family patterns may presage or accompany PIU. It follows from these data that psychosocial interventions at the school or family level and attempts to strengthen family functioning and promote positive family relationships might help prevent PIU or mitigate its effects.

Cognitive Factors

Individuals with PIU may have difficulty with offline decision making and urge suppression. Several studies have investigated decision making and related impulsivity in PIU. A study using the Iowa Gambling Task, a measure of decision making, found deficits (chiefly, a strategy learning lag) in individuals with PIU (Sun et al., 2009). However, these individuals showed better performance on a go/no-go task, which measures prepotent response inhibition (i.e., a response for which immediate reinforcement—positive or negative—is available or has been previously associated with that response). Also, a study by Ko et al. (2010) showed that students with PIU exhibited better decision making on the Iowa Gambling Task compared with substance users and gamblers, whereas their performance on the Balloon Analog Risk Task, which measures impulsivity, indicated that they were not more likely to engage in risk-taking behaviors than the two other groups. The subjects' better performance on the Iowa Gambling Task was seen as potentially differentiating PIU from substance use disorders and pathological gambling. In another study, individuals with PIU performed poorly on a computerized stop signal test, which measures inhibitory function, and scored highly on impulsivity and novelty seeking (Choi et al., 2014). Finally, a resting-state fast-wave brain activity pattern, which has been linked to impulsivity, was also described in PIU and suggested as a possible neurobiological marker for PIU (Choi et al., 2014).

Executive control ability is another measure of cognition and has been explored in several PIU studies. In a study of 17 male students with PIU and 17 control subjects, executive control was assessed by recording event-related brain potentials during a color-word Stroop task (Dong et al., 2011). The Stroop task measures response to words in congruent (e.g., the word "red" in red color) and noncongruent colors (e.g., the word "red" in green color), where the incongruent words cause an interference, presumably due to divided attention. In response to incongruent conditions, students with PIU had a longer reaction time, more response errors, and reduced activity of event-related potentials in the medial frontal area. These results suggest possible executive control impairment in PIU. A subsequent brain imaging study using the Stroop task in PIU showed increased brain activity compared with control subjects in several areas (superior temporal gyrus, bilateral insula, and bilateral precuneus areas) during switching from easy to difficult and difficult to easy tasks (Dong et al., 2014). This finding might suggest better flexibility, which would contradict the suggestion that individuals with PIU may have deficits in executive control. Also, a study by Dong et al. (2013a) showed increased brain activity on functional magnetic resonance imaging (fMRI) in several brain areas (the inferior frontal cortex, insula, and the anterior cingulate cortex) during decision-making tasks, although attention capacity was reduced.

The Erikson Flanker Task is a response inhibition test used to assess the ability to suppress responses that are inappropriate in a particular context. The target is flanked by nontarget stimuli, which correspond to the same directional response as the target (congruent flankers), to the opposite response (incongruent flankers), or to neither (neutral flankers). Zhou et al. (2013) used a modified Erikson Flanker Task and measured event-related potentials in subjects with PIU. Results showed that they had more total error rates while displaying shorter reaction times and reduced activity in frontal and central areas of the brain. In another study using a gambling task in fMRI, Dong et al. (2014) showed that subjects with gambling-focused PIU displayed an enhanced sensitivity to gains and reduced sensitivity to losses, as indicated by the activation of the superior frontal gyrus after continuous wins and decreased activation of the posterior cingulate after continuous losses; this may explain continuing gambling despite apparent losses. Finally, while performing a fast Stroop task, subjects with PIU showed impaired error-monitoring ability, which was associated with increased anterior cingulate activation on fMRI (Dong et al., 2013b).

Taken together, these studies show increased brain activity during performance of the Stroop and the decision-making tasks in the fMRI scanner. This may indicate that these brain areas have to work harder to enable the participants to provide accurate responses.

Finally, a study compared 59 PIU students with 43 non-PIU students using an IQ test (Park et al., 2011). Compared to healthy controls, students with PIU had significantly lower comprehension scores, suggesting a possible relationship between PIU and lower intelligence. Also, earlier onset and longer duration of PIU were associated with poorer performance in areas related to attention (Park et al., 2011). The cross-sectional nature of this study, however, limits its value.

TREATMENT

There are no established treatments for PIU, and clinical interventions are largely based on psychotherapeutic and psychopharmacological strategies that have been used in conditions that share a resemblance with PIU, namely OCD, impulse control disorders, and substance use disorders. A careful initial evaluation is key to making the diagnosis and identifying any comorbid conditions. Those should then be addressed according to established treatment guidelines. Beyond that, treatment of PIU can consist of psychotherapy (individual, group, family-based, or school-based), psychopharmacology, or a combination.

Both psychotherapy and psychopharmacology approaches that have been tested are reviewed below, but the overall quality of the studies precludes strong treatment recommendations. King et al. (2011) evaluated PIU treatment research based on eight published studies and noted a number of important limitations in the extant literature, including inconsistencies in the definition and diagnosis of "Internet addiction"; lack of randomization and blinding techniques; lack of adequate controls or other comparison groups; and insufficient information concerning recruitment, sample characteristics, and treatment effect sizes.

Psychological Treatment

Psychotherapeutic approaches, especially cognitive-behavioral therapy (CBT), appear to be a mainstay of treatment. CBT usually requires approximately 3 months of treatment or 12 weekly sessions. The early stage of therapy tends to be behavioral, focusing on situations where the disorder causes the greatest difficulty. As therapy progresses, there is growing focus on confronting the cognitive assumptions and distortions that accompany and encourage the problematic behavior, such as the exaggerated belief that the person can control the amount of time spent online. This often involves assessment of the type of distortions present, analysis of thought records, problem-solving skills training, coping strategies training, modeling in therapy, and support groups (Young, 2007).

In the largest CBT study to date, conducted in 114 adults with PIU, most subjects were able to manage their presenting complaints by the eighth session, with improvement maintained at a 6-month follow-up (Young, 2007). A study of group CBT in 56 Chinese adolescents aged 12 to 17 years, randomized 32 subjects to active treatment and 24 to a wait list control (Du et al., 2010). Participants in the active treatment group were treated with an eight-session, multimodal, school-based group CBT. Therapy included learning principles of effective communication with parents, learning how to manage online relationships, techniques for controlling impulses, and techniques for recognizing and stopping the problematic behavior. Treatment also included teaching parents to recognize a child's emotional state and improve communication among family members. Both groups were assessed at baseline, immediately after the intervention, and at the 6-month follow-up in terms of Internet use; time management ability; and emotional, cognitive, and behavioral measures. Internet use decreased in both groups, but only subjects receiving the multimodal, school-based group CBT demonstrated an improvement in time management skills and a decrease in emotional, cognitive, and behavioral symptoms postintervention. Treatment gains were maintained at the 6-month follow-up.

Given the associated family, relationship, and interpersonal difficulties discussed, couple or family therapy may also be beneficial. Other strategies may include self-help books and tapes (Shaw and Black, 2008), self-imposed bans on computer use and Internet access (Shaw and Black, 2008), and "initiated absti-nence" programs such as the ones tested in students in Austria, Germany, and Italy (Kalke and Raschke, 2004). Typically very expensive and restrictive residential treatment programs that are often featured in the media lack generally indepen-dent long-term treatment outcome data to recommend them (Aboujaoude, 2010).

Pharmacological Treatment

A pharmacotherapeutic study tested escitalopram, an SSRI known to be effective in OCD, based on the observation of shared features between PIU and OCD and their occasional coexistence (Dell'Osso et al., 2007). The discontinuation study was conducted in 19 adults with "impulsive-compulsive Internet use." A significant decrease in the number of hours spent online was seen in the 10-week open-label phase of treatment with escitalopram, 20 mg/day. However, when responders were randomized to 9 weeks of either continued escitalopram or placebo, both groups did similarly well. The authors hypothesized that 9 weeks may not have been enough to lose the response in the placebo group, but it is also possible that the initial open-label response may have been due to the placebo effect.

Given that PIU often coexists with ADHD, an open-label treatment study tested extended-release methylphenidate in 62 South Korean children with "Internet video game addiction" and comorbid ADHD. After 8 weeks of treatment (aver-age dose 30.5 mg/day), Internet use was significantly reduced and the improve-ment was positively correlated with improvement in measures of attention (Han et al., 2009). These findings led the investigators to suggest that online video games might have an analogous effect to stimulants in ADHD (Han et al., 2009)—both methylphenidate and video game playing might regulate dopamine levels.

Isolated reports suggest that other medications might also be beneficial and deserve to be rigorously tested in controlled trials. For example, a case study (Bostwich and Bucci, 2008) reported successful treatment of a 31-year-old male with compulsive cybersexual behavior using naltrexone (150 mg/day), a medica-tion that has shown promise in impulse control disorders (Aboujaoude, 2010). Another case study reported on the beneficial addition of the atypical antipsy-chotic quetiapine (200 mg/day) to citalopram, an SSRI that alone was not ade-quately treating a 23-year-old patient with PIU (Atmaca, 2007).

CONCLUSION

Much remains to be elucidated about the definition, biopsychosocial causes, course, and treatment of PIU. Nearly 20 years into the Internet revolution, there is still no agreement about the existence of PIU, the "gold standard" for its diagnosis, valid and reliable instruments to help identify and track it, or treatment guidelines. Without diagnostic clarity, it is not surprising that PIU prevalence rates have been inconsistent, although younger individuals and males seem to be at higher risk. Once a diagnosis of PIU is made, it is likely that other psychiatric disorders will also be present, even if it is unclear whether PIU preceded or resulted from the coexisting conditions. Besides comorbid disorders, PIU has been associated with deficits in social skills and parental attachment, personality dimensions such as novelty seeking and harm avoidance, and possible impairment in cognitive processes involved in decision making and executive function. The nature of these associations, however, is also unclear, especially regarding any causality between PIU and the various variables. Preliminary evidence exists for the efficacy of psychological interventions, especially CBT, and certain pharmacotherapies, but in treatment, too, much more research is needed to allow for strong recommendations and data-driven guidelines.

DISCLOSURE STATEMENT

Dr. Aboujaoude is cofounder of eTherapi, a telemental health platform. Dr. Weinstein discloses no relationships with commercial entities and professional activities that may bias his views.

REFERENCES

Aboujaoude E (2010). Problematic Internet use: an overview. World Psychiatry 9: 85–90.

Aboujaoude E (2011). Virtually You: The Dangerous Powers of the e-Personality. W.W. Norton, New York, NY.

Aboujaoude E, Koran LM, Gamel N, Large MD, Serpe RT (2006). Potential markers for problematic Internet use: a telephone survey of 2,513 adults. CNS Spectrums 11: 750–755.

Achab S, Nicolier M, Mauny F, et al (2011). Massively multiplayer online role-playing games: comparing characteristics of addict vs non-addict online recruited gamers in a French adult population. BMC Psychiatry 11: 144.

Alavi SS, Alaghemandan H, Maracy MR, Jannatifard F, Eslami M, Ferdosi M (2010). Impact of addiction to Internet on a number of psychiatric symptoms in students of Isfahan universities, Iran. International Journal of Preventive Medicine 3: 122–127.

American Psychiatric Association (2013). Diagnostic and Statistical Manual of Mental Disorders, Fifth Edition. American Psychiatric Publishing, Arlington, VA.

Atmaca M (2007). A case of problematic Internet use successfully treated with an SSRI-anti-psychotic combination. Progress in Neuropsychopharmacology and Biological Psychiatry 31: 961–962.

Bakken IJ, Wenzel HG, Götestam KG (2009). Internet addiction among Norwegian adults: a stratified probability sample study. Scandinavian Journal of Psychology 50: 121–127.

Bener A, Bhugra D (2013). Lifestyle and depressive risk factors associated with problematic Internet use in adolescents in an Arabian Gulf culture. Journal of Addiction Medicine 7: 236–242.

Bernardi S, Pallanti S (2009). Internet addiction: a descriptive clinical study focusing on comorbidities and dissociative symptoms. Comprehensive Psychiatry 50: 510–516.

Billieux J, Chanal J, Khazaal, et al (2011). Psychological predictors of problematic involvement in massively multiplayer online role-playing games: illustration in a sample of male cybercafé players. Psychopathology 44: 165–171.

Black DW, Belsare G, Schlosser S (1999). Clinical features, psychiatric comorbidity, and health related quality of life in persons reporting compulsive computer use behavior. Journal of Clinical Psychiatry 60: 839–844.

Block JJ (2008). Issues for DSM-V: Internet addiction. American Journal of Psychiatry165: 306–307.

Botswich JM, Bucci JA (2008). Internet sex addiction treated with naltrexone. Mayo Clinic Proceedings 83: 226–230.

Bozoglan B, Demirer V, Sahin I (2013). Loneliness, self-esteem, and life satisfaction as predictors of Internet addiction: a cross-sectional study among Turkish university students. Scandinavian Journal of Psychology 54: 313–319.

Byun S, Ruffini C, Mills JE, et al (2009). Internet addiction: metasynthesis of 1996–2006 quantitative research. Cyberpsychology and Behavior 12: 203–207.

Campbell AJ, Cumming SR, Hughes I (2006). Internet use by the socially fearful: addiction or therapy? Cyberpsychology and Behavior 9: 69–81.

Canan F, Ataoglu A, Ozcetin A, Icmeli C (2012). The association between Internet addiction and dissociation among Turkish college students. Comprehensive Psychiatry 53: 422–426.

Canan F, Yildirim O, Ustunel TY, et al (2014). The relationship between Internet addiction and Body Mass Index in Turkish adolescents. Cyberpsychology, Behavior, and Social Networking 17: 40–45.

Cao F, Su L, Liu T, Gao X (2007). The relationship between impulsivity and Internet addiction in a sample of Chinese adolescents. European Psychiatry 22: 466–471.

Cao H, Sun Y, Wan Y, Hao J, Tao F (2011). Problematic Internet use in Chinese adolescents and its relation to psychosomatic symptoms and life satisfaction. BMC Public Health 11: 802.

Carli V, Durkee T, Wasserman D, et al (2013). The association between pathological Internet use and comorbid psychopathology: a systematic review. Psychopathology 46: 1–13.

Cheung LM, Wong WS (2011). The effects of insomnia and Internet addiction on depression in Hong Kong Chinese adolescents: an exploratory cross-sectional analysis. Journal of Sleep Research 20: 311–317.

Cho SC, Kim JW, Kim BN, Lee JH, Kim EH (2008). Biogenetic temperament and character profiles and attention deficit hyperactivity disorder symptoms in Korean adolescents with problematic Internet use. Cyberpsychology and Behavior 11: 735–737.

Cho SM, Sung MJ, Shin KM, Lim KY, Shin YM (2013). Does psychopathology in childhood predict Internet addiction in male adolescents? Child Psychiatry and Human Development 44: 549–555.

Choi JS, Park SM, Roh MS, et al (2014). Dysfunctional inhibitory control and impulsivity in Internet addiction. Psychiatry Research 215: 424–428.

Choi K, Son H, Park M (2009). Internet overuse and excessive daytime sleepiness in adolescents. Psychiatry and Clinical Neurosciences 63: 455–462.

Christakis DA, Moreno MM, Jelenchick L, Myaing MT, Zhou C (2011). Problematic Internet usage in US college students: a pilot study. BMC Medicine 22: 77.

De Berardis, D, D'Albenzio A, Gambi F, et al (2009). Alexithymia and its relationships with dissociative experiences and Internet addiction in a nonclinical sample. Cyberpsychology and Behavior 12: 67–69.

Dell'Osso B, Altamura C, Allen A, Marazziti D, Hollander E (2006). Epidemiological and clinical updates on impulse control disorders: a critical review. European Archives of Psychiatry and Clinical Neuroscience 256: 464–475.

Dell'Osso B, Altamura AC, Hadley SJ, Baker BR, Hollander E (2007). An open-label trial of escitalopram in the treatment of impulsive-compulsive Internet usage disorder. European Neuropsychopharmacology 16: S82–S83.

Deng YX, Hu M, Hu GQ, Wang LS, Sun ZQ (2007). An investigation on the prevalence of Internet addiction disorder in middle school students of Hunan province [in Chinese]. Zhonghua Liu Xing Bing Xue Za Zhi 28: 445–448.

Dong G, Hu Y, Lin X, Lu Q (2013a). What makes Internet addicts continue playing online even when faced by severe negative consequences? Possible explanations from an fMRI study. Biological Psychology 94: 282–289.

Dong G, Lin X, Zhou H, Lu Q (2014). Cognitive flexibility in Internet addicts: fMRI evidence from difficult-to-easy and easy-to-difficult switching situations. Addictive Behaviors 39: 677–683.

Dong G, Shen Y, Huang J, Du X (2013b). Impaired error-monitoring function in people with Internet addiction disorder: an event-related fMRI study. European Addiction Research 19: 269–275.

Dong G, Zhou H, Zhao X (2011). Male Internet addicts show impaired executive control ability: evidence from a color-word Stroop task. Neuroscience Letters 499: 114–118.

Du YS, Jiang W, Vance A (2010). Longer term effect of randomized, controlled group cognitive behavioural therapy for Internet addiction in adolescent students in Shanghai. Australian and New Zealand Journal of Psychiatry 44: 129–134.

Durkee T, Kaess M, Carli V, et al (2012). Prevalence of pathological Internet use among adolescents in Europe: demographic and social factors. Addiction 107: 2210–2222.

Fischer G, Brunner R, Parzer P, et al (2012). Depression, deliberate self-harm and suicidal behaviour in adolescents engaging in risky and pathological Internet use. Praxis der Kinderpsychologie und Kinderpsychiatrie 61: 16–31. [Article in German]

Fortson BL, Scotti JR, Chen YC, Malone J, Del Ben KS (2007). Internet use, abuse, and dependence among students at a southeastern regional university. Journal of American College Health 56: 137–144.

Fu KW, Chan WS, Wong PW, Yip PS (2010). Internet addiction: prevalence, discriminant validity and correlates among adolescents in Hong Kong. British Journal of Psychiatry 196: 486–492.

Goel D, Subramanyam A, Kamath R (2013). A study on the prevalence of Internet addiction and its association with psychopathology in Indian adolescents. Indian Journal of Psychiatry 55: 140–143.

Grant JE, Potenza MN, Weinstein A, Gorelick DA (2010). Introduction to behavioral addictions. American Journal of Drug and Alcohol Abuse 36: 233–241.

Greenfield DN (1999). Psychological characteristics of compulsive Internet use: a preliminary analysis. Cyberpsychology and Behavior 2: 403–412.

Griffiths M (1998). Internet addiction: does it really exist? In Gackenbach J, Editor. Psychology and the Internet. Academic Press, Waltham, MA, pp. 61–75.

Griffiths M (2000). Internet addiction—Time to be taken seriously? Addiction Research 8: 413–418.

Grusser SM, Thalemann R, Albrecht U, Thalemann CN (2005). Excessive computer usage in adolescents—results of a psychometric evaluation [in German]. Die Wiener Klinische Wochenschrift 117: 188–195.

Guo J, Chen L, Wang X, et al (2012). The relationship between Internet addiction and depression among migrant children and left-behind children in China. Cyberpsychology, Behavior, and Social Networking 15: 585–590.

Ha JH, Kim SY, Bae SC, et al (2007). Depression and Internet addiction in adolescents. Psychopathology 40: 424–430.

Han D, Lee Y, Na C, et al (2009). The effect of methylphenidate on Internet video game play in children with attention-deficit/hyperactivity disorder. Comprehensive Psychiatry 50: 251–256.

Hetzel-Riggin MD, Pritchard JR (2011). Predicting problematic Internet use in men and women: the contributions of psychological distress, coping style, and body esteem. Cyberpsychology, Behavior, and Social Networking 14: 519–525.

Israelashvili M, Kim T, Bukobza G (2012). Adolescents' over-use of the cyber world. Internet addiction or identity exploration? Journal of Adolescence 35: 417–424.

Jang KS, Hwang SY, Choi JY (2008). Internet addiction and psychiatric symptoms among Korean adolescents. Journal of School Health 78: 165–171.

June KJ, Sohn SY, So AY, Yi GM, Park SH (2007). A study of factors that influence Internet addiction, smoking, and drinking in high school students [in Korean]. Taehan Kanho Hakhoe Chi 37: 872–882.

Kalke J, Raschke P (2004). Learning by doing: "initiated abstinence," a school-based programme for the prevention of addiction. Results of an evaluation study. European Addiction Research 10: 88–94.

Kim K (2013). Association between Internet overuse and aggression in Korean adolescents. Pediatrics International 55: 703–709.

Kim K, Ryu E, Chon MY, et al (2006). Internet addiction in Korean adolescents and its relation to depression and suicidal ideation: a questionnaire survey. International Journal of Nursing Studies 43: 185–192.

King DL, Delfabbro PH, Griffiths MD, Gradisar M (2011). Assessing clinical trials of Internet addiction treatment: a systematic review and CONSORT evaluation. Clinical Psychology Review 31: 1110–1116.

Kittinger R, Correia CJ, Irons JG (2012). Relationship between Facebook use and problematic Internet use among college students. Cyberpsychology, Behavior, and Social Networking 15: 324–327.

Ko CH, Hsiao S, Liu GC, Yen JU, Yang MJ, Yen CF (2010). The characteristics of decision making, potential to take risks, and personality of college students with Internet addiction. Psychiatry Research 170: 121–125.

Ko CH, Yen JY, Chen CS (2008a). Psychiatric comorbidity of Internet addiction in college students: an interview study. CNS Spectrums 13: 147–153.

Ko CH, Yen JY, Chen CC, Chen SH, Wu K, Yen CF (2006). Tridimensional personality of adolescents with Internet addiction and substance use experience. Canadian Journal of Psychiatry 51: 887–894.

Ko CH, Yen JY, Yen CF, Chen CS, Weng CC, Chen CC (2008b). The association between Internet addiction and problematic alcohol use in adolescents: the problem behavior model. Cyberpsychology and Behavior 11: 571–576.

Kormas G, Critselis E, Janikian M, Kafetzis D, Tsitsika A (2011). Risk factors and psychosocial characteristics of potential problematic Internet use among adolescents: a cross-sectional study. BMC Public Health 11: 595.

Kratzer S, Hegerl U (2008). Is "Internet Addiction" a disorder of its own? A study on subjects with excessive Internet use [in German]. Psychiatriche Praxis 35: 80–83.

Kuss DJ, Griffiths MD, Karila L, Billieux J (2014). Internet addiction: a systematic review of epidemiological research for the last decade. Current Pharmaceutical Design 20:4026–4052.

Lai CM, et al (2013). Psychometric properties of the internet addiction test in Chinese adolescents. Journal of Pediatric Psychology 38: 794–807.

Lam LT, Peng ZW, Mai JC, Jing J (2009). Factors associated with Internet addiction among adolescents. Cyberpsychology and Behavior 12: 551–555.

Lee BW, Stapinski LA (2012). Seeking safety on the Internet: relationship between social anxiety and problematic Internet use. Journal of Anxiety Disorders 26: 197–205.

Lee YS, Han DH, Yang KC, Daniels MA, et al (2008) Depression like characteristics of 5HTTLPR polymorphism and temperament in excessive Internet users. Journal of Affective Disorders 109: 165–169.

Leménager T, Gwodz A, Richter A, et al (2013). Self-concept deficits in massively multiplayer online role-playing games addiction. European Addiction Research 19: 227–234.

Li D, Liau A, Khoo A (2011). Examining the influence of actual-ideal self-discrepancies, depression, and escapism, on pathological gaming among massively multiplayer online adolescent gamers. Cyberpsychology, Behavior, and Social Networking 14: 535–539.

Li M, Deng Y, Ren Y, Guo S, He X (2014a). Obesity status of middle school students in Xiangtan and its relationship with Internet addiction. Obesity (Silver Spring) 22: 482–487.

Li Y, Zhang X, Lu F, Zhang Q, Wang Y (2014b). Internet addiction among elementary and middle school students in China: a nationally representative sample study. Cyberpsychology, Behavior, and Social Networking 17: 111–116.

Liberatore KA, Rosario K, Colón-De Martí LN, Martínez KG (2011). Prevalence of Internet addiction in Latino adolescents with psychiatric diagnosis. Cyberpsychology, Behavior, and Social Networking 14: 399–402.

Mazhari S (2012). Association between problematic Internet use and impulse control disorders among Iranian university students. Cyberpsychology, Behavior, and Social Networking 15: 270–273.

Mehroof M, Griffiths MD (2010). Online gaming addiction: the role of sensation seeking, self-control, neuroticism, aggression, state anxiety, and trait anxiety. Cyberpsychology, Behavior, and Social Networking 13: 313–316.

Montag C, Kirsch P, Sauer C, Markett S, Reuter M (2012). The role of the CHRNA4 gene in Internet addiction: a case-control study. Journal of Addiction Medicine 6: 191–195.

Moreno MA, Jelenchick L, Cox E, Young H, Christakis DA (2011). Problematic Internet use among US youth: a systematic review. Archives of Pediatric and Adolescent Medicine 165: 797–805.

Morrison CM, Gore H (2010). The relationship between excessive Internet use and depression: a questionnaire-based study of 1,319 young people and adults. Psychopathology 43: 121–126.

Mottram AJ, Fleming MJ (2009). Extraversion, impulsivity, and online group membership as predictors of problematic Internet use. Cyberpsychology and Behavior 12: 319–321.

Ni X, Yan H, Chen S, Liu Z (2009). Factors influencing Internet addiction in a sample of freshmen university students in China. Cyberpsychology and Behavior 12: 327–330.

Niemz K, Griffiths M, Banyard P (2005). Prevalence of pathological Internet use among university students and correlations with self-esteem, the General Health Questionnaire (GHQ) and disinhibition. Cyberpsychology and Behavior 8: 562–570.

Pallanti S, Bernardi S, Quercioli L (2006). The Shorter PROMIS Questionnaire and the Internet Addiction Scale in the assessment of multiple addictions in a high-school population: prevalence and related disability. CNS Spectrums 11: 966–974.

Park MH, Park EJ, Choi J, et al (2011). Preliminary study of Internet addiction and cognitive function in adolescents based on IQ tests. Psychiatry Research 190: 275–281.

Park SK, Kim JY, Cho CB (2008). Prevalence of Internet addiction and correlations with family factors among South Korean adolescents. Adolescence 43: 895–909.

Petersen KU, Weymann N, Schelb Y, Thiel R, Thomasius R (2009). Pathological Internet use: epidemiology, diagnostics, co-occurring disorders and treatment [in German]. Fortschritte der Neurologie Psychiatrie 77: 263–271.

Pies R (2009). Should DSM-V designate "Internet addiction" a mental disorder? Psychiatry (Edgmont) 6: 31–37.

Poli R, Agrimi E (2012). Internet addiction disorder: prevalence in an Italian student population. Nordic Journal of Psychiatry 66: 55–59.

Ricquebourg M, Bernède-Bauduin C, Mété D, et al (2013). Internet and video games among students of Reunion Island in 2010: uses, misuses, perceptions and associated factors. Revue Epidemiologique Santé Publique 61: 503–512. [Article in French]

Rodgers RF, Melioli T, Laconi S, Bui E, Chabrol H (2013). Internet addiction symptoms, disordered eating, and body image avoidance. Cyberpsychology, Behavior, and Social Networking 16: 56–60.

Rumpf HJ, Vermulst AA, Bischof A, et al (2014). Occurence of internet addiction in a general population sample: a latent class analysis. European Addiction Research 20: 159–166.

Senormanci O, Senormanci G, Güçlü O, Konkan R (2014). Attachment and family functioning in patients with Internet addiction. General Hospital Psychiatry 36: 203–207.

Seo M, Kang HS, Yom YH (2009). Internet addiction and interpersonal problems in Korean adolescents. Computers Informatics Nursing 27: 226–233.

Shapira NA, Goldsmith TD, Keck PE (2000). Psychiatric features of individuals with problematic Internet use. Journal of Affective Disorders 57: 267–272.

Shaw M, Black DW (2008). Internet addiction: definition, assessment, epidemiology and clinical management. CNS Drugs 22: 353–365.

Shin SE, Kim NS, Jang EY (2011). Comparison of problematic Internet and alcohol use and attachment styles among industrial workers in Korea. Cyberpsychology, Behavior, and Social Networking 14: 665–672.

Siomos K, Paradeisioti A, Hadjimarcou M, et al (2013). The impact of Internet and PC addiction in school performance of Cypriot adolescents. Studies in Health Technology Information 191: 90–94.

Smahel D, Brown BB, Blinka L (2012). Associations between online friendship and Internet addiction among adolescents and emerging adults. Developmental Psychology 48: 381–388.

Southern S (2008). Treatment of compulsive cybersex behavior. Psychiatric Clinics of North America 31: 697–712.

Stavropoulos V, Alexandraki K, Motti-Stefanidi F (2013). Recognizing Internet addiction: prevalence and relationship to academic achievement in adolescents enrolled in urban and rural Greek high schools. Journal of Adolescence 36: 565–576.

Sun DL, Chen ZJ, Ma N, Zhang XC, Fu XM, Zhang DR (2009). Decision-making and prepotent response inhibition functions in excessive Internet users. CNS Spectrums 14: 75–81.

Tang J, Yu Y, Du Y, Ma Y, Zhang D, Wang J (2014). Prevalence of Internet addiction and its association with stressful life events and psychological symptoms among adolescent Internet users. Addictive Behaviors 39: 744–747.

Tao R, Huang X, Wang J, Zhang H, Zhang Y, Li M (2010). Proposed diagnostic criteria for Internet addiction. Addiction 105: 556–564.

te Wildt BT, Putzig I, Zedler M, Ohlmeier MD (2007). Internet dependency as a symptom of depressive mood disorders [in German]. Psychiatrische Praxis 34(Suppl 3): S318–S322.

Tosun LP, Lajunen T (2009). Why do young adults develop a passion for Internet activities? The associations among personality, revealing "true self" on the Internet, and passion for the Internet. Cyberpsychology and Behavior 12: 401–406.

Tsai HF, Cheng SH, Yeh TL, et al (2009). The risk factors of Internet addiction—a survey of university freshmen. Psychiatry Research 167: 294–299.

Tsitsika A, Critselis E, Kormas G, et al (2009). Internet use and misuse: a multivariate regression analysis of the predictive factors of Internet use among Greek adolescents. European Journal of Pediatrics 168: 655–665.

Tsitsika A, Critselis E, Louizou A, et al (2011). Determinants of Internet addiction among adolescents: a case-control study. Scientific World Journal 11: 866–874.

Wang H, Zhou X, Lu C, Wu J, Deng X, Hong L (2011). Problematic Internet use in high school students in Guangdong province, China. PLoS One 6: e19660.

Wei HT, Chen MH, Huang PC, Bai YM (2012). The association between online gaming, social phobia, and depression: an Internet survey. BMC Psychiatry 12: 92.

Weinstein A, Lejoyeux M (2010). Internet addiction or excessive Internet use. American Journal of Drug and Alcohol Abuse 36: 277–283.

Weinstein AM, Lejoyeux M (2013). New developments in the psychobiology of video game addiction. American Journal of Addiction 20: 1–9.

Weinstein AM, Weizman A (2012). Emerging association between addictive gaming and attention-deficit/hyperactivity disorder. Current Psychiatry Reports 14: 590–597.

Whang LS, Lee S, Chang G (2003). Internet over-users' psychological profiles: a behavior sampling analysis on Internet addiction. Cyberpsychology and Behavior 6: 143–150.

Wu X, Chen X, Han J, et al (2013). Prevalence and factors of addictive Internet use among adolescents in Wuhan, China: interactions of parental relationship with age and hyperactivity-impulsivity. PLoS One 8: e61782.

Xiuqin H, Huimin Z, Mengchen L, Jinan W, Ying Z, Ran T (2010). Mental health, personality, and parental rearing styles of adolescents with Internet addiction disorder. Cyberpsychology, Behavior, and Social Networking 13: 401–406.

Xu J, Shen LX, Yan CH, et al (2012). Personal characteristics related to the risk of adolescent Internet addiction: a survey in Shanghai, China. BMC Public Health 12: 1106.

Yadav P, Banwari G, Parmar C, Maniar R (2013). Internet addiction and its correlates among high school students: apreliminary study from Ahmedabad, India. Asian Journal of Psychiatry 6: 500–505.

Yao B, Han W, Zeng L, Guo X (2013). Freshman year mental health symptoms and level of adaptation as predictors of Internet addiction: a retrospective nested case-control study of male Chinese college students. Psychiatry Research 210: 541–547.

Yates TM, Gregor MA, Haviland MG (2012). Child maltreatment, alexithymia, and problematic Internet use in young adulthood. Cyberpsychology, Behavior, and Social Networking 15: 219–225.

Yellowlees PM, Marks S (2007). Problematic Internet use or Internet addiction? Computers in Human Behavior 23: 1447–1453.

Yen CF, Ko CH, Yen JY, Chang YP, Cheng CP (2009a). Multi-dimensional discriminative factors for Internet addiction among adolescents regarding gender and age. Psychiatry and Clinical Neurosciences 63: 357–364.

Yen JY, Ko CH, Yen CF, Chen CS, Chen CC (2009b). The association between harmful alcohol use and Internet addiction among college students: comparison of personality. Psychiatry and Clinical Neurosciences 63: 218–224.

Yen JY, Ko CH, Yen CF, Chen SH, Chung WL, Chen CC. (2008). Psychiatric symptoms in adolescents with Internet addiction: comparison with substance use. Psychiatry and Clinical Neurosciences 62: 9–16.

Yen JY, Ko CH, Yen CF, Wu HY, Yang MJ (2007).The comorbid psychiatric symptoms of Internet addiction: attention deficit and hyperactivity disorder (ADHD), depression, social phobia, and hostility. Journal of Adolescent Health 41: 93–98.

Yen JY, Yen CF, Chen CS, Tang TC, Ko CH (2009c). The association between adult ADHD symptoms and Internet addiction among college students: the gender difference. Cyberpsychology and Behavior 12: 187–191.

Yen JY, Yen CF, Wu HY, Huang CJ, Ko CH (2011). Hostility in the real world and online: the effect of Internet addiction, depression, and online activity. Cyberpsychology, Behavior, and Social Networking 14: 649–655.

Yoo YS, Cho OH, Cha KS (2014). Associations between overuse of the Internet and mental health in adolescents. Nursing Health Science 16:193–200.

Yoo HJ, Cho SC, Ha J (2004). Attention deficit hyperactivity symptoms and Internet addiction. Psychiatry and Clinical Neuroscience 58: 487–494.

Young KS (1998). Caught in the Net. Wiley, New York, NY.

Young KS (2007). Cognitive behavior therapy with Internet addicts: treatment outcomes and implications. Cyberpsychology and Behavior 10: 671–679.

Young KS (2004). Internet addiction. A new clinical phenomenon and its consequences. American Behavioral Scientist 48: 402–415.

Zanetta Dauriat F, Zermatten A, Billieux J, et al (2011). Motivations to play specifically predict excessive involvement in massively multiplayer online role-playing games: evidence from an online survey. European Addiction Research 17: 185–189.

Zhou Z, Li C, Zhu H (2013). An error-related negativity potential investigation of response monitoring function in individuals with Internet addiction disorder. Frontiers in Behavioral Neuroscience 7: 131.

2 An Overview of Problematic Gaming

Mark D. Griffiths, Orsolya Király,
Halley M. Pontes, and Zsolt Demetrovics

INTRODUCTION

During the past decade, as the video game industry has grown to $93 billion world-wide (Gartner, 2013) and as the average age of gamers has increased to 30 years (Entertainment Software Association, 2013), video game addiction has become a topic of increasing research interest. But despite the growth in published studies, there is a lack of consensus regarding whether problematic gaming exists and whether it constitutes an "addiction." A wide range of different terms have been used to describe what is essentially the same phenomenon, including problem video game playing (King et al., 2011c), problematic online game use or gaming (Kim and Kim, 2010; Demetrovics et al., 2012), video game addiction (Griffiths and Davies, 2005; Skoric et al., 2009; King et al., 2010a), pathological video game use or gaming (Gentile, 2009; Lemmens et al., 2011), online gaming addiction (Charlton and Danforth, 2007; Griffiths, 2010), compulsive Internet use (van Rooij et al., 2011), Internet gaming addiction (Kuss and Griffiths, 2012), and Internet gaming disorder (American Psychiatric Association, 2013).

Prior to the publication in 2013 of the fifth edition of the *Diagnostic and Statistical Manual of Mental Disorders* (DSM-5; American Psychiatric Association, 2013), there had been some debate about whether "Internet addiction" should be introduced into the text as a separate disorder (Petry and O'Brien, 2013). In parallel, there has also been debate regarding whether those conducting online addiction research should be studying general Internet use or the potentially addictive specific activities that can be engaged in online (e.g., gambling, video gaming, sex, shopping). Ultimately, the Substance Use Disorder Work Group recommended that the DSM-5 include a subtype of problematic Internet use (i.e., Internet gaming disorder [IGD]) in Section III ("Emerging Measures and Models") as an area that required further research before possible inclusion in future editions of the manual (Petry and O'Brien, 2013). The implications of this decision will be returned to later in the chapter.

For the sake of consistency, this chapter will use the term "problematic gaming" as the umbrella term to describe the phenomenon of problematic video game use. It has both online and offline manifestations. The chapter briefly examines a number of key areas in the study of problematic gaming, including (1) history of problematic gaming research, (2) offline versus online problematic gaming, (3) prevalence of problematic gaming, (4) factors associated with problematic gaming, and (5) the treatment of problematic gaming. This chapter does not address the instruments developed to assess problematic gaming as those are reviewed elsewhere (see Chapter 3).

HISTORY OF PROBLEMATIC GAMING

The first reports of problematic gaming predate the Internet. They appeared in the psychological literature in the early 1980s and included cases of "*Space Invaders* obsession" (Ross et al., 1982), "computer catatonia" (Nilles, 1982), and "video game addiction" (Soper and Miller, 1983). Other early articles on the topic also reported the use of cognitive-behavioral therapy (CBT) to treat adolescents addicted to arcade video games (Kuczmierczyk et al., 1987; Keepers, 1990). However, these reports were mostly observational, anecdotal case studies that were primarily based on teenage males and featured a particular type of video game in a particular medium (i.e., "pay-to-play" arcade video games). Shotton (1989) conducted the first empirical study of problematic gaming in a sample of male teenagers and young adults (N = 127) who claimed to be "hooked on" video console games. The study's only criterion for being "addicted" to gaming was the individual's own admission of being "hooked." Shotton reported only few negative consequences in her sample. However, given that no instrument was used to assess problematic gaming, it is possible that participants were preoccupied with gaming rather than addicted to it.

In the 1990s, research into problematic gaming became more systematic, but almost all the published studies were relatively small surveys conducted in British schools and involving children and teenagers aged 10 to 15 years (e.g., Brown and Robertson, 1993; Fisher, 1994; Griffiths and Hunt, 1995, 1998; Phillips et al., 1995; Griffiths, 1997). These studies mainly examined nonarcade video games (i.e., home console games, handheld games, personal computer [PC] gaming). However, these studies had many methodological limitations, especially the use of nonpsychometrically validated scales to assess problematic gaming (typically, scales adapted from the DSM-III-R [American Psychiatric Association, 1987] or DSM-IV [American Psychiatric Association, 1994] criteria for pathological gambling). These studies were later criticized by Charlton (2002) as more likely assessing gaming preoccupation rather than gaming addiction.

Since 2000, the academic gaming field has seen substantial growth in studies of problematic gaming. This is most likely due to the rise of online gaming (e.g., massively multiplayer online role-playing games [MMORPGs] such as *World of Warcraft* and *Everquest*). Unlike traditional offline video games that are typically played alone and against the computer, online video games are usually played with, or against, other gamers (i.e., multiplayer games) in large, sophisticated, detailed, and evolving worlds based in different narrative environments (Griffiths et al., 2004). These games offer a rich three-dimensional world that is populated by thousands of players. In MMORPGs, the focus is on role playing; these games usually allow the player to choose from a variety of races, professions, moralities, and genders (Ghuman and Griffiths, 2012) and provide vast virtual environments in which to explore. Game play is based around gaining skills and abilities through completing quests and defeating opponents. The player is encouraged to "level-up" the character to broaden the environment of the game. Social interactions are a big part of the game and may be considered obligatory in order to complete objectives (Ghuman and Griffiths, 2012).

Between 2000 and 2010, approximately 60 empirical studies were published on various aspects of (mainly) MMORPG addiction (Kuss and Griffiths, 2012). Unlike previous studies, most gamers were adults (i.e., older than age 18 years) and some studies were nationally representative. Also, researchers tended to collect their data online or via non–self-report methods, including polysomnographic measures and visual and verbal memory tests (Dworak et al., 2007); medical evaluations, including the patient's history and physical examination and radiological, intraoperative, or pathological findings (Cultrara and Har-El, 2002); functional magnetic resonance imaging (Hoeft et al., 2008; Ko et al., 2009; Han et al., 2010); electroencephalography (Thalemann et al., 2007); and genotyping (Han et al., 2007).

OFFLINE VERSUS ONLINE PROBLEMATIC GAMING

As noted earlier, video gaming that is problematic, pathological, or addictive lacks a widely accepted definition. Some researchers consider video games as the starting point for examining the characteristics of this specific disorder, whereas others consider the Internet as the main platform that unites different and disparate addictive Internet activities, including online games (see Chapter 3). Recent studies (Kim and Kim, 2010; Demetrovics et al., 2012) have made an effort to integrate both approaches. Consequently, online problematic gaming can be viewed as a specific type of video game addiction, as a variant of Internet addiction, or as an independent condition.

Griffiths (2005) has argued that although all chemical and behavioral addictions have specific and idiosyncratic characteristics, they share more commonalities than differences (i.e., salience, mood modification, tolerance and withdrawal symptoms, conflict, and relapse), and that these commonalities most likely reflect a common etiology for addictive behavior. Consequently, online game addiction is viewed as a specific type of video game addiction. Similarly, Porter et al. (2010) do not differentiate between problematic video game use and problematic online game use. They conceptualize problematic video game use as excessive use of one or more video games (regardless of platform), resulting in a preoccupation with, and a loss of control over, playing video games, along with various negative psychosocial or physical consequences. However, unlike Griffiths (2005), their criteria for problematic video game use do not include other features commonly associated with dependence or addiction (e.g., tolerance, physical symptoms of withdrawal), because they do not see clear evidence that problematic gaming is associated with such phenomena. Other researchers (e.g., Young, 1998) view online problematic gaming as a subtype of Internet addiction. They see the Internet itself as providing situation-specific characteristics that can make gaming problematic or addictive (i.e., the fact that players can theoretically play all day every day is a situational characteristic that may facilitate excessive gaming).

Kim and Kim's (2010) Problematic Online Game Use Model takes a more integrative approach, viewing both the game and the medium as contributory factors in the development of problematic gaming. It claims that neither of the approaches outlined above adequately captures the unique features of online games such as MMORPGs. They argue that the Internet itself has features that may facilitate excessive use but also that the Internet is just one channel where people may access the content they want (e.g., gambling, shopping, sex) and that such users may become addicted to the particular content rather than the channel itself. This is analogous to the argument by Griffiths (2000) that there is a fundamental difference between addiction to the Internet and addictions on the Internet. However, MMORPGs differ from traditional stand-alone video games because there are social and/or role-playing dimensions that allow interaction with other gamers. The Problematic Online Game Use Model stresses five underlying dimensions of addictive game play: euphoria, health problems, conflict (with other activities or relationships), failure of self-control, and preference of virtual relationship.

Demetrovics et al. (2012) also support the integrative approach and stress the need to include all types of online games in addiction models to make comparisons between genres and gamer populations possible, such as those who play online real-time strategy (RTS) games and online first-person shooter (FPS) games, in addition to the widely researched MMORPG players. FPS games portray three-dimensional environments that are viewed as if through the eyes of the character, with usually only the weapon being depicted. The majority of FPS games produced (eg, *Return to Castle Wolfenstein*) have both a "single player mode" and a "multiplayer mode" (Ghuman and Griffiths, 2012). The RTS genre differs from "turn-based" strategy games (such as chess) in that players have to respond to events as they occur. RTS games differ from FPS games in that the camera angle is positioned in a "birds-eye view" of the virtual environment. Players control many characters (units) at the same time. As in FPS games, these games often have both a "single player mode" and a "multiplayer mode."

The model by Demetrovics et al. (2012) has six dimensions: preoccupation, overuse, immersion, social isolation, interpersonal conflicts, and withdrawal. But irrespective of approach or model, the components and dimensions for online problematic gaming outlined above are very similar to the criteria for IGD in Section III of the DSM-5. For instance, Griffiths' six addiction components (2005; in brackets below) directly map onto the nine proposed criteria for IGD (of which five or more need to be endorsed, resulting in clinically significant impairment). They are as follows: (1) preoccupation with Internet games [salience]; (2) withdrawal symptoms when Internet gaming is taken away [withdrawal]; (3) the need to spend increasing amounts of time engaged in Internet gaming [tolerance]; (4) unsuccessful attempts to control participation in Internet gaming [relapse/loss of control]; (5) loss of interest in hobbies and entertainment as a result of, and with the exception of, Internet gaming [conflict]; (6) continued excessive use of Internet games despite knowledge of psychosocial problems [conflict]; (7) deception of family members, therapists, or others regarding the amount of Internet gaming [conflict]; (8) use of the Internet gaming to escape or relieve a negative mood [mood modification]; and (9) loss of a significant relationship, job, or educational or career opportunity because of participation in Internet games [conflict].

THE PREVALENCE OF PROBLEMATIC GAMING

Table 2.1 presents a summary of prevalence studies examining problematic gaming (or its conceptual equivalent). The studies were selected on the basis of (1) having at least 300 subjects and (2) using a screening instrument to assess problematic gaming (rather than self-diagnosis). The results show large variation in the prevalence rates, ranging from 0.2% to 34%. However, the populations differ widely in type of gaming played (i.e., some studies just examined online gaming, whereas others examined console gaming or a mixture of both), size, age range, type (i.e., some studies assessed gamers only, whereas others assessed general population), and instrument used to assess gaming. These differences are the likely reason for the variation in rates. Five of the published studies, all of which were conducted in adolescents, used nationally representative samples. The prevalence rates in these studies were as follows: 1.7% in Germany (Rehbein et al., 2010); 4.2% in Norway (Brunborg et al., 2013); 4.6% in Hungary (Pápay et al., 2013); 8.5% in the United States (Gentile, 2009); and 9% in Singapore (Gentile et al., 2011). The studies also indicate that males are significantly more likely than females to develop problematic gaming. However, many studies failed to assess prior problematic gaming (i.e., lifetime prevalence) and the presence of comorbid psychopathology (King et al., 2012). Furthermore, because they used different screening instruments or cutoff criteria, it cannot be ascertained whether prevalence differences are real.

The instruments used to assess problematic gaming, discussed elsewhere, represent a key challenge in the field (see Chapter 3). A recent comprehensive review by King et al. (2013) of 63 quantitative studies involving 58,415 participants reported that the main weaknesses among the 18 screens they identified were (1) inconsistency of core addiction indicators across studies, (2) a general lack of any temporal dimension, (3) inconsistent cutoff scores relating to clinical status, (4) poor and/or inadequate interrater reliability and predictive validity, and (5) inconsistent and/or untested dimensionality. There are also questions about the appropriateness of certain screens for certain settings, because those used in clinical practice milieus may require a different emphasis than those used in epidemiological, experimental, or neurobiological research settings (Koronczai et al., 2011; King et al., 2013).

Table 2.1 Prevalence of Problematic Gaming in the Largest Survey Studies

Study	Year	Country	Sample	Age (years)	Assessment Screen	Problematic Gaming Prevalence (%)	Gender Ratio
Fisher	1994	England	467 secondary school children	11–16	DSM-IV[a]	6.0	M = F
Phillips et al.	1995	England	868 secondary school children	11–16	DSM-III-R	5.7	M = F
Griffiths and Hunt	1998	England	387 adolescents	12–16	DSM-III	19.9	M > F (3:1)
Johansson and Götestam	2004	Norway	3237 adolescents	12–18	Young's DQ	2.7	M = F
Grüsser et al.	2005	Germany	323 schoolchildren	11–12	DSM-IV[a]/ICD-10[b]	9.3	M > F (3:1)
Grüsser et al.	2007	Germany	7069 gamers	15+	ICD-10[b]	11.9	Not reported
Lee and Han	2007	South Korea	2584 students	5th/6th grade	DSM-IV[a]	2.5	Not reported
Wan and Chiou	2007	Taiwan	416 adolescents	17–24	OAST	34.0	Not reported
Gentile	2009	United States	1178 students	8–18	DSM-IV[a]	8.5	M > F (4:1)
Batthyány et al.	2009	Austria	1068 students	13–18	CSVK-R	2.7	M > F (3:1)
Lemmens et al.	2009	Holland	721 adolescents	12–18	GASA	1.4–9.4	Not reported
Arnesen	2010	Norway	2500 young adults	16–40	DSM-IV[a]	0.6–4.0	M > F (4:1)
Choo et al.	2010	Singapore	2998 children and adolescents	9–13	DSM-IV[a]	8.7	M > F (3:1)
Rehbein et al.	2010	Germany	15,168 schoolchildren	14–16	KFN-CSAS-II	1.7	M = F
Thomas and Martin	2010	Australia	(a) 1326 school students (b) 705 university students	12–54	Young DQ (adaptation)	5.0	(a) M = F (b) M < F (1:3)
Porter et al.	2010	Australia	1945 gamers	14–40+	DSM-IV[a] and others	8.0	M > F (9:1)
Zamani et al.	2010	Iran	564 students	"Students"	QACG	17.1	M > F
Wölfling et al.	2010	Germany	1710 adolescents	13–18	ICD-10[b]	7.5–8.4	Not reported
Van Rooij et al.	2011	Holland	3048 adolescent gamers	13–16	DSM-IV[a]	3.0	M > F (4:1)

Study	Year	Country	Sample	Age	Measure/Criteria	Prevalence (%)	Gender
Achab et al.	2011	France	448 MMORPG gamers	18–54	DSM-IV[a] Substance Dependence Adapted Scale (DAS)	27.5	M > F (4:1)
Jeong and Kim	2011	South Korea	600 students	12–18	IAT (adapted version)	2.2	M = F
Lemmens et al.	2011	Holland	543 adolescent gamers	11–17	GASA	4.0–6.0	M > F (7:3)
Mentzoni et al.	2011	Norway	816 individuals	15–40	GASA	4.1 problem 0.6 addicted	M > F
Gentile et al.	2011	Singapore	3034 students	12–18	DSM-IV[a]	9.0	M > F (3:1)
Stetina et al.	2011	Germany	486 online gamers	11–67	ISS-20 (adapted version)	8.0	M > F (9:1)
Zanetta Dauriat et al.	2011	Switzerland	696 gamers	13–54	Self-developed MMORPG addiction scale (no name)	11.2	M > F (9:1)
Hussain et al.	2012	England	1420 gamers	12–62	DSM-IV[a]	3.6 (monothetic)	M > F (4:1)
Demetrovics et al.	2012	Hungary	3415 online gamers	21 (mean)	POGQ	3.4	M > F (9:1)
Walther et al.	2012	Germany	2553 students	12–25	KFN-CSAS-II	3.3 at risk 1.1 addicted	M = F
Xu et al.	2012	China	623 adolescents	13–18	DSM-IV[a] and others	21.5	Not reported
Brunborg et al.	2013	Norway	1320 adolescents	14 (mean)	GASA	4.2	M = F
Festl et al.	2013	Germany	4382 adolescents and adults	14–90	GASA	3.7 problem 0.2 addicted	M > F (3:2)
Pápay et al.	2013	Hungary	5045 adolescents	16 (mean)	POGQ-SF	4.6	M = F
Spekman et al.	2013	Holland	1004 secondary school adolescent boys	11–18	Components model of addiction	8.6	Not applicable

Abbreviations: CSVK-R, Fragebogen zum Computerspielverhalten bei Kindern und Jugendlichen; GASA, Game Addiction Scale for Adolescents; IAT, Internet Addiction Test; ISS-20, Die Internetsuchtskala-20; KFN-CSAS-II, Video Game Dependency Scale; N/A, not applicable; POGQ, Problematic Online Gaming Questionnaire; POGQ-SF, Problematic Online Gaming Questionnaire Short Form; QACG, Questionnaire of Addiction to Computer Games; Young's DQ, Young's Diagnostic Questionnaire.

[a] Specific DSM-IV criteria varied across studies. Adapted DSM-IV criteria for pathological gambling were used in several studies.

[b] Refers to symptoms of dependence described in the International Classification of Disease, tenth revision (ICD-10).

With regard to the demographic characteristics, the data allow for some basic conclusions. As mentioned, adolescent males and young male adults appear to be at greater risk for problematic gaming. However, the course and severity of their symptoms is not well known (King et al., 2012), and the finding that this group is more at risk may be a consequence of sampling bias and the fact that this group plays video games more frequently than other sociodemographic groups. It has also been suggested that university students may be vulnerable to developing problematic video gaming (King et al., 2012). Reasons for this include their flexible timetables and study hours (i.e., nonstandard working days), ready access to high-speed broadband around the clock, and multiple stressors associated with adjusting to new social obligations or living away from home for the first time (Young, 1998; King et al., 2012).

FACTORS ASSOCIATED WITH PROBLEMATIC GAMING

A number of studies have examined the association between problematic gaming and various personality factors, comorbidity factors, and biological factors. Although some studies have examined the relationship between personality traits and Internet addiction, studies specifically examining online problematic gaming have shown it to be associated with neuroticism (Peters and Malesky, 2008; Mehroof and Griffiths, 2010), aggression and hostility (Chiu et al., 2004; Kim et al., 2008; Caplan et al., 2009; Mehroof and Griffiths, 2010), avoidant and schizoid tendencies (Allison et al., 2006), loneliness and introversion (Caplan et al., 2009), social inhibition (Porter et al., 2010), boredom inclination (Chiu et al., 2004), sensation-seeking (Chiu et al., 2004; Mehroof and Griffiths, 2010), diminished agreeableness (Peters and Malesky, 2008), diminished self-control and narcissistic personality traits (Kim et al., 2008), low self-esteem (Ko et al., 2005), state and trait anxiety (Mehroof and Griffiths, 2010), and low emotional intelligence (Parker et al., 2008). It is difficult, however, to assess the etiological significance of these associations because they may not be unique to problematic gaming. Further research is therefore needed to understand their true relevance.

Research has also shown online problematic gaming to be associated with a variety of comorbid disorders, including attention deficit hyperactivity disorder (Allison et al., 2006; Chan and Rabinowitz, 2006; Batthyány et al., 2009; Han et al., 2009), symptoms of generalized anxiety disorder, panic disorder, depression, and social phobia (Allison et al., 2006), and various psychosomatic symptoms (Batthyány et al., 2009). The much discussed association with offline violence is addressed in Chapter 5.

Through use of functional magnetic resonance imaging, biological research has shown that online gaming addicts show similar neural processes and activity in brain areas associated with substance use disorders and behavioral addictions such as pathological gambling (significant activation in the left occipital lobe, parahippocampal gyrus, dorsolateral prefrontal cortex, nucleus accumbens, right orbitofrontal cortex, bilateral anterior cingulate, medial frontal cortex, and the caudate nucleus [Hoeft et al., 2008; Ko et al., 2009; Han et al., 2010]). It has also been reported that gaming addicts, like substance addicts, have a higher prevalence of two specific polymorphisms of the dopaminergic system: Taq1A1 allele of the dopamine D2 receptor and the Val158Met in the catecholamine-O-methyltransferase enzyme (Han et al., 2007). Most biological data, however, come from small nonrepresentative studies and should be considered preliminary. More research is needed to replicate them, understand their relevance, and ascertain that they are not by-products of coexisting conditions (see Chapter 4).

TREATMENT OF PROBLEMATIC GAMING

The evidence base on the treatment of problematic or addictive gaming is limited. Clinical interventions vary considerably in the literature, but most of the very few published studies (Table 2.2) use some type of CBT, pharmacotherapy, or self-devised psychological interventions (Griffiths and Meredith, 2009; Han et al., 2009, 2010; King et al., 2010b, 2012; Young, 2013; Thorens et al., 2014). The lack of consistent approaches to treating problematic gaming makes it difficult to produce definitive conclusions about efficacy and, consequently, to generate treatment guidelines, although CBT does appear to show good preliminary support. There remains a need for controlled, comparative studies of psychological and pharmacological treatments, administered individually and in combination with each other, to determine the optimal treatment approach.

The lack of comparative treatment studies might suggest that there is a general lack of demand for psychological and psychiatric services for problematic gaming (King et al., 2010b), but this is not necessarily the case. For instance, Woog (2004) surveyed a random sample of 5000 US mental health professionals. Although only 229 participants completed the questionnaire, two-thirds had treated someone with excessive computer use problems in the year prior to the survey. Survey results showed that problematic gaming was most common among 11- to 17-year-old clients. However, this client group may be more likely to present in therapy; anecdotal evidence suggests that they are typically forced by concerned parents to seek treatment. Adult gaming addicts may not seek treatment, or seek treatment at a later stage for other psychological problems, such as depression, which may develop after experiencing the negative consequences of gaming.

There appears to be significant demand for treatment of online-related problems, including problematic gaming, in Southeast Asia. Besides governmental funds for research into problematic gaming, this is evidenced by the government-supported establishment in South Korea of a network of more than 140 counseling centers devoted to treating online addiction (Kim, 2008). Problematic gaming clinics have also started to emerge in Western countries such as Holland and the United Kingdom (Griffiths and Meredith, 2009; King et al., 2011b). Treatment groups modeled on 12-step self-help programs (e.g., Online Gamers Anonymous) have also appeared (Griffiths and Meredith, 2009), but little is known about their treatment protocols or efficacy.

Table 2.2 Selected Characteristics of Treatment Studies for Problematic Online Gaming (or Internet Use)

Study	Assessment Instrument and/or Criteria for Inclusion	Extent of Gaming Problem	Treatment Conditions	N	Age Range (years)	Treatment Outcome	Treatment Effect Size
Young (2007)	IAT (score not specified)	10% reported a video gaming problem	1. CBT (12 sessions)	114	Not reported	CBT reduced most clients' thoughts and behaviors related to compulsive Internet use at 6-month follow-up	Not reported
Kim (2008)	K-IAS (score not specified)	Unclear	1. R/T group counseling (5 weeks) 2. Control	25	Not reported	10 counseling sessions reduced addiction symptoms and increased self-esteem, compared to the control group	Not reported
Han et al. (2009)	YIAS-K score ≥ 50	100% reported a video gaming problem	1. Methylphenidate (8 weeks)	62	8–12	Methylphenidate significantly reduced severity of Internet addiction symptoms and overall Internet usage	Not reported
Shek et al. (2009)	YIAS-10 score of 4; YIAS-8 score of 5; YIAS-7 score of 3; CIAS score of 3	Unclear	1. Multimodal counselling (15 to 19 months)	59	11–18	Counseling produced a decrease in symptoms of Internet addiction. Participants reported high satisfaction with the program	Not reported
Du et al. (2010)	Beard's Diagnostic Questionnaire	Unclear	1. CBT (eight sessions) 2. Control	56	12–17	CBT reduced Internet overuse and associated symptoms and improved time management skills. Treatment gains were observed at 6-month follow-up	Cohen's d = 1.08 (post) and 1.35 (6-month follow-up)
Han et al. (2010)	>4 hours per day/30 hours per week; YIAS score ≥ 50; DSM-IV criteria for substance abuse	100% reported a video gaming problem	1. Bupropion (6 weeks) 2. Control	19	17–29	Bupropion reduced cravings for video game play, total game play time, and cue-induced brain activity	Not reported
Su et al. (2011)	YDQ score of 5; Internet use ≥14 hours per week	Unclear	1. HOSC-NE (one session) 2. HOSC-LE (one session) 3. HOSC-NI (one session) 4. Control	65	Not reported	All treatment groups demonstrated significant decreases in online activity and YDQ scores after 1 month. The "expert system" treatments were the most effective.	Cohen's d = 0.72–0.82 (YDQ score); Cohen's d = 0.75–0.98 (activity)

Study	Criteria	Sample	Intervention	N	Age	Outcomes	
Han et al. (2012)	> 30 hours per week; YIAS score > 50; impaired behaviors/distress due to gaming measured by modifying the DSM-IV criteria for substance abuse	Not reported	1. Family therapy (seven sessions) 2. Control	30	Not reported	Family therapy over seven sessions reduced gaming addiction severity	Not reported
Han and Renshaw (2013)	>4 hours per day/30 hours per week; YIAS score > 50; impaired behaviors/distress due to gaming measured by modifying the DSM-IV criteria for substance abuse	100% reported video gaming problem	1. Bupropion (8 weeks) plus education for Internet use 2. Placebo (8 weeks) plus education for Internet use	50	13–42	Bupropion significantly reduced levels of gaming addiction during the 8 weeks and also at a follow-up period of 4 weeks	Not reported
Marco and Choliz (2013)	TDV (score not specified); DSM-IV-TR criteria for substance abuse	Patient (100%) reported a video gaming problem	1. CBT (19 sessions)	1	22	CBT improved patient's sense of control over games and decreased the level of gaming addiction. Positive outcomes were not steady during the 19 sessions. The positive results of CBT lasted during a 3-month follow-up period	Not reported
Taquet and Hautekeete (2013)	PVP (score not specified); QAJV (score not specified)	Patient (100%) reported a video gaming problem	1. CBT (17 sessions over 11 months)	1	19	After 6 months of CBT, the patient could effectively control his game behavior and after 10 months, PVP score was 0 (out of 9) and QAJV score was 6 (out of 380)	Not reported

Abbreviations: CBT, cognitive-behavior therapy; CIAS, Chinese Internet Addiction Scale; HOSC, Healthy Online Self-Helping Center [NE, Natural Environment; LE, Learning Environment; NI, Noninteractive]; IAT, Internet Addiction Test; K-IAS, Korean Internet Addiction Scale; PVP, problem video gaming playing; QAJV, Questionnaire sur l'addiction aux JV; R/T, reality training; TDV, Test de Dependencia de Videojuegos; YDQ, Young's Diagnostic Questionnaire; YIAS, Young Internet Addiction Scale; YIAS-K, Young Internet Addiction Scale–Korean Version.

CONCLUSION AND FUTURE DIRECTIONS

Based on available data, and particularly studies published in the past decade, it appears that in extreme cases, excessive gaming displays compulsive or addictive properties similar to more traditional addictions and can have damaging effects on individuals. However, the field continues to be seriously hindered by the use of inconsistent and nonstandardized criteria to identify and assess addictive gaming as well as by research recruitment methods that have sampling biases due to overreliance on self-selected samples. The result is significant gaps in the understanding of the incidence and demographic characteristics of problematic gaming. For epidemiological purposes, research by Koronczai et al. (2011) asserts that the most appropriate measures in assessing problematic Internet use (including Internet gaming) should satisfy six requirements: (1) brevity (to help overcome question fatigue), (2) comprehensiveness (to examine all core aspects of problematic gaming), (3) reliability and validity across age groups (e.g., adolescents, adults), (4) reliability and validity across data collection methods (e.g., online, face-to-face interview, paper-and-pencil), (5) reliability and validity across cultures, and (6) clinical validation. More research is needed to arrive at such an instrument, because it could yield more accurate prevalence rates and better quality phenomenological data. Other deficits in the knowledge of problematic gaming relate to its comorbidity with other disorders, neurobiology, natural course, and treatment.

Moreover, studies tend to examine addictive gaming from the perspective of the gamer. Yet a small body of research suggests that structural characteristics of the video games themselves may have a role in the development and maintenance of problematic gaming (Wood et al., 2004; Westwood and Griffiths, 2010; King et al., 2011a). More empirical research into those characteristics might help explain why some individuals may be protected from developing excessive playing habits or simply mature out of their problematic gaming behavior, whereas others may be vulnerable to addiction and relapse. Further, the suspected strong links between online gaming, gambling, nongambling fantasy games, role-playing games, board games, and card games remain largely unexplored (Griffiths et al., 2014a). These deserve close study, in part due to the concern that youths may migrate from free gaming sites to online gambling.

Finally, the recent explosion in mobile gaming is transforming the gaming landscape but has received little research scrutiny so far. Given the growth in mobile technology, including mobile gaming apps, it is important for future research to focus on those as well. But despite these shortcomings, several promising trends can be drawn from the research conducted so far.

- There has been a significant increase in empirical research decade by decade since the early 1980s.
- A noticeable shift in researching the mode of video game play has occurred in an attempt to keep up with rapidly advancing technology. In the 1980s, research mainly concerned "pay-to-play" arcade video games. In the 1990s, research

focus shifted to stand-alone (offline) video games played at home on consoles, PCs, or handheld devices. In the 2000s, research mainly concerned online massively multiplayer video games.

- Survey study sample sizes have generally increased. In the 1980s and 1990s, sample sizes were typically in the low hundreds. In the 2000s, sample sizes in the thousands—even if unrepresentative—are not uncommon.
- There has been a diversification in the way data are collected, including experiments, physiological investigations, secondary analysis of existing data (such as that collected from online forums), and behavioral tracking studies.
- Research in adult (i.e., nonchild and nonadolescent) samples has increased, reflecting the fact that the demographics of gaming have changed.
- The assessment and measurement of problematic gaming has become more sophisticated. In recent years, instruments with more robust psychometric properties, including better reliability and validity, have been developed. However, many of the most widely used screening instruments were adapted from adult screens of nongaming behaviors, and much of the gaming literature has examined children and adolescents.

Together, these trends point toward progress in the understanding of problematic gaming. Inclusion of IGD in Section III of the DSM-5 has come as a result of this progress. This inclusion appears to have been well received by researchers and clinicians in the problematic gaming field (Griffiths et al., 2014b) and by those who have sought treatment for such disorders and who may now feel more validated and less stigmatized. However, for problematic gaming to be included in the section on substance-related and addictive disorders, alongside the newly included "gambling disorder," the problematic gaming field must unite around a diagnostic definition and assessment measures so that comparisons can be made across different demographic groups and cultures. According to Petry and O'Brien (2013), problematic gaming will not be included as a separate mental disorder until (1) its defining features have been identified, (2) reliability and validity of the specific criteria have been obtained cross-culturally, (3) prevalence rates have been determined in representative epidemiological samples across the world, and (4) etiology and associated biological features have been evaluated. Fortunately, research does appear to be leading toward an emerging consensus. For example, King et al. (2013) note that across many different studies, problematic gaming is commonly defined by (1) withdrawal, (2) loss of control, and (3) conflict. More such examples of unity and methodological consistency are required for sufficient empirical evidence to accumulate in support of an official DSM problematic gaming diagnosis.

DISCLOSURE STATEMENT

The authors disclose no relationships with commercial entities and professional activities that may bias their views.

REFERENCES

Achab S, Nicolier M, Mauny F, et al (2011). Massively multiplayer online role-playing games: comparing characteristics of addict vs non-addict online recruited gamers in a French adult population. BMC Psychiatry 11: 144.

Allison SE, von Wahlde L, Shockley T, Gabbard GO (2006). The development of the self in the era of the Internet and role-playing fantasy games. American Journal of Psychiatry 163: 381–385.

American Psychiatric Association (1987). Diagnostic and Statistical Manual of Mental Disorders. Third Edition, Revised. American Psychiatric Association, Washington, DC.

American Psychiatric Association (1994). Diagnostic and Statistical Manual of Mental Disorders. Fourth Edition. American Psychiatric Association, Washington, DC.

American Psychiatric Association (2013). Diagnostic and Statistical Manual of Mental Disorders. Fifth Edition. American Psychiatric Association, Washington, DC.

Arnesen AA (2010). Video game addiction among young adults in Norway: prevalence and health. Unpublished manuscript. University of Bergen, Faculty of Psychology. Bergen, Norway.

Batthyány D, Müller KW, Benker F, Wölfling K (2009). Computer game playing: clinical characteristics of dependence and abuse among adolescents. Wiener Klinische Wochenschrift 121: 502–509.

Brown RIF, Robertson S (1993). Home computer and video game addictions in relation to adolescent gambling: conceptual and developmental aspects. In Eadington WR, Cornelius J, Editors. Gambling Behavior and Problem Gambling. University of Nevada Press, Reno, NV, pp. 451–471.

Brunborg GS, Mentzoni RA, Melkevik, et al (2013). Gaming addiction, gaming engagement, and psychological health complaints among Norwegian adolescents. Media Psychology 16: 115–128

Caplan SE, Williams D, Yee N (2009). Problematic Internet use and psychosocial well-being among MMO players. Computers in Human Behavior 25: 1312–1319.

Chan PA, Rabinowitz T (2006). A cross-sectional analysis of video games and attention deficit hyperactivity disorder symptoms in adolescents. Annals of General Psychiatry 5: 16–26.

Charlton JP (2002). A factor-analytic investigation of computer "addiction" and engagement. British Journal of Psychology 93: 329–344.

Charlton JP, Danforth IDW (2007). Distinguishing addiction and high engagement in the context of online game playing. Computers in Human Behavior 23: 1531–1548.

Chiu SI, Lee JZ, Huang DH (2004). Video game addiction in children and teenagers in Taiwan. Cyberpsychology and Behavior 7: 571–581.

Choo H, Gentile DA, Sim T, Li D, Khoo A, Liau AK (2010). Pathological video-gaming among Singaporean youth. Annals Academy of Medicine Singapore 39: 822–829.

Cultrara A, Har-El G (2002). Hyperactivity-induced suprahyoid muscular hypertrophy secondary to excessive video game play: a case report. Journal of Oral and Maxillofacial Surgery 60: 326–327.

Demetrovics Z, Urbán R, Nagygyörgy K, et al (2012). The development of the Problematic Online Gaming Questionnaire (POGQ). PLoS ONE 7: e36417.

Du Y, Jiang W, Vance A (2010). Longer term effect of randomized, controlled group cognitive behavioral therapy for Internet addiction in adolescent students in Shanghai. Australian and New Zealand Journal of Psychiatry 44: 129–134.

Dworak M, Schierl T, Bruns T, Struder HK (2007). Impact of singular excessive computer game and television exposure on sleep patterns and memory performance of school-aged children. Pediatrics 120: 978–985.

Entertainment Software Association (2013). Essential facts about the video game industry: 2013 sales, demographic and usage data. Available at http://www.theesa.com/facts/pdfs/esa_ef_2013.pdf Retrieved on April 22, 2014.

Festl R, Scharkow M, Quandt T (2013). Problematic computer game use among adolescents, younger and older adults. Addiction 108: 592–599.

Fisher SE (1994). Identifying video game addiction in children and adolescents. Addictive Behaviors 19: 545–553.

Gartner (2013). Gartner says worldwide video game market to total $93 Billion in 2013. Available at http://www.gartner.com/newsroom/id/2614915 Retrieved on April 21, 2014.

Gentile DA (2009). Pathological video-game use among youth ages 8 to 18: a national study. Psychological Science 20: 594–602.

Gentile DA, Choo H, Liau A, et al (2011). Pathological video game use among youths: a two-year longitudinal study. Pediatrics 127: E319–E329.

Ghuman D, Griffiths MD (2012). A cross-genre study of online gaming: player demographics, motivation for play, and social interactions among players. International Journal of Cyber Behavior, Psychology and Learning 2: 13–29.

Griffiths MD (1997). Computer game playing in early adolescence. Youth and Society 29: 223–237.

Griffiths MD (2000). Internet addiction—Time to be taken seriously? Addiction Research 8: 413–418.

Griffiths MD (2005). A "components" model of addiction within a biopsychosocial framework. Journal of Substance Use 10: 191–197.

Griffiths MD (2010). The role of context in online gaming excess and addiction: some case study evidence. International Journal of Mental Health and Addiction 8: 119–125.

Griffiths MD, Davies MNO (2005). Videogame addiction: does it exist? In Goldstein J, Raessens J, Editors. Handbook of Computer Game Studies. MIT Press, Boston, MA, pp. 359–368.

Griffiths MD, Davies MNO, Chappell D (2004). Demographic factors and playing variables in online computer gaming. Cyberpsychology and Behavior 7: 479–487.

Griffiths MD, Hunt N (1995) Computer game playing in adolescence: prevalence and demographic indicators. Journal of Community and Applied Social Psychology 5: 189–193.

Griffiths MD, Hunt N (1998). Dependence on computer games by adolescents. Psychological Reports 82: 475–480.

Griffiths MD, King DL, Delfabbro PH (2014a). The technological convergence of gambling and gaming practices. In Richard DCS, Blaszczynski A, Nower L, Editors. The Wiley-Blackwell Handbook of Disordered Gambling. Wiley, Chichester, UK, pp. 327–346.

Griffiths MD, King DL, Demetrovics Z (2014b). DSM-5 Internet gaming disorder needs a unified approach to assessment. Neuropsychiatry 4: 1–4.

Griffiths MD, Meredith A (2009). Videogame addiction and treatment. Journal of Contemporary Psychotherapy 39: 47–53.

Grüsser SM, Thalemann R, Albrecht U, Thalemann CN (2005). Exzessive Computernutzung im Kindesalter—Ergebnisse einer psychometrischen Erhebung. Wiener Klinische Wochenschrift 117: 188–195.

Grüsser SM, Thalemann R, Griffiths MD (2007). Excessive computer game playing: evidence for addiction and aggression? Cyberpsychology and Behavior 10: 290–292.

Han DH, Hwang JW, Renshaw PF (2010). Bupropion sustained release treatment decreases craving for video games and cue-induced brain activity in patients with Internet video game addiction. Experimental and Clinical Psychopharmacology 18: 297–304.

Han DH, Kim SM, Lee YS, Renshaw PF (2012). The effect of family therapy on the changes in the severity of on-line game play and brain activity in adolescents with on-line game addiction. Psychiatry Research: Neuroimaging 202: 126–131.

Han DH, Lee YS, Na C, et al (2009). The effect of methylphenidate on Internet video game play in children with attention-deficit/hyperactivity disorder. Comprehensive Psychiatry 50: 251–256.

Han DH, Lee YS, Yang KC, Kim EY, Lyoo IK, Renshaw PF (2007). Dopamine genes and reward dependence in adolescents with excessive Internet video game play. Journal of Addiction Medicine 1: 133–138.

Han DH, Renshaw PF (2013). Bupropion in the treatment of problematic online game play in patients with major depressive disorder. Journal of Psychopharmacology 26: 689–696.

Hoeft F, Watson CL, Kesler SR, Bettinger KE, Reiss AL (2008). Gender differences in the mesocorticolimbic system during computer game-play. Journal of Psychiatric Research 42: 253–258.

Hussain Z, Griffiths MD, Baguley T (2012). Online gaming addiction: classification, prediction and associated risk factors. Addiction Research and Theory 20: 359–371.

Jeong EJ, Kim DW (2011). Social activities, self-efficacy, game attitudes, and game addiction. Cyberpsychology, Behavior, and Social Networking 14: 213–221.

Johansson A, Gotestam KG (2004). Problems with computer games without monetary reward: similarity to pathological gambling. Psychological Reports 95: 641–650.

Keepers G (1990). Pathological preoccupation with video games. Journal of the American Academy of Child and Adolescent Psychiatry 29: 49–50.

Kim EJ, Namkoong K, Ku T, Kim SJ (2008). The relationship between online game addiction and aggression, self-control and narcissistic personality traits. European Psychiatry 23: 212–218.

Kim J (2008). The effect of a R/T group counselling program on the Internet addiction level and self-esteem of Internet addiction university students. International Journal of Reality Therapy 17: 4–12.

Kim MG, Kim J (2010). Cross-validation of reliability, convergent and discriminant validity for the problematic online game use scale. Computers in Human Behavior 26: 389–398.

King DL, Delfabbro PH, Griffiths MD (2012). Clinical interventions for technology-based problems: excessive Internet and video game use. Journal of Cognitive Psychotherapy 26: 43–56.

King DL, Delfabbro PH, Griffiths MD (2010b). Cognitive behavioural therapy for problematic video game players: conceptual considerations and practice issues. Journal of CyberTherapy and Rehabilitation 3: 261–273.

King DL, Delfabbro PH, Griffiths MD (2010a). Recent innovations in video game addiction research and theory. Global Media Journal 4(1). Available at http://www.commarts.uws.edu.au/gmjau/v4_2010_1/daniel_king_RA.html Retrieved on April 22, 2014.

King DL, Delfabbro PH, Griffiths MD (2011a). The role of structural characteristics in problematic video game play: an empirical study. International Journal of Mental Health and Addiction 9: 320–333.

King DL, Delfabbro PH, Griffiths MD, Gradisar M (2011b). Assessing clinical trials of Internet addiction treatment: a systematic review and CONSORT evaluation. Clinical Psychology Review 31: 1110–1116.

King DL, Delfabbro PH, Zajac IT (2011c). Preliminary validation of a new clinical tool for identifying problem video game playing. International Journal of Mental Health and Addiction 9: 72–87.

King DL, Haagsma MC, Delfabbro PH, Gradisar MS, Griffiths MD (2013). Toward a consensus definition of pathological video-gaming: a systematic review of psychometric assessment tools. Clinical Psychology Review 33: 331–342.

Ko CH, Liu GC, Hsiao SM, et al (2009). Brain activities associated with gaming urge of online gaming addiction. Journal of Psychiatric Research 43: 739–747.

Ko CH, Yen JY, Chen CC, Chen SH, Yen CF (2005). Gender differences and related factors affecting online gaming addiction among Taiwanese adolescents. Journal of Nervous and Mental Disease 193: 273–277.

Koronczai B, Urban R, Kokonyei G, et al (2011). Confirmation of the three-factor model of problematic Internet use on off-line adolescent and adult samples. Cyberpsychology, Behavior, and Social Networking 14: 657–664.

Kuczmierczyk AR, Walley PB, Calhoun KS (1987). Relaxation training, in vivo exposure and response-prevention in the treatment of compulsive video-game playing. Scandinavian Journal of Behaviour Therapy 16: 185–190.

Kuss DJ, Griffiths MD (2012). Online gaming addiction: a systematic review. International Journal of Mental Health and Addiction 10: 278–296.

Lee C, Han S (2007). Development of the scale for diagnosing online game addiction. Paper presented at the Third WSEAS/IASME International Conference on Educational Technologies, Arcachon, France.

Lemmens JS, Valkenburg PM, Peter J (2011). Psychosocial causes and consequences of pathological gaming. Computers in Human Behavior 27: 144–152.

Marco C, Choliz M (2013). Tratamiento cognitivo-conductual en un caso de adicción a Internet y videojuegos. International Journal of Psychology and Psychological Therapy 13: 125–141.

Mehroof M, Griffiths MD (2010). Online gaming addiction: the role of sensation seeking, self-control, neuroticism, aggression, state anxiety, and trait anxiety. Cyberpsychology and Behavior 13: 313–316.

Mentzoni RA, Brunborg GS, Molde H, et al (2011). Problematic video game use: estimated prevalence and associations with mental and physical health. Cyberpsychology, Behavior, and Social Networking 14: 591–596.

Nilles JM (1982). Exploring the World of the Personal Computer. Prentice Hall, Englewood Cliffs, NJ.

Pápay O, Urbán R, Griffiths MD, et al (2013). Psychometric properties of the Problematic Online Gaming Questionnaire Short-Form (POGQ-SF) and prevalence of problematic online gaming in a national sample of adolescents. Cyberpsychology, Behavior, and Social Networking 16: 340–348.

Parker JDA, Taylor RN, Eastabrook JM, Schell SL, Wood LM (2008). Problem gambling in adolescence: relationships with Internet misuse, gaming abuse and emotional intelligence. Personality and Individual Differences 45: 174–180.

Peters CS, Malesky LA (2008). Problematic usage among highly-engaged players of massively multiplayer online role playing games. Cyberpsychology and Behavior 11: 480–483.

Petry NM, O'Brien CP (2013). Internet gaming disorder and the DSM-5. Addiction 108: 1186–1187.

Phillips CA, Rolls S, Rouse A, Griffiths MD (1995). Home video game playing in school-children: a study of incidence and pattern of play. Journal of Adolescence 18: 687–691.

Porter G, Starcevic V, Berle D, Fenech P (2010). Recognizing problem video game use. Australian and New Zealand Journal of Psychiatry 44: 120–128.

Rehbein F, Kleimann M, Mossle T (2010). Prevalence and risk factors of video game dependency in adolescence: results of a German nationwide survey. CyberPsychology, Behavior, and Social Networking 13: 269–277.

Ross DR, Finestone DH, Lavin GK (1982). Space Invaders obsession. Journal of the American Medical Association 248: 1117.

Shek DTL, Tang VMY, Lo CY (2009). Evaluation of an Internet addiction treatment program for Chinese adolescents in Hong Kong. Adolescence 44: 359–373.

Shotton M. (1989). Computer Addiction? A Study of Computer Dependency. Taylor and Francis, London, UK.

Skoric MM, Teo LLC, Neo RL (2009). Children and video games: addiction, engagement, and scholastic achievement. Cyberpsychology and Behavior 12: 567–572.

Soper WB, Miller MJ (1983). Junk time junkies: an emerging addiction among students. School Counsellor 31: 40–43.

Spekman MLC, Konijn EA, Roelofsma PHMP, Griffiths MD (2013). Gaming addiction, definition and measurement: a large-scale empirical study. Computers in Human Behavior 29: 2150–2155.

Stetina BU, Kothgassner OD, Lehenbauer M, Kryspin-Exner I (2011). Beyond the fascination of online-games: probing addictive behavior and depression in the world of online-gaming. Computers in Human Behavior 27: 473–479.

Su W, Fang X, Miller JK, Wang Y (2011). Internet-based intervention for the treatment of online addiction for college students in China: a pilot study of the Healthy Online Self-Helping Center. Cyberpsychology, Behavior, and Social Networking 14: 497–503.

Taquet P, Hautekeete M (2013). A CBT intervention of a video game addiction: Gaming experience helps the therapy. Journal de Thérapie Comportementale et Cognitive 23: 102–112.

Thalemann R, Wölfling K, Grüsser SM (2007). Specific cue reactivity on computer game-related cues in excessive gamers. Behavioral Neuroscience 12: 614–618.

Thomas NJ, Martin FH (2010). Video-arcade game, computer game and Internet activities of Australian students: participation habits and prevalence of addiction. Australian Journal of Psychology 62: 59–66.

Thorens G, Achab S, Billieux J, et al (2014). Characteristics and treatment response of self-identified problematic Internet users in a behavioral addiction outpatient clinic. Journal of Behavioral Addictions 3: 78–81.

van Rooij AJ, Schoenmakers TM, van de Eijnden R, van de Mheen, D (2011). Compulsive Internet use: the role of online gaming and other Internet applications. Journal of Adolescent Health 47: 51–57.

Walther B, Morgenstern M, Hanewinkel R (2012). Co-occurrence of addictive behaviours: personality factors related to substance use, gambling and computer gaming. European Addiction Research 18: 167–174.

Wan CS, Chiou WB (2007). The motivations of adolescents who are addicted to online games: a cognitive perspective. Adolescence 42: 179–197.

Westwood D, Griffiths MD (2010). The role of structural characteristics in video game play motivation: a Q-methodology study. Cyberpsychology, Behavior, and Social Networking 13: 581–585.

Wood RTA, Griffiths MD, Chappell D, Davies MNO (2004). The structural character-istics of video games: a psycho-structural analysis. Cyberpsychology and Behavior 7: 1–10.

Woog K (2004). A survey of mental health professionals' clinical exposure to problematic computer use. Unpublished study. Available at http://www.wooglabs.com. Retrieved on August 18, 2011.

Wölfling K, Müller K, Beutel M (2010). Reliabilität und Validität der Skala zum Computerspielverhalten (CSV-S). Psychotherapie, Psychosomatik, Medizinische Psychologie 61: 216–224.

Xu Z, Turel O, Yuan Y (2012). Online game addiction among adolescents: motivation and prevention factors. European Journal of Information Systems 21: 321–340.

Young K (1998). Caught in the Net. Wiley, Chichester, UK.

Young K (2007). Cognitive behavior therapy with Internet addicts: treatment outcomes and implications. Cyberpsychology and Behavior 10: 671–679.

Young K (2013). Treatment outcomes using CBT-IA with Internet-addicted patients. Journal of Behavioral Addictions 2: 209–214.

Zamani E, Kheradmand A, Cheshmi M, Abedi A, Hedayati N (2010). Comparing the social skills of students addicted to computer games with normal students. Journal of Addiction and Health 2: 59–69.

Zanetta Dauriat F, Zermatten A, Billieux J, Thorens G, Bondolfi G, Khazaal Y (2011). Motivations to play specifically predict excessive involvement in massively mul-tiplayer online role-playing games: evidence from an online survey. European Addiction Research 17: 185–189.

3 Assessment of Problematic Internet Use and Online Video Gaming

Orsolya Király, Katalin Nagygyörgy, Beatrix Koronczai, Mark D. Griffiths, and Zsolt Demetrovics

INTRODUCTION

Although "digital natives" (sometimes referred to as "screenagers") have never known a world without the Internet (Griffiths, 2010b), the enormous growth in informational connectivity has occurred only recently. Nevertheless, excessive and potentially problematic Internet use was reported shortly after it became widely available (Griffiths, 1998; Young, 1998b). Since the growth of the World Wide Web in the mid-1990s, the Internet has developed substantially and become more wide-ranging in terms of the types of activities that can be engaged in online. Although articles addressing problematic Internet use (PIU) before 2000 focused on general use (e.g., surfing, communicating), another trend has emerged in the empirical literature—treating the Internet as an all-embracing channel or medium for numerous and independently existing activities such as gambling, shopping, sex, gaming, and social networking. This approach appears to imply that the content and/or activity are more important than the medium. However, Király et al. (2014) point out that the Internet not only mediates but also changes some essential aspects of the original activity, so that both the content and the channel become essential ingredients of the emerging online activity.

Online gaming serves as an excellent example of this phenomenon. Adding the Internet to stand-alone offline games has led to the development of entire living game worlds (i.e., massively multiplayer online role-playing games) where social connectivity is both a real and global experience. Consequently, this combination has proven to be so appealing (and, in some cases, addictive) that online gaming is now the only Internet-based activity included in the Section III of the fifth edition of the *Diagnostic and Statistic Manual of Mental Disorders* (DSM-5; "conditions for further study") as a behavior with a potential to become excessive and cause detrimental effects, thus leading to a disorder (American Psychiatric Association, 2013).

The assessment of PIU and problematic online gaming (POG) reflects well the development of these technologies and the changing approaches to the question of what makes online activities problematic and potentially addictive. The instruments that were developed first assessed the degree of problems related to excessive and general use of the Internet on the basis of the DSM-IV criteria for pathological gambling or substance dependence (e.g., Brenner, 1997; Young, 1998a, 1998b). Instruments for the specific assessment of POG were developed later and followed three different approaches. The first approach does not differentiate between offline and online video games. It views online gaming addiction as a subtype of video game addiction and assesses problematic gaming based on Brown's behavioral addiction criteria (e.g., Charlton and Danforth, 2007, 2010; Porter et al., 2010) or criteria for pathological gambling (e.g., Gentile, 2009; Lemmens et al., 2009; Porter et al., 2010) (1991). The second approach views online gaming as a subtype of online activity and assesses problematic online gaming based on instruments for PIU (e.g., Kim et al., 2008; Jeong and Kim, 2011; van Rooij et al., 2011). The third approach is more integrative and stresses the importance of both the content and the channel; it has created instruments based on the specific characteristics of online games as a starting point while still accepting that online gaming addiction is a type of video game addiction (e.g., Kim and Kim, 2010; Demetrovics et al., 2012).

As a result of these different conceptualizations, one essential question regarding the assessment of both problematic behaviors is the theoretical background on which this assessment is based. This is closely related to the psychometric properties and dimensional structure that underpin the assessment instruments. The present chapter makes an attempt to review and evaluate the most important instruments created to assess both PIU and POG to assist clinicians and serve as a recommended guide for further research.

Although it can be argued that both PIU and POG represent behavioral addictions (Király et al., 2014), the authors of this chapter use the terms "problematic Internet use," or PIU, and "problematic online gaming," or PIG, instead of other terms encountered in the literature, such as "addiction," "dependency," "pathological," or "disorder." The word "problematic" clearly describes the quintessence of the phenomenon (i.e., the behavior, besides being excessive, causes problems in functioning). Additionally, putting aside other terms is justified until an agreement on a precise definition and diagnostic criteria for these behaviors is reached.

ASSESSMENT OF PROBLEMATIC INTERNET USE

Although research on PIU has a brief history, many assessment tools have already been developed (Laconi et al., 2014). However, all tools developed so far are self-report instruments (i.e., there are no clinician-administered interviews). Considering the limited scope of this chapter and the fact that systematic reviews of the instruments assessing PIU are available (Lortie and Guitton, 2013; Laconi et al., 2014), this chapter provides a selective review of the most important and most frequently used instruments published in English. Table 3.1 presents data regarding the initial development of the instruments. Further empirical studies that used these measures (e.g., validation studies, studies that assess the correlates of PIU) have not been included for reasons of both simplicity and conciseness.

Theoretical Basis, Description, and Format

Almost all of the PIU instruments constructed to date have been developed using a theoretical basis. The majority of the instruments are based on the DSM-IV criteria for pathological gambling and/or substance dependence (American Psychiatric Association, 1994). A cognitive-behavioral model of the pathological Internet use (Davis, 2001) and the concept of behavioral addictions (Brown, 1991, 1993; Griffiths, 1999) were also used as theoretical starting points. Meerkerk et al. (2009) included empirical data in the process of scale development by comparing the theoretically derived dimensions with the results of a previous qualitative study with self-declared Internet users. Demetrovics et al. (2008) also took into consideration previous research results when developing instrument items.

The questionnaires that have been developed and tested are relatively short and thus easy to administer in both research and clinical settings. The number of items ranges from 8 to 36, and the response options are either dichotomous ("yes" or "no") or dimensional (on up to a 10-point Likert scale). Some scales, such as the Problematic Internet Use Questionnaire (Koronczai et al., 2011), have a long (18 items) and a short (6 or 9 items) version. Criteria for problematic use and related cutoff points have only been reported in very few studies. Thus, the Internet Addiction Diagnostic Questionnaire (Young, 1998b) and the Internet Addiction Test (Young, 1998a) have ad hoc cutoff points (i.e., they were not based on empirical analyses), whereas the developers of the Problematic Internet Use Questionnaire recommended a cutoff based on a latent profile analysis of the sample. Unfortunately, none of these studies used clinical validation techniques to obtain an accurate cutoff value for discriminating problematic from nonproblematic Internet users.

The studies presented in Table 3.1 were conducted in a wide variety of samples of students (majority) and adults. Student samples consisted of both university and high school students. Other samples comprised members of the general population, including, in particular, heavy Internet users. Only one study was conducted in a nationally representative sample (Koronczai et al., 2011). Either online or offline (i.e., paper-and-pencil) data collection methods were used.

Table 3.1 Measurement Instruments Assessing Problematic Internet Use

Source	Measure	Theoretical Basis	Number of Items[a]	Criteria for Problematic Use	Sample and Assessment Method	Factor Structure	Psychometric Properties
Young (1998b)	Internet Addiction Diagnostic Questionnaire (IADQ)	DSM-IV pathological gambling criteria	8	Five or more "Yes" responses (ad-hoc)	496 Internet users 396 classified as "dependent" (39.6% male) 100 classified as "nondependent" (64% male) Online survey and telephone interview	Not reported	Not reported
Young (1998a)	Internet Addiction Test/Scale (IAT/ IAS)	DSM-IV pathological gambling criteria	20	Score > 70 associated with significant problems (ad hoc)	Not reported	Not reported	Not reported
Armstrong et al. (2000)	Internet Related Problem Scale (IRPS)	DSM-IV criteria for substance abuse	20	Not reported	52 Internet users (55.8% male) Online survey	Not reported	Cronbach's alpha = 0.88 Concurrent validity (time spent online) Convergent validity (MMPI-2 Addiction Potential Scale)

(continued)

Table 3.1 Continued

Source	Measure	Theoretical Basis	Number of Items[a]	Criteria for Problematic Use	Sample and Assessment Method	Factor Structure	Psychometric Properties
Caplan (2002)	Generalized Problematic Internet Use Scale (GPIUS)	Cognitive-behavioral model of problematic Internet use (Davis, 2001)	29	Not reported	386 college students (31.1% male) Paper-and-pencil survey	1. Mood alteration 2. Perceived social benefits available online 3. Negative outcomes associated with Internet use 4. Compulsive Internet use 5. Excessive amounts of time spent online 6. Withdrawal symptoms when away from the Internet 7. Perceived social control available online	Cronbach's alpha of the seven subscales = 0.78–0.85 Convergent validity (depression, loneliness, shyness, self-esteem)
Davis et al, (2002)	Online Cognition Scale (OCS)	Literature on problematic Internet use and related measures of procrastination, depression, impulsivity, and pathological gambling	36	Not reported	211 college students (49.3% male) Paper-and-pencil survey	1. Loneliness/depression 2. Diminished impulse control 3. Social comfort 4. Distraction	Cronbach's alpha = 0.94 Item-total correlations = 0.47–0.81 Concurrent validity (time spent online) Convergent validity (impulsivity, depression, loneliness, procrastinatory cognitions, rejection sensitivity, Internet Behavior and Attitude Scale [IBAS; Morahan-Martin and Schumacher, 2000]) Factor structure confirmed by confirmatory factor analysis

Reference	Measure	Basis	Items	Cutoff	Sample	Factors	Psychometric properties
Demetrovics et al. (2008); Koronczai et al. (2011)	Problematic Internet Use Questionnaire (PIUQ)	Internet Addiction Test (IAT; Young, 1998a) and literature review	18	Score ≥ 41 (LPA-based)	1037 adults, high school students, and college students (54.1% male); Online survey (Demetrovics et al., 2008); 438 high school students (44.5% male); 963 adults representing the Hungarian adult population (49.9% male); Paper-and-pencil survey (Koronczai et al., 2011)	1. Obsession 2. Neglect 3. Control disorder	Cronbach's alpha = 0.87; Item-total correlations = 0.32–0.69; Test-retest reliability = 0.90; Factor structure confirmed by confirmatory factor analysis
Meerkerk et al. (2009)	Compulsive Internet Use Scale (CIUS)	DSM-IV criteria for substance dependence and pathological gambling, concept of behavioral addiction (Brown, 1991, 1993; Griffiths, 1999), and qualitative study with self-declared Internet users	14	Not reported	Sample 1 at T1: 447 adult heavy Internet users (49.4% male); Sample 2 at T2: 229 adults; Sample 3 with 16,925 adult and adolescent normal users (77.4% male); Online survey	Single factor	Cronbach's alpha = 0.89 (Samples 1 and 2), 0.90 (Sample 3); Concurrent validity (time spent online, self-reported problems concerning Internet use); Convergent validity (Online Cognition Scale [OCS; Davis et al., 2002]); Factor structure confirmed by confirmatory factor analysis; Factorial invariance over time and across gender, age, and heavy and nonheavy Internet users

(continued)

Table 3.1 Continued

Source	Measure	Theoretical Basis	Number of Items[a]	Criteria for Problematic Use	Sample and Assessment Method	Factor Structure	Psychometric Properties
Caplan (2010)	Generalized Problematic Internet Use Scale 2 (GPIUS2)	Generalized Problematic Internet Use Scale (GPIUS; Caplan, 2002), the concepts of preference for online social interaction (Caplan, 2003) and deficient self-regulation (LaRose et al, 2003)	15	Not reported	785 adults (69.2% male) Paper-and-pencil survey	1. Preference for online social interaction 2. Mood alteration 3. Cognitive preoccupation 4. Compulsive use 5. Negative outcomes	Cronbach's alpha = 0.91 Factor structure confirmed by confirmatory factor analysis
Koronczai et al. (2011)	Problematic Internet Use Questionnaire–Short Form (PIUQ-SF)	Problematic Internet Use Questionnaire (PIUQ; Demetrovics et al., 2008)	9	Score ≥ 22 (LPA-based)	438 high school students (44.5% male) 963 adults representing the Hungarian adult population (49.9% male) Paper-and-pencil survey	1. Obsession 2. Neglect 3. Control disorder	Cronbach's alpha = 0.84 (adult sample), 0.87 (adolescent sample)

Abbreviation: LPA, latent profile analysis.

[a]Responses are on a Likert scale for all measures except for the Internet Addiction Diagnostic Questionnaire, which only has "Yes" and "No" response options.

Factor Structure

The latent factor structure was not reported for three instruments, whereas the other six measures reported either one or up to seven latent factors (Table 3.1). However, many instrument items loaded on similar factors were labeled differently in different studies. By reclassifying scale items, items assessing the following PIU components appeared in all the instruments: loss of control, withdrawal, and conflict associated with relationships. Items assessing preoccupation with the Internet and conflict associated with work or school were also included in the majority of the instruments reviewed. Other PIU components frequently assessed by the individual items were escape and mood enhancement, neglecting other activities such as household duties, reduced sleep, perceived social benefits of the Internet, and deception (e.g., lying to hide the amount of time spent online). Although tolerance is an important component of addiction, items assessing this component appeared in only two instruments.

Psychometric Properties

In relation to the psychometric properties of the instruments for PIU, the main analyses presented by the authors in their original studies are reported here. Because different researchers reported the same type of analysis using different terms (e.g., a strong association between the scores on the instrument measuring PIU and time spent online has been reported as suggesting "criterion validity," "discriminant validity," or "construct validity"), the chapter authors have decided to integrate the findings relying on the definitions of reliability, validity, and factor structure provided below.

Reliability concerns the consistency of the measure across different circumstances and at different points in time (Howitt and Cramer, 2011). One of the most frequently used types of reliability is the Cronbach's alpha indicator. This measures the internal consistency of a scale—namely, how closely related a set of items are as a group. Item-total correlation shows the degree of consistency of the individual items of the instrument with the total scale score. The test-retest reliability examines consistency over time by administering the instrument to the same set of people on two separate occasions and then comparing the scores. Finally, cross-validation of reliability refers to the administration of the instrument to two independent samples and assessing whether the hypothesized dimensional structure of the scale holds true for both samples.

Validity is usually defined as the degree to which a test measures what it is intended to measure. Criterion validity assesses how well the instrument correlates with an external criterion for the construct that it measures (assessed at the same time in the case of concurrent validity or later in the case of predictive validity) (Barker et al., 2002). Testing whether a measure can predict membership of two separate criterion groups (e.g., whether a depression scale can distinguish between depressed and nondepressed patients) also indicates concurrent validity (Barker et al., 2002). For instance, a positive association of the scale score with time spent online was considered an indicator of concurrent validity because several studies reported a strong correlation between the amount of time spent online and PIU or POG, although excessive use is not by itself a sufficient criterion for problematic use (Griffiths, 2010a; Király et al., 2014; Laconi et al., 2014). Construct validity measures how the construct in question relates to other constructs and measures. Convergent validity measures how strongly the instrument correlates with measures of related constructs (e.g., other instruments, psychological health variables), whereas discriminant validity measures the extent to which items correlate with measures of unrelated constructs (Barker et al., 2002).

Finally, a scale's factor structure refers to the number and nature of the variables reflected in its items (Furr, 2011). It can be assessed using exploratory data analyses (exploratory factor analysis or principal component analysis). Usually, a confirmatory factor analysis is needed to confirm whether the hypothesized theoretical factor model fits the empirical data, providing factorial validity to the instrument (Groth-Marnat, 2003).

As shown in Table 3.1, the majority of studies examining instruments for PIU only assessed a few of the psychometric properties. Assessing reliability through internal consistency was the most frequent method. Cronbach's alpha values were excellent (above 0.90) for the Online Cognition Scale and the Generalized Problematic Internet Use Scale 2, but the Internet Related Problem Scale, the Generalized Problematic Internet Use Scale, the Problematic Internet Use Questionnaire, the Problematic Internet Use Questionnaire–Short Form, and the Compulsive Internet Use Scale all performed well (Cronbach's alpha above 0.80). Concurrent validity was assessed for three instruments (Internet-Related Problem Scale, Online Cognition Scale, and Compulsive Internet Use Scale) by measuring the association between PIU scores and time spent online. The association was significant for all three instruments, with a moderate effect size. Convergent validity for some measures was demonstrated through the correlation with the scores on other instruments for PIU or with psychological health variables such as depression, loneliness, self-esteem, and impulsivity. Item-total correlations were assessed for two measures (Online Cognition Scale and Problematic Internet Use Questionnaire) and were very good (above 0.40) for both instruments. Test-retest reliability was reported for only one instrument (Problematic Internet Use Questionnaire) and was found to be excellent (0.90). Factor structure was reported for six instruments using exploratory or confirmatory factor analyses, or both methods. Confirmatory factor analysis was used to establish that for four measures (Online Cognition Scale, Compulsive Internet Use Scale, Generalized Problematic Internet Use Scale 2, and Problematic Internet Use Questionnaire) the theoretical factor model fitted the empirical data, thus providing factorial validity to these instruments.

Although the Internet Addiction Test did not undergo psychometric validation in the original publication (Young, 1998a) and was developed on an ad hoc basis, it is by far the most widely used instrument. It has also been translated into many languages. The psychometric properties of the Internet Addiction Test were tested only later, and results vary, as suggested by one systematic review (Laconi et al., 2014). The test-retest reliability appeared to be satisfactory, between 0.73 and 0.88 in the different studies. Convergent validity and concurrent validity (i.e., correlation with time spent online) have been shown to be good to excellent. However, the factor structure of the Internet Addiction Test is highly inconsistent. Models with one to six factors have been reported in several studies that subsequently attempted to validate the instrument.

Of all the instruments, the Compulsive Internet Use Scale (Meerkerk et al., 2009) and the Online Cognition Scale (Davis et al., 2002) have been the most thoroughly explored psychometrically. Both have high internal consistency; their factor structure has been confirmed; and they seem to be valid measures of PIU based on their association with related variables. However, of these two instruments, only the Compulsive Internet Use Scale has been developed using a considerable sample size. Furthermore, its original findings were replicated in another sample. The factor structure of the Problematic Internet Use Questionnaire (Demetrovics et al., 2008) has also been confirmed in two different samples (an adolescent sample and a nationally representative adult sample), which suggests the stability of its dimensions. The reliability indicators of this instrument are also very good. Therefore, based on their psychometric properties, three measures are recommended for the assessment of PIU: the Compulsive Internet Use Scale; the Problematic Internet Use Questionnaire; and the Online Cognition Scale. Considering the global nature of PIU, it is important that these assessment tools as well as any instruments developed in the future make cross-cultural comparisons possible and assess different age groups adequately.

ASSESSMENT OF PROBLEMATIC ONLINE VIDEO GAME USE

With regard to the instruments for POG, the issues are almost identical to those pertaining to the measures of PIU. Although research in this area has been carried out over a relatively brief period, a large number of assessment tools have been developed (King et al., 2013). This chapter provides a selective review of the most important instruments as it focuses on tools that have been used in two or more studies, of the instruments involving considerable sample sizes in their development, or the measures that have shown good psychometric properties. Table 3.2 presents data regarding the initial development of the instruments for POG. For a comprehensive and systematic review of the measures of POG, the reader is referred to the article by King et al. (2013), which reviewed 18 instruments tested in more than 54,000 participants.

In some studies, POG was assessed by using an instrument for PIU and measuring time spent on online gaming (Meerkerk et al., 2006, 2010; Lee et al., 2007; Han et al., 2010; van Rooij et al., 2010, 2011). The theoretical basis for this method is that the authors viewed POG as a form of PIU, which allowed its assessment by means of an instrument measuring PIU. However, this method may underestimate the number of problematic online gamers because some gamers do not consider

Table 3.2 Measurement Instruments Assessing Problematic Online Gaming

Source	Measure	Theoretical basis	Number of Items[a]	Criteria for Problematic Use	Sample and Assessment Method	Factor Structure	Psychometric Properties
Young (1998b)	Internet Addiction Diagnostic Questionnaire (IADQ)	DSM-IV pathological gambling criteria	8	Five or more "Yes" responses (ad hoc)	496 Internet users 396 classified as "dependent" (39.6% male) 100 classified as "nondependent" (64% male) Online survey and telephone interview	Not reported	Not reported
Young (1998a)	Internet Addiction Test (IAT)	DSM-IV pathological gambling criteria	20	Score > 70 associated with significant problems (ad hoc)	Not reported	Not reported	Not reported
Tejeiro Salguero and Moran (2002)	Problem Video Game Playing (PVP)	DSM-IV criteria for substance dependence and pathological gambling and literature on addictions	9	Not reported	223 high school students (53% male) Paper-and-pencil survey	Single factor	Cronbach's alpha = 0.69 Item-total correlations = 0.21–0.54 Concurrent validity (time spent gaming, self and parents' perception of playing excessively) Convergent validity (Severity of Dependence Scale [SDS; Gossop et al., 1995])

Authors	Scale	Based on	Items	Cutoff	Sample	Components	Psychometric properties
Wan and Chiou (2006, 2007)	Online Games Addiction Scale for Adolescents in Taiwan (OAST)	Internet Addiction Scale for high schoolers in Taiwan (IAST; Lin and Tsai, 1999)	29	80th percentile (ad-hoc)	199 high school and college students Paper-and-pencil survey	1. Compulsive use and withdrawal 2. Tolerance 3. Related problems of family, school, and health 4. Related problems of peer interaction and finance	Cronbach's alpha = 0.92 Item-total correlations = 0.69–0.84 Concurrent validity ("addicts" selected with in-depth interview screening scored significantly higher than "nonaddicts" on OAST) Factor structure confirmed by confirmatory factor analysis
Charlton and Danforth (2007, 2010)	Addiction–Engagement Questionnaire (A-EQ)	General Computing Questionnaire (Charlton, 2002)	29 (2007) 24 (2010)	Four or more "core" criteria associated with addiction (ad hoc)	442 adult online gamers (85.7% male) Online survey (Charlton and Danforth, 2007) 388 adult online gamers (86% male) Online survey (Charlton and Danforth, 2010)	1. Addiction 2. Engagement	Concurrent validity (time spent gaming) (Charlton and Danforth, 2007) Cronbach's alpha = 0.79 for addiction subscale, 0.80 for engagement subscale (Charlton and Danforth, 2010) Convergent validity (negativity on five personality dimensions: extraversion, agreeableness, emotional stability, attractiveness, and negative valence) (Charlton and Danforth, 2010)

(continued)

Table 3.2 Continued

Source	Measure	Theoretical basis	Number of Items[a]	Criteria for Problematic Use	Sample and Assessment Method	Factor Structure	Psychometric Properties
Gentile (2009)	Pathological Gaming Scale (PGS)	DSM-IV pathological gambling criteria	11	Six or more criteria met (ad hoc): (Yes = 1, Sometimes = 0.5, No = 0)	1178 adolescents National representative sample (United States) Online survey	Not reported	Concurrent validity (time spent gaming, school performance, attention deficit disorder, health problems, self and friends' perception of being addicted to games, being involved in physical fights, possessing a video game system in their bedrooms) Discriminant validity (age, frequency of using the Internet to do homework, having a television in the bedroom, type of school attended)
Lemmens et al. (2009)	Game Addiction Scale for Adolescents (GAS-21) and its short form (GAS-7)	DSM-IV pathological gambling criteria	7 or 21	Two different approaches (ad hoc): monothetic (score ≥ 3 on all 7 criteria) Polythetic (score ≥ 3 on at least 4 criteria)	Two independent samples of high school students who had played video games in the last month N_1 = 352 (67% male) N_2 = 369 (68% male) Paper-and-pencil survey	1. Salience 2. Tolerance 3. Mood modification 4. Relapse 5. Withdrawal 6. Conflict 7. Problems	Cronbach's alpha for GAS-21 = 0.94 (Sample 1), 0.92 (Sample 2) Cronbach's alpha for GAS-7 = 0.86 (Sample 1), 0.81 (Sample 2) Cross-validation of reliability Concurrent validity (time spent online) - Convergent validity (loneliness, life satisfaction, aggression, and social competence) - Factor structure confirmed by confirmatory factor analysis

Study	Measure	Items	Cutoff	Sample/Method	Dimensions	Psychometric properties
Kim and Kim (2010)	Problematic Online Game Use Scale (POGU)	20	Not reported	Sample 1 with 1422 high school students; Sample 2 with 199 high school students; Sample 3 with 393 high school students; Paper-and-pencil survey	1. Euphoria 2. Health problem 3. Conflict 4. Failure of self-control 5. Preference of virtual relationship	Cronbach's alpha: not reported (Sample 1), 0.91 (Sample 2), 0.95 (Sample 3); Cross-validation of reliability; Convergent validity (life satisfaction, academic self-efficacy, anxiety, and loneliness); Factor structure confirmed by confirmatory factor analysis
Rehbein et al. (2010)	Video Game Dependency Scale (KFN-CSAS-II)	14	Scores between 35 and 41 associated with risk of dependency (ad hoc); Score ≥ 42 associated with dependency (ad hoc)	15,168 high school students (51.3% male); National representative sample (Germany); Paper-and-pencil survey	1. Preoccupation/salience 2. Conflict 3. Loss of control 4. Withdrawal symptoms 5. Tolerance	Cronbach's alpha = 0.92; Concurrent validity (time spent gaming, self-evaluation of being dependent, school achievement, school absenteeism, sleep time, sleep disturbance, participating regularly in other leisure-time activities, thoughts of committing suicide)
Demetrovics et al. (2012)	Problematic Online Gaming Questionnaire (POGQ)	18	Score ≥ 66; (LPA-based: sensitivity and specificity analyses)	3415 high school and college student and adult online gamers (90% male); Online survey	1. Preoccupation 2. Overuse 3. Immersion 4. Social isolation 5. Interpersonal conflicts 6. Withdrawal	Cronbach's alpha = 0.91; Factor structure confirmed by confirmatory factor analysis

(continued)

Table 3.2 Continued

Source	Measure	Theoretical basis	Number of Items[a]	Criteria for Problematic Use	Sample and Assessment Method	Factor Structure	Psychometric Properties
van Rooij et al. (2012)	Video Game Addiction Test (VGAT)	Compulsive Internet Use Scale (CIUS; Meerkerk et al., 2009)	14	Not reported	2894 high school students who played video games (62% male) National representative sample of Dutch secondary school students Paper-and-pencil survey	1. Loss of control 2. Intra- and interpersonal conflict 3. Preoccupation/salience 4. Coping/mood modification 5. Withdrawal symptoms	Cronbach's alpha = 0.93 Concurrent validity (time spent on various game types) Convergent validity (Game Addiction Scale [Lemmens et al., 2009], Compulsive Internet Use Scale [Meerkerk et al., 2009], depressive mood, negative self-esteem, loneliness, and social anxiety) Factor structure confirmed by confirmatory factor analysis
Papay et al. (2013)	Problematic Online Gaming Questionnaire–Short Form (POGQ-SF)	Problematic Online Gaming Questionnaire (POGQ; Demetrovics et al., 2012)	12	Score ≥ 32; (LPA-based: sensitivity and specificity analyses)	2804 high school students who played video games (65% male) National representative sample of Hungarian 9th–10th graders Paper-and-pencil survey	1. Preoccupation 2. Overuse 3. Immersion 4. Social isolation 5. Interpersonal conflicts 6. Withdrawal	Cronbach's alpha = 0.91 Concurrent validity (time spent gaming, school performance) Convergent validity (self-esteem, depressive symptoms) Factor structure confirmed by confirmatory factor analysis

Abbreviation: LPA, latent profile analysis.

[a]Responses are on a Likert scale for all measures except for the Internet Addiction Diagnostic Questionnaire, which only has "Yes" and "No" response option.

online gaming as an Internet activity, but rather as gaming per se; for them, the content is more important than the medium in which they play. A need to assess POG and PIU separately is in line with a finding by Rehbein and Mößle (2013) that Internet addiction and video game addiction can be regarded as distinct problems.

Theoretical Basis, Description, and Format

Similar to the instruments for PIU, scales measuring POG were mostly developed on a theoretical basis using (1) the DSM-IV criteria for pathological gambling or substance dependence (American Psychiatric Association, 1994); (2) the contemporary literature on addiction, including PIU and POG; and (3) the concept of behavioral addictions (Brown, 1991, 1993; Griffiths, 1999). In addition, several tools relied on existing instruments for PIU. Empirical data derived from the interviews with online gamers were also used in the development of the Problematic Online Gaming Questionnaire (Demetrovics et al., 2012).

The questionnaires for POG are short and therefore appropriate for surveys and assessment. The number of scale items ranges from 8 to 29. Some scales have both long and short versions. Cutoff scores that differentiated problematic from normal gamers have been reported in the majority of the studies. However, most of these cutoffs are of an ad hoc nature (i.e., they were not based on empirical analyses). The cutoff scores for only two instruments—the Problematic Online Gaming Questionnaire and its short form (Pápay et al., 2013)—were empirically tested using the sensitivity and specificity analyses.

The studies reporting on the instruments for POG were conducted in both adolescent and adult samples. The sample sizes ranged from small (N = 199) to large (N = 15,168). Among the 12 instruments listed in Table 3.2, 4 were used in the nationally representative samples of adolescents in the United States (Gentile, 2009), Germany (Rehbein et al., 2010), the Netherlands (van Rooij et al., 2012), and Hungary (Pápay et al., 2013). Data were collected either online or in a traditional (paper-and-pencil) manner.

Content and Factor Structure of the Instruments for Problematic Online Gaming Compared to the DSM-5 Internet Gaming Disorder Criteria

The instruments show a great variability both in terms of their factor structure and the symptoms of POG that they include. Some of the scales appear to be unidimensional, with all their items measuring one construct or dimension, whereas others measure two, four, five, six, or seven distinct dimensions. Because POG is now included in the DSM-5 Section III under the name of Internet gaming disorder (IGD), it is useful to compare the proposed criteria for IGD with items of various instruments. The DSM-5 symptoms of IGD are as follows: (1) preoccupation with online gaming (cognitive and behavioral); (2) withdrawal symptoms when it is not possible to play online games; (3) tolerance (the need to spend increasing amounts of time engaged in online gaming); (4) loss of control (unsuccessful attempts to control the participation in online gaming); (5) loss of interests in previous hobbies and entertainment activities; (6) continued excessive online gaming despite knowledge of psychosocial problems; (7) deception (i.e., deceiving family members, therapists, or others regarding the amount of time spent online gaming); (8) online gaming for the purpose of escaping or relieving a negative mood, and (9) conflicts in the domains of relationships, work, or school.

No instrument presented in Table 3.2 covers all the IGD criteria as defined in the DSM-5. However, both the 21-item version of the Game Addiction Scale for Adolescents (Lemmens et al., 2009) and the Problem Video Game Playing (Tejeiro Salguero and Moran, 2002) achieve the closest coverage. The Pathological Gaming Scale (Gentile, 2009) and the Internet Addiction Diagnostic Questionnaire (Young, 1998b) also cover the majority of the diagnostic criteria. The most poorly covered IGD criteria are loss of interests in previous hobbies and entertainment activities and continued excessive online gaming despite knowledge of psychosocial problems. In contrast, the criterion concerning interpersonal, work-related, or school-related conflicts is assessed by all the questionnaires, and the criteria pertaining to preoccupation, withdrawal symptoms, and loss of control are also included in all but one instrument. Tolerance is not assessed by three instruments, and four scales do not have items assessing escapism and relieving a negative mood. Some instruments have items that do not refer to any of the criteria for IGD but relate to other aspects that might be associated with problematic gaming such as euphoria (a "buzz" or "high" that is experienced during online gaming), health-related problems, reduced sleep, and/or neglect of household chores.

Overall, none of the previously developed instruments is recommended to test the DSM-5 criteria for IGD because the instruments do not fully cover the nine proposed criteria and because they have been developed on the basis of theoretical approaches different from IGD. However, the inclusion of IGD in the Section III of the DSM-5 is likely to stimulate further research in this area and lead to the development of new instruments specifically assessing the DSM-5 criteria.

Psychometric Properties

Regarding psychometric properties, the same terms and definitions as for PIU were used due to similar inconsistencies in the studies of measures used to assess POG. Psychometric analyses of the instruments for POG also show mixed results (Table 3.2). Internal consistency measured by the Cronbach's alpha was excellent (above 0.90) for the majority of the studies (Online Games Addiction Scale for Adolescents in Taiwan, Game Addiction Scale for Adolescents, Problematic Online Game Use Scale, Video Game Dependency Scale, Video Game Addiction Test, and Problematic Online Gaming Questionnaire–Short Form), whereas it was good (around 0.80) for the Addiction-Engagement Questionnaire and the short form of the Game Addiction Scale for Adolescents, and acceptable (around 0.70) for the Problem Video Game Playing instrument. Item-total correlations were excellent for the Online Games Addiction Scale for Adolescents in Taiwan and acceptable (above 0.20) for Problem Video Game Playing instrument. Reliability of the Game Addiction Scale for Adolescents and the Problematic Online Game Use Scale was cross-validated in two and three samples, respectively.

In terms of validation, concurrent validity was assessed for the majority of the instruments by correlating their scores with time spent gaming, self-evaluation of excessive or problematic use, and school performance. Convergent validity was tested by measuring the association with indicators of psychological well-being (i.e., loneliness, life satisfaction, self-esteem, depressive symptoms), other addiction measures, and personality traits. Discriminant validity of the Pathological Gaming Scale was demonstrated by reporting the lack of association with non-related variables such as age and type of school attended. Factor structure for eight instruments was determined by means of exploratory or confirmatory factor analyses, or both. Six studies used confirmatory factor analysis to confirm the factorial validity of the Game Addiction Scale for Adolescents, Problematic Online Game Use Scale, Online Games Addiction Scale for Adolescents in Taiwan, Video Game Addiction Test, Problematic Online Gaming Questionnaire, and Problematic Online Gaming Questionnaire–Short Form.

The Internet Addiction Test is also one of the most frequently used scales for assessing POG. Some studies used it without modification (e.g., Billieux et al., 2011), considering online gaming a type of Internet activity. However, this approach might distort the results, as argued above. Other researchers modified the Internet Addiction Test to measure POG by replacing the word "Internet" from its items with "online games" (Wang and Chu, 2007), "Internet gaming" (Jeong and Kim, 2011), and "WoW" (derived from the popular online game *World of Warcraft*) (Snodgrass et al., 2011a, 2011b). Given the inconsistencies in the psychometric properties of the original Internet Addiction Test, cautious use is recommended, especially when assessing online gaming, which is different from the general Internet use in important respects (Rehbein and Mößle, 2013).

Of the instruments reviewed here, the Game Addiction Scale for Adolescents (Lemmens et al., 2009) and the Video Game Addiction Test (van Rooij et al., 2012) used the widest range of psychometric analyses in their development process and both show good psychometric characteristics. However, some of the other instruments also look promising. The factor structure of the Problematic Online Game Use Scale (Kim and Kim, 2010) was confirmed in three different samples and showed association with POG-related variables. The Video Game Dependency Scale (Rehbein et al., 2010) was developed in a large sample; it has good internal consistency and its concurrent validity has been assessed thoroughly. The Problematic Online Gaming Questionnaire (Demetrovics et al., 2012) and the Problematic Online Gaming Questionnaire–Short Form (Pápay et al., 2013) were developed both on a theoretical basis and empirically (i.e., through interviews with online gamers). Their factor structures appear to be stable across both adolescent and adult samples and with different data collection methods, and they also appear to have concurrent and convergent validity. The Addiction-Engagement Questionnaire (Charlton and Danforth, 2007) has the potential to distinguish between addiction and high engagement and also shows association with different POG-related variables.

In summary, the authors would recommend the use of any of the aforementioned instruments for assessing POG, taking into account the nature of the sample, the data collection method, and the cultural setting when deciding which instrument to choose.

CONCLUSION

In spite of the relative novelty of PIU and POG, a large number of measurement instruments have been developed to assess these related but different behaviors. However, most of the tools were used in only one or two studies, which makes drawing solid conclusions regarding their quality rather difficult.

Findings of the research concerning instruments for PIU and POG can be characterized as inconsistent. The main reason for this is the lack of a consensual definition and solid theoretical background regarding both PIU and POG. Without common criteria to describe problematic behavior and distinguish it from normal behavior, it is difficult to create truly valid instruments.

The advantages of many of the existing scales are their brevity, ease of use, and good psychometric properties in terms of internal consistency, concurrent validity, and convergent validity (King et al., 2013). However, few of the instruments have had their factor structure confirmed, which is essential for exploring the latent content of these scales. Overall, very few of the instruments have undergone a comprehensive psychometric evaluation.

In addition to rigorous reliability and validity requirements, other important aspects need to be kept in mind in the process of developing new assessment instruments. According to Koronczai et al. (2011), a good measurement instrument should meet all of the following criteria:

(1) Comprehensiveness (i.e., examining many and possibly all aspects of PIU and POG)
(2) Brevity, so that the instrument can be used by the more impulsive individuals and fit time-limited surveys
(3) Reliability and validity for different data collection methods (e.g., online, paper-and-pencil, self-rating, and face-to-face);
(4) Reliability and validity for different age groups (e.g., adolescents and adults);
(5) Cross-cultural reliability and validity
(6) Validation on clinical samples so that cutoff scores could be determined for problematic use and possibly for addiction

To date, none of the instruments for PIU or POG outlined in this chapter fulfills these six key criteria. Clinical validation (with clinically established cutoff scores) is almost entirely missing. Some of the measures (e.g., the Compulsive Internet Use Scale, Online Cognition Scale, Problematic Internet Use Questionnaire, Video Game Addiction Test, Problematic Online Gaming Questionnaire, and Game

Addiction Scale for Adolescents) are promising but must be further validated in order to meet all the aforementioned criteria and be considered appropriate tools for assessment of PIU and POG.

ACKNOWLEDGMENTS

The present work was supported by the Hungarian Scientific Research Fund (83884). Zsolt Demetrovics acknowledges financial support of the János Bolyai Research Fellowship awarded by the Hungarian Academy of Science.

DISCLOSURE STATEMENT

The authors disclose no relationships with commercial entities and professional activities that may bias their views.

REFERENCES

American Psychiatric Association (1994). Diagnostic and Statistical Manual of Mental Disorders. Fourth Edition. American Psychiatric Association, Washington, DC.

American Psychiatric Association. (2013). Diagnostic and Statistical Manual of Mental Disorders. Fifth Edition. American Psychiatric Association, Washington, DC.

Armstrong L, Phillips JG, Saling LL (2000). Potential determinants of heavier Internet usage. International Journal of Human-Computer Studies 53: 537–550.

Barker C, Pistrang N, Elliott R (2002). Research Methods in Clinical Psychology. Second Edition. Wiley, Oxford, UK.

Billieux J, Chanal J, Khazaal Y, et al (2011). Psychological predictors of problematic involvement in massively multiplayer online role-playing games: illustration in a sample of male cybercafé players. Psychopathology 44: 165–171.

Brenner V (1997). Psychology of computer use: XLVII. Parameters of Internet use, abuse and addiction: the first 90 days of the Internet Usage Survey. Psychological Reports 80: 879–882.

Brown RIF (1991). Gaming, gambling and other addictive play. In Kerr JH, Apter MJ, Editors. Adult Play: A Reversal Theory Approach. Swets & Zeitlinger, Amsterdam, The Netherlands, pp. 101–118.

Brown RIF (1993). Some contributions of the study of gambling to the study of other addictions. In Eadington WR, Cornelius JA, Editors. Gambling Behavior and Problem Gambling. University of Nevada, Reno, NV, pp. 241–272.

Caplan SE (2002). Problematic Internet use and psychosocial well-being: development of a theory-based cognitive-behavioral measurement instrument. Computers in Human Behavior 18: 553–575.

Caplan SE (2003). Preference for online social interaction: a theory of problematic Internet use and psychosocial well-being. Communication Research 30: 625–648.

Caplan SE (2010). Theory and measurement of generalized problematic Internet use: a two-step approach. Computers in Human Behavior 26: 1089–1097.

Charlton JP (2002). A factor-analytic investigation of computer "addiction" and engagement. British Journal of Psychology 93: 329–344.

Charlton JP, Danforth IDW (2007). Distinguishing addiction and high engagement in the context of online game playing. Computers in Human Behavior 23: 1531–1548.

Charlton JP, Danforth IDW (2010). Validating the distinction between computer addiction and engagement: online game playing and personality. Behaviour & Information Technology 29: 601–613.

Davis RA (2001). A cognitive-behavioral model of pathological Internet use. Computers in Human Behavior 17: 187–195.

Davis RA, Flett GL, Besser A (2002). Validation of a new scale for measuring problematic Internet use: implications for preemployment screening. Cyberpsychology and Behavior 5: 331–345.

Demetrovics Z, Szeredi B, Rozsa S (2008). The three-factor model of Internet addiction: the development of the Problematic Internet Use Questionnaire. Behavior Research Methods 40: 563–574.

Demetrovics Z, Urbán R, Nagygyörgy K, et al (2012). The development of the Problematic Online Gaming Questionnaire (POGQ). PLoS ONE 7: e36417.

Furr M (2011). Scale Construction and Psychometrics for Social and Personality Psychology. Sage, London, UK.

Gentile DA (2009). Pathological video-game use among youth ages 8 to 18: a national study. Psychological Science 20: 594–602.

Gossop M, Darke S, Griffiths P, et al (1995). The Severity of Dependence Scale (SDS): psychometric properties of the SDS in English and Australian samples of heroin, cocaine and amphetamines users. Addiction 90: 607–614.

Griffiths MD (1998). Internet addiction: does it really exist? In Gackenbach J, Editor. Psychology and the Internet: Intrapersonal, Interpersonal, and Transpersonal Implications Academic Press, New York, NY, pp. 61–75.

Griffiths MD (1999). Internet addiction: fact or fiction? Psychologist 12: 246–250.

Griffiths MD (2010a). The role of context in online gaming excess and addiction: some case study evidence. International Journal of Mental Health and Addiction 8: 119–125.

Griffiths MD (2010b). Trends in technological advance: implications for sedentary behaviour and obesity in screenagers. Education and Health 28: 35–38.

Groth-Marnat G (2003). Handbook of Psychological Assessment. Fourth Edition. Wiley, New York, NY.

Hahn A, Jerusalem M (2001). Internetsucht: Validierung eines Instruments und explorative Hinweise auf personale Bedingungen [Internet addiction: validation of an instrument and explorative evidence on personal causes]. In Theobald A, Dreyer M, Starsetzki T, Editor. Handbuch zur Online-Marktforschung. Beiträge aus Wissenschaft und Praxis. Gabler, Wiesbaden, Germany, pp. 213–233.

Han DH, Hwang JW, Renshaw PF (2010). Bupropion sustained release treatment decreases craving for video games and cue-induced brain activity in patients with Internet video game addiction. Experimental and Clinical Psychopharmacology 18: 297–304.

Howitt D, Cramer D (2011). Introduction to Research Methods in Psychology. Third Edition. Pearson Education, Essex, UK.

Jeong EJ, Kim DH (2011). Social activities, self-efficacy, game attitudes, and game addiction. Cyberpsychology, Behavior, and Social Networking 14: 213–221.

Kim EJ, Namkoong K, Ku T, Kim SJ (2008). The relationship between online game addiction and aggression, self-control and narcissistic personality traits. European Psychiatry 23: 212–218.

Kim MG, Kim J (2010). Cross-validation of reliability, convergent and discriminant validity for the Problematic Online Game Use Scale. Computers in Human Behavior 26: 389–398.

King DL, Haagsma MC, Delfabbro PH, Gradisar M, Griffiths MD (2013). Toward a consensus definition of pathological video-gaming: a systematic review of psychometric assessment tools. Clinical Psychology Review 33: 331–342.

Király O, Nagygyörgy K, Griffiths MD, Demetrovics Z (2014). Problematic online gaming. In Rosenberg K, Feder L, Editors. Behavioral Addictions: Criteria, Evidence and Treatment. Elsevier, New York, NY, pp. 61–97.

Koronczai B, Urban R, Kokonyei G, et al (2011). Confirmation of the three-factor model of problematic Internet use on off-line adolescent and adult samples. Cyberpsychology, Behavior, and Social Networking 14: 657–664.

Laconi S, Rodgers RF, Chabrol H (2014). The measurement of Internet addiction: a critical review of existing scales and their psychometric properties. Computers in Human Behavior 41: 190–202.

LaRose R, Lin CA, Eastin MS (2003). Unregulated Internet usage: addiction, habit, or deficient self-regulation? Media Psychology 5: 225–253.

Lee MS, Ko YH, Song HS, et al (2007). Characteristics of Internet use in relation to game genre in Korean adolescents. Cyberpsychology and Behavior 10: 278–285.

Lemmens JS, Valkenburg PM, Peter J (2009). Development and validation of a game addiction scale for adolescents. Media Psychology 12: 77–95.

Lin SSJ, Tsai C-C (1999). Internet addiction among high schoolers in Taiwan. Paper presented at the American Psychological Association Annual Meeting, Boston, MA.

Lortie CL, Guitton MJ (2013). Internet addiction assessment tools: dimensional structure and methodological status. Addiction 108: 1207–1216.

Meerkerk GJ, van den Eijnden RJ, Franken IHA, Garretsen HF (2010). Is compulsive Internet use related to sensitivity to reward and punishment, and impulsivity? Computers in Human Behavior 26: 729–735.

Meerkerk GJ, van den Eijnden RJ, Garretsen HF (2006). Predicting compulsive Internet use: it's all about sex! Cyberpsychology and Behavior 9: 95–103.

Meerkerk GJ, van den Eijnden RJ, Vermulst AA, Garretsen HF (2009). The Compulsive Internet Use Scale (CIUS): some psychometric properties. Cyberpsychology and Behavior 12: 1–6.

Morahan-Martin J, Schumacher P (2000). Incidence and correlates of pathological Internet use among college students. Computers in Human Behavior 16: 13–29.

Pápay O, Urbán R, Griffiths MD, et al (2013). Psychometric properties of the Problematic Online Gaming Questionnaire—Short Form (POGQ-SF) and prevalence of problematic online gaming in a national sample of adolescents. Cyberpsychology, Behavior, and Social Networking 16: 340–348.

Porter G, Starcevic V, Berle D, Fenech P (2010). Recognizing problem video game use. Australian and New Zealand Journal of Psychiatry 44: 120–128.

Rehbein F, Mößle T (2013). Video game and Internet addiction: is there a need for differentiation? SUCHT—Zeitschrift für Wissenschaft und Praxis/Journal of Addiction Research and Practice 59: 129–142.

Rehbein F, Psych G, Kleimann M, Mediasci G, Mößle T (2010). Prevalence and risk factors of video game dependency in adolescence: results of a German nationwide survey. Cyberpsychology, Behavior, and Social Networking 13: 269–277.

Snodgrass JG, Lacy MG, Dengah HJF II, Fagan J (2011a). Enhancing one life rather than living two: playing MMOs with offline friends. Computers in Human Behavior 27: 1211–1222.

Snodgrass JG, Lacy MG, Dengah HJF II, Fagan J, Most DE (2011b). Magical flight and monstrous stress: technologies of absorption and mental wellness in Azeroth. Culture, Medicine and Psychiatry 35: 26–62.

Tejeiro Salguero RA, Moran RM (2002). Measuring problem video game playing in adolescents. Addiction 97: 1601–1606.

van Rooij AJ, Schoenmakers TM, van den Eijnden RJ, van der Mheen D (2010). Compulsive Internet use: the role of online gaming and other Internet applications. Journal of Adolescent Health 47: 51–57.

van Rooij AJ, Schoenmakers TM, van den Eijnden RJ, Vermulst AA, van der Mheen D (2012). Video Game Addiction Test (VAT): validity and psychometric characteristics. Cyberpsychology, Behavior, and Social Networking 15: 507–511.

van Rooij AJ, Schoenmakers TM, Vermulst AA, van den Eijnden RJ, van der Mheen D (2011). Online video game addiction: identification of addicted adolescent gamers. Addiction 106: 205–212.

Wan CS, Chiou WB (2006). Psychological motives and online games addiction: a test of flow theory and humanistic needs theory for Taiwanese adolescents. Cyberpsychology and Behavior 9: 317–324.

Wan CS, Chiou WB (2007). The motivations of adolescents who are addicted to online games: a cognitive perspective. Adolescence 42: 179–197.

Wang CC, Chu YS (2007). Harmonious passion and obsessive passion in playing online games. Social Behavior and Personality 35: 997–1005.

Young KS (1998a). Caught in the Net: How to Recognize the Signs of Internet Addiction and a Winning Strategy for Recovery. Wiley, New York, NY.

Young KS (1998b). Internet addiction: the emergence of a new clinical disorder. Cyberpsychology and Behavior 1: 237–244.

4 Neurobiological Aspects of Problematic Internet and Video Game Use

Sun Mi Kim and Doug Hyun Han

INTRODUCTION

Problematic Internet and video game use is a growing public health and social problem that has received research attention worldwide. In 2013, Internet gaming disorder was introduced in Section III of the fifth edition of the *Diagnostic and Statistical Manual of Mental Disorders* (DSM-5; American Psychiatric Association, 2013) as a condition for further research. Until recently, individuals from clinical settings with problematic Internet and video game use have often been diagnosed with an impulse control disorder, not otherwise specified (Shapira et al., 2000), because no specific diagnosis for these conditions existed in the fourth edition of the DSM (DSM-IV) (American Psychiatric Association, 1994). This was based on the repetitive, impulse-driven behaviors exhibited by individuals with problematic Internet and video game use, also seen in pathological gambling and other impulse control disorders. Some clinicians and researchers also conceptualized problematic Internet and video game use as an "addiction," with similarities to the DSM-IV diagnostic definition for substance dependence; this included continued use, leading to significant functional impairment, at school, work, or home, despite health, social, or interpersonal problems (Ko et al., 2009, 2013; Han et al., 2010b).

Thus, research on the neurobiological aspects of problematic Internet and video game use has focused on comparing these conditions with other impulse control disorders or substance dependence. Understanding the neurobiological aspects of problematic Internet and video game use by means of neuroimaging studies, neurophysiological studies, as well as genetic studies, may provide insight into their pathogenesis and consequences. In addition, understanding the underlying biological vulnerability is important to develop treatment strategies and interventions.

This chapter reviews the research performed so far in neuroimaging, neuro-physiological, and genetic aspects of problematic Internet and video game use. It initially discusses the functional and structural brain changes in response to Internet and video game use and then addresses treatment-related brain changes. Finally, the chapter discusses the neurophysiological and genetic research into problematic Internet and video game use. To the extent possible and to help with the conceptual clarification and distinction, the text addresses problematic Internet use and problematic online gaming separately.

NEUROIMAGING STUDIES OF PROBLEMATIC VIDEO GAME AND INTERNET USE

The neuroimaging research of Internet use and video game play can be summarized as follows: (1) studies of functional brain changes in response to video game play in healthy individuals, (2) studies of anatomic brain changes in healthy individuals with long-term continuous video game play, and (3) studies of functional or anatomic brain changes in individuals with problematic Internet or video game use.

The brain activity in response to video game play has been investigated via functional neuroimaging studies conducted in nonproblematic gamers and healthy volunteers who are able to control their game use and do not have marked distress or functional impairment as a result of it. Functional neuroimaging research includes functional magnetic resonance imaging (fMRI), positron emission tomography (PET), and single-photon emission computed tomography (SPECT). All three techniques provide information regarding brain activity in different areas as indicated by cerebral blood flow levels. Researchers use fMRI to estimate blood oxygenation levels (Huettel et al., 2009). They use PET and SPECT, which involve an injection of a small amount of radioactive tracer, to assist with locating functionally activated brain regions where the radioactive material is taken up more readily (Rahmim and Zaidi, 2008).

Long-term continuous video game play may lead to structural brain changes. Those have been assessed in structural neuroimaging studies using voxel-based morphometry (VBM) and cortical thickness analysis. With VBM, the structural comparison of white and gray matter volume between an experimental group and a control group is possible (Ashburner and Friston, 2000). Cortical thickness is typically calculated based on the gray matter in segmented neuroimaging data. It coarsely correlates with the number of neurons and tends to be considered an indicator of cognitive abilities (Hutton et al., 2008).

Brain changes related to problematic Internet and video game use have been investigated using both functional and structural brain imaging techniques. Finally, functional neuroimaging studies have been used to assess treatment-related brain changes.

Frontoparietal Network: Visuospatial Attention

Studies using fMRI studies conducted in nonproblematic game users or healthy volunteers have reported that video game use may improve visuospatial attention and alter the visuomotor network (Granek et al., 2010). Bavelier et al. (2012) investigated functional brain changes during the engagement of the attentional network for processing irrelevant or distracting stimuli. The frontoparietal network displayed increased engagement as demands on attentional effort increased in nonaction video game players, relative to action video game players. On the other hand, the decreased activity within the frontoparietal network in action video game players suggests that they may have a more effective and automatic strategy for attentional resource allocation (i.e., more selective attention than nonaction video game players). Granek et al. (2010) examined the neural control of complex eye-hand coordination tasks using fMRI techniques. In experienced gamers, reduced frontoparietal activity was involved in processing a standard level of visuomotor tasks in comparison to nongamers. Furthermore, during a more complex visuomotor task, additional prefrontal activity that may have association with planning for the task was concomitantly engaged in experienced gamers but not in nongamers.

Long-term continuous game play may eventually be associated with structural brain changes in the brain region related to visuospatial attention (Kühn et al., 2011; Tanaka et al., 2013). A VBM study by Tanaka et al. (2013) demonstrated an increased gray matter volume in the right posterior parietal cortex in expert action video game players relative to nongamers. Larger gray matter volume in the right posterior parietal cortex is positively correlated with superior capacity for visuospatial working memory performance in game experts. In a study using VBM analysis in healthy male adults, Kühn and Gallinat (2014) reported that in addition to the changes in the frontoparietal network, there were changes in gray matter volume in other brain regions related to visual attention. This study also suggested that the amount of lifetime video gaming was positively related to gray matter volume in brain regions associated with navigation and visual attention, such as bilateral hippocampal, entorhinal, and occipital regions.

In summary, studies using cognitive measures have consistently reported that playing video games, especially action video games, enhances visuospatial attention and speed of processing of tasks (Granek et al., 2010; Bavelier et al., 2012). Neurobiological evidence has increasingly shown that long-term, extensive video game use is associated with significant changes in the brain regions related to visuospatial attention and visuomotor function, specifically the frontoparietal network.

Corticolimbic Circuit: Reward System

Neuroimaging studies conducted with healthy volunteers have shown that video game use engages the reward systems of the brain. Studies with fMRI in healthy volunteers using a cue-induced paradigm have reported that the gaming cues activate the dopaminergic circuit (including midbrain, striatum, amygdala, and prefrontal cortical regions), which is involved in the brain rewards system (Hoeft et al., 2008; Mathiak et al., 2011; Kätsyri et al., 2012). In a PET study, increased dopamine neurotransmission, especially in the ventral striatum, was observed during video game play (Koepp et al., 1998). Functional changes in the corticolimbic circuit have also been consistently reported in studies conducted with participants with problematic video game use (Ko et al., 2009; Han et al., 2011; Sun et al., 2012; Lorenz et al., 2013).

Studies using fMRI have demonstrated that gaming cues activate the anterior cingulate, orbitofrontal cortex (OFC), nucleus accumbens, dorsal striatum, dorsolateral prefrontal cortex (DLPFC) and parahippocampus in participants with problematic video game use (Ko et al., 2009; Han et al., 2011; Lorenz et al., 2013). In addition, the participants' rating of craving for Internet video games was positively correlated with the activation of the above brain areas (Han et al., 2011; Sun et al., 2012; Lorenz et al., 2013). In another cue-induced fMRI study conducted with participants who had both problematic Internet game use and nicotine dependence, Ko et al. (2013) suggested that problematic Internet game use and nicotine dependence might share a similar neurobiological mechanism in the frontolimbic network, especially for the cue-induced reactivity in the anterior cingulate and parahippocampus. In a resting state MRI study in problematic game use (Ding et al., 2013), connectivity with the posterior cingulate cortex was positively correlated with the severity of problematic game use in the right precuneus, thalamus, caudate, nucleus accumbens, supplementary motor area, and lingual gyrus. These alterations in resting state functional connectivity are also partially consistent with those found in patients with substance dependence (Tanabe et al., 2011; Zhang et al., 2011; Janes et al., 2012). The results of these studies support a hypothesis that problematic video game use and substance dependence may share common mechanisms.

Cingulate Cortex: Cognition and Emotional Regulation

The anterior cingulate cortex, along with the OFC and amygdala, is implicated in neural networks for drive, cognition, and emotional regulation (Davidson et al., 2000). Also, the posterior cingulate cortex plays a role in cognitive control, including visuospatial and sensorimotor processes (Leech et al., 2011; Pearson et al., 2011). Using fMRI, Weber et al. (2006) studied brain activation in healthy volunteers as they played a video game with some violent content. Participants' brain activation patterns were analyzed as a function of the violent content of their on-screen activities. The results showed that virtual violence during video game playing was associated with decreased activity in regions related to positive emotion, such as the rostral anterior cingulate cortex and the amygdala, as well as increased activity in the dorsal anterior cingulate cortex, which is the region related to cognition. Virtual violence during video game playing may lead to neural patterns in the anterior cingulate cortex and the amygdala similar to those elicited by aggressive behavior. In addition, the authors suggested that virtual violence might also involve a defensive component due to fear of losing the player's virtual life, which could explain fear reactions in the amygdala. See Chapter 5 for discussion of the effects of video game violence in more detail.

Structural Brain Changes

The findings of functional neuroimaging studies conducted in healthy volunteers and individuals with problematic video game use indicate that similar brain regions related to the brain reward system are activated in response to gaming cues in both groups. However, the structural neuroimaging studies have shown differences between individuals with problematic video game use and healthy volunteers. Thus, in comparison with healthy participants, adolescents with problematic video game use had decreased cortical thickness within the OFC (Yuan et al., 2013) and gray matter atrophy in the right OFC, bilateral insula, and right supplementary motor area (Weng et al., 2013). The decreased cortical thickness of the OFC was also associated with impaired cognitive control ability in adolescents with problematic Internet game use (Yuan et al., 2013). The impaired gray and white matter integrity of the right OFC and bilateral insula was positively correlated with the Young's Internet Addiction Scale scores in individuals with problematic Internet game use (Naqvi and Bechara, 2009).

These studies suggest dysfunction in the OFC and insula in problematic video game use. The dysfunction of the OFC and insula has been known to be a neurobiological marker of addictive disorders and to be related to impaired abilities in impulse control, cognitive flexibility, and reward-related decision making (Rolls, 2000; Rolls and Grabenhorst, 2008; Naqvi and Bechara, 2009).

Brain Changes in Response to Problematic Internet Use

Corticolimbic Circuit: Reward System

In a resting-state MRI study, Hong et al. (2013b) suggested that problematic Internet use was related to decreased functional connectivity in corticostriatal circuits, especially in the bilateral putamen. A PET study showed that participants with problematic Internet use showed decreased dopamine D2 receptor availability in the right putamen and bilateral dorsal caudate (Kim et al., 2011). In a study using SPECT in participants with problematic Internet use, decreased dopamine transporter expression in the striatum and reduced volume and weight of the corpus striatum were observed (Hou et al., 2012). Finally, structural neuroimaging studies have reported that in comparison with healthy participants, adolescents with problematic Internet use had decreased cortical thickness in the right OFC (Hong et al., 2013a). It seems that problematic Internet use, like problematic video game use, may share some common mechanisms with substance dependence in terms of engaging the brain reward system.

Cingulate Cortex: Cognition and Emotional Regulation

Cue-induced fMRI studies using working memory tasks for assessing cognitive process in individuals with problematic Internet use have reported increased responses in the anterior cingulate cortex, posterior cingulate cortex, inferior frontal cortex, and insula (Dong et al., 2012, 2013). These researchers evaluated the brain activity associated with response inhibition by using a cue-induced fMRI and the Stroop task in participants with problematic Internet use. The Stroop task measures response to words in congruent (e.g., the word "blue" in blue color) and non-congruent colors (e.g., the word "blue" in red color), where the incongruent words cause an interference, presumably due to divided attention. Participants with problematic Internet use showed increased activity in response to the Stroop task in the anterior cingulate cortex and posterior cingulate cortex compared to healthy participants. These results suggest reduced effectiveness of response inhibition processes in participants with problematic Internet use.

In a cue-induced fMRI study using the continuous-wins and continuous-losses task, Dong et al. (2013) also evaluated neural correlates of decision-making processes. Individuals with problematic Internet use showed increased brain activity compared to healthy controls in both continuous-wins and continuous-losses tasks in the inferior frontal cortex, insula, and anterior cingulate cortex. This finding seems to suggest that individuals with problematic Internet use need greater engagement to complete a decision-making task. This may translate into possible impairment in executive functioning.

In a study using VBM analysis, Zhou et al. (2011) reported that adolescents with problematic Internet use had lower gray matter density in the left anterior cingulate cortex, left posterior cingulate cortex, left insula, and left lingual gyrus— regions thought to be responsible for modulating emotional behavior. These results are consistent with the findings that adolescents with problematic Internet use exhibit more behavioral or emotional problems, compared to those without problematic Internet use.

The Question of Causality

Due to the cross-sectional nature of these structural studies, it is not possible to determine a causal relationship between structural abnormalities of the brain and problematic Internet and video game use. As part of the effort to investigate the causality in this relationship, some researchers have compared the regional brain volumes of individuals with problematic game with those of professional gamers. Professional gamers play games extensively, but they are able to control their gaming and are not distressed about this activity. In a study using VBM analysis, Han et al. (2012b) reported that professional gamers demonstrated a larger gray matter volume in the left cingulate gyrus compared to problematic Internet game users, as well as healthy controls. Furthermore, the gray matter volume of the left cingulate gyrus in professional gamers had a negative correlation with levels of impulsivity and perseverative errors. Thus, an increase in gray matter volume in the left anterior cingulate may be implicated in executive functioning and attentional control, which could be a correlate of successful gaming in professional gamers. There is clearly a need for further research in this domain.

Another issue in terms of the causality is the role of the conditions that frequently coexist with problematic Internet and video game use, including attention deficit hyperactivity disorder (ADHD), major depression, and social phobia (Yen et al., 2007; Ko et al., 2008). These disorders can be characterized by brain changes similar to those found in individuals with problematic Internet and video game use (e.g., dysfunction in the OFC and the insula). Therefore, it is an open question whether such brain changes are the result of problematic Internet and video game use, preexisting or coexisting psychiatric disorders, or other causes altogether.

NEUROIMAGING STUDIES OF TREATMENT-RELATED CHANGES

There have been only a few studies investigating the functional brain changes in response to therapeutic intervention in individuals with problematic video game use. The chapter will review the studies regarding functional brain changes following treatment with bupropion (Han et al., 2010a) and family therapy (Han et al., 2012a), as well as changes occurring following abstinence from online gaming (Kim et al., 2012).

Han et al. (2010a) investigated whether treatment with bupropion would affect the level of craving for Internet video games and gaming cue-induced brain activity in individuals with problematic online gaming. At baseline, subjects exhibited increased brain activity in the left occipital lobe cuneus, left DLPFC, and left parahippocampal gyrus during exposure to visual gaming cues. After bupropion treatment for 6 weeks, the intensity of craving for online gaming, the time spent gaming, and the level of reactivity in the DLPFC to gaming cues were all decreased. In addition, the changes in the reactivity in the DLPFC were positively correlated with the changes in the intensity of craving. These results could potentially be explained by the effects of bupropion as a norepinephrine-dopamine reuptake inhibitor that increases extracellular concentrations of catecholamines (Page and Lucki, 2002). An increase of norepinephrine and dopamine in the DLPFC, mediated by bupropion (Dazzi et al., 2002), may attenuate the positive reinforcing properties of gaming and consequently reduce craving for gaming. Additionally, an increased extracellular concentration of dopamine caused by bupropion may replace dopamine release that occurs during gaming.

Han et al. (2012a) subsequently investigated effects of a 3-week family therapy intervention on brain activity in adolescents with considerable family dysfunction. During fMRI assessments, participants were exposed to visual cues depicting scenes of parental affection as well as scenes of online video gaming. Participants with problematic Internet use demonstrated reduced activity in the caudate, middle temporal gyrus, and occipital lobe in response to cues related to parental affection and increased activity in the middle frontal and inferior parietal regions in response to gaming cues. At follow-up, participants with problematic

Internet use reported an improvement in perceived level of family cohesion; this improvement was shown to be positively associated with an increase in the activity of the caudate nucleus in response to cues related to parental affection and was negatively correlated with changes in time spent gaming. Han et al. (2012a) suggested that adolescents with low level of perceived family cohesion seemed to play games to compensate for striatal dopamine deficits caused by poor parental care during early life (Bartels and Zeki, 2004; Pruessner et al., 2004; Aron et al., 2005). Improvement in the perception of family cohesion during family therapy could conceivably facilitate dopaminergic neurotransmission in the brain reward system and consequently reduce the level of craving for gaming.

Kim et al. (2012) investigated the effect of four weeks of abstinence from online gaming on brain activity in response to simple and complex working memory tasks in adolescents with problematic video game use. At baseline, individuals with problematic video game use demonstrated increased activity during working memory tasks in the right middle occipital gyrus, left cerebellum posterior lobe, left premotor cortex, and left middle temporal gyrus. After abstaining from gaming, individuals with problematic video game use demonstrated increased activity in the right DLPFC and left occipital fusiform gyrus during exposure to working memory tasks. Additionally, a decrease in the severity of problematic video game use was correlated with an increase in activity in the right DLPFC in response to complex working memory tasks. Kim et al. (2012) suggested that the dysfunction of working memory in individuals with problematic video game use might be similar to that observed in individuals with substance use disorders (Pope et al., 2001; Tapert et al., 2004). In a finding that seems reversible, excessive game playing may inhibit the function of the DLPFC, which appears to play a major role in working memory.

In summary, an increase in the activity in the DLPFC and in dopaminergic neurotransmission in the corticostriatal reward pathway seems to be associated with positive therapeutic outcomes. However, no firm conclusions can be made about the treatment-related brain changes in problematic Internet and video game use because of the very limited number of studies.

NEUROPHYSIOLOGICAL STUDIES OF PROBLEMATIC INTERNET AND VIDEO GAME USE

The neurophysiological research on Internet and video game use can be categorized into three types: (1) studies in individuals with long-term nonproblematic gaming, (2) studies in individuals with problematic gaming, and (3) studies of instantaneous effects of gaming on the brain.

The effects of gaming on neurophysiology have been investigated by means of a power spectral analysis of the electroencephalography (EEG), event-related potentials, and evoked potentials. EEG measures electrical activity of the brain along the scalp using surface electrodes. Electrical activity measured by EEG results from ionic current flows within the neurons. A power spectrum analysis evaluates the distribution of signal power over frequency bands that reflect pathological brain lesions or certain mental states (e.g., being relaxed, alert, anxious, or actively think-ing) (Blanco et al., 1995). Event-related potentials are a stereotyped electrophysio-logical response to certain events, including a sensory stimulus and recognition of a target stimulus or the omission of a stimulus. Event-related potentials can reflect a perception and cognitive process, including attention, memory, expectation, or alterations in mental state (Donchin, 1979). Evoked potentials are a subclass of event-related potentials and they are thought to reflect the direct processing of the simple physical stimulus, such as a flashing light, a click/tone, or tactile stimula-tion (Sutton et al., 1967). Event-related potentials, including evoked potentials, are measured by EEG during exposure to stimuli that are usually auditory or visual.

Neurophysiological Studies in Individuals with Long-Term Nonproblematic Game Use

As already noted, video game experience has been found to have a beneficial effect on visuospatial attention and cognition. In a study observing steady-state visual-evoked potentials and event-related potentials, action video game players showed better target detection capabilities than non–video game players (Mishra et al., 2011). Also, the amplitude of target-elicited P300 component was increased in action video game players compared to non–video game players, suggesting that action video game players can make perceptual decisions with greater accuracy and confidence under conditions of high perceptual load (Mishra et al., 2011). Another study assessed neurophysiological differences by measuring steady-state visual-evoked potentials in fast-action video game players (playing first-person shooter games) and nonaction players (playing role-playing games) during a visual search task (Krishnan et al., 2013). The first-person shooter players tended to engage an active suppression mechanism to organize selective attention, whereas players of role-playing games primarily engaged a signal enhancement mechanism. These electrophysiological findings suggest that fast-action gaming may cause changes in neural strategies with regard to attention, possibly by means of training in sup-pressing the information at irrelevant locations during gaming.

Neurophysiological Studies in Individuals with Problematic Internet and Video Game Use

Several neurophysiological studies have suggested that individuals with prob-lematic Internet and video game use may have electrophysiological characteris-tics similar to individuals with substance dependence, such as incentive salience, poor error processing, and impulsivity. Incentive salience is defined as a strong motivation for rewarding stimuli, and it is thought to be mediated by the dopa-mine reward system (Berridge and Robinson, 1998). This process converts neutral stimuli into desirable and "wanted" stimuli that command attention.

In a study using event-related potentials, amplitudes of the late positive com-plex evoked by gaming cues in participants with problematic gaming were found to be stronger in parietal regions, relative to casual players (Thalemann et al., 2007).

This result suggested increased emotional processing, implying incentive salience of specific cues, as in addictive disorders. Another study using event-related potentials reported that participants with problematic gaming showed reduced error-related negativity amplitudes in response to incorrect trials in comparison with correct trials, which suggests poor error processing (Littel et al., 2012).

In a study using power spectral analysis of EEG, participants with problematic Internet use showed lower absolute power on the beta band and higher absolute power on the gamma band compared to control participants (Choi et al., 2013). In addition, resting-state fast-wave brain activities were positively related to the severity of Internet overuse as well as to the level of impulsivity. In a study measuring using event-related potentials during a go/no-go task, individuals with problematic Internet use demonstrated lower NoGo-N2 amplitude, higher NoGo-P3 amplitude, and longer NoGo-P3 peak latency than casual users (Dong et al., 2010). Individuals with problematic Internet use also showed lower activation in the conflict detection stage than casual users (Dong et al., 2010). These results suggest that individuals with problematic Internet use may need to make greater cognitive efforts to carry out an inhibition task, implying less proficiency in processing information and impaired impulse control compared to casual users.

Neurophysiological Studies of Instantaneous Effects of Gaming on the Brain

Effects of Presleep Video Game Playing on Sleep Physiology

Higuchi et al. (2005) investigated the effect of pre-sleep video game playing on sleep variables. Levels of self-reported sleepiness and relative theta power measured by EEG were reduced after playing computer games compared to control conditions of passive exposure to bright or dark displays. Increased sleep latency and decreased rapid eye movement (REM) sleep were also found after playing games compared to control conditions. Neither playing computer games nor being exposed to bright displays showed an effect on slow-wave sleep. Thus, playing a computer game before going to sleep may have an influence on sleep latency and REM sleep, but being passively exposed to bright displays does not seem to have any influence on sleep physiology.

Weaver et al. (2010) compared the effects of presleep video game playing and passive DVD watching on sleep in adolescents. Presleep video game playing was slightly related to increased sleep latency and decreased levels of self-reported sleepiness; it was also associated with increased alertness as assessed by the relative alpha power of EEGs. However, REM sleep was not affected by presleep video game playing. These inconsistent results call for further research.

Video Game–Related Seizures

Many cases of epileptic seizures triggered by playing video games have been reported since the first report by Rushton (1981). Although some of these individuals had photosensitive epilepsy, seizures in others were unrelated to photosensitivity (Bureau et al., 2004). Chuang et al. (2006) compared the clinical characteristics and the results of EEG and brain MRI assessment in patients who experienced seizures exclusively while playing games (group I) and patients who experienced both game-induced and spontaneous seizures (group II). In group I, there were associations with (1) middle-age onset of seizures (mean age of 39.1 years); (2) nonspecific abnormalities on EEG or brain MRI (60% of participants); and (3) partial-onset seizures (30% of participants). In group II, associations were found with (1) adolescent-onset of seizures (mean age of 16.3 years); (2) epileptiform discharge on EEG (42% of participants); and (3) generalized tonic-clonic seizures, myoclonic seizures, and absence seizures (most participants).

Photosensitivity has been suggested as the most important pathophysiological factor for seizures triggered by playing video games (Fylan et al., 1999; Bureau et al., 2004). In addition, increased cognitive activities, emotional intensity, mental stress, fatigue, and lack of sleep seem to be precipitants of game-related seizures (Chuang, 2006). According to European collaborative studies, a distance of more than 2 meters from the screen and 100-Hz TV screens as opposed to 50-Hz TV screens may be less likely to induce paroxysmal seizures during video game play (Kasteleijn-Nolst Trenite et al., 1999, 2002; Bureau et al., 2004).

GENETICS OF PROBLEMATIC INTERNET AND VIDEO GAME USE

Genetic studies are still preliminary but suggest that there may be a genetic predisposition to problematic Internet and video game use. Han et al. (2007) compared adolescents with problematic and casual Internet use in terms of reward dependence measured by Cloninger's Temperament and Character Inventory and the frequencies of two dopamine polymorphisms: Taq1A1 allele of the dopamine D2 receptor (DRD2 Taq1A1) and Val158Met in the catecholamine-O-methyltransferase (COMT) genes. Adolescents with problematic Internet use showed higher reward dependence and increased prevalence of the DRD2 Taq1A1 and COMT alleles relative to controls.

Another study compared adolescents with problematic and casual Internet use in terms of the genetic polymorphisms of the serotonin transporter gene and novelty seeking and harm avoidance measured by Cloninger's Temperament and Character Inventory (Lee et al., 2008). Adolescents with problematic Internet use showed higher homozygous short allelic variant of the serotonin transporter gene (SS-5HTTLPR) frequencies, greater harm avoidance, and higher Beck Depression Inventory scores. Among the adolescents with problematic Internet use, those who expressed SS-5HTTLPR showed greater harm avoidance and greater severity of problematic Internet use than those expressing the other serotonin transporter gene allele variants. These results suggest that individuals with problematic Internet use may have genetic predispositions and personality traits similar to individuals with depression and anxiety disorders.

The role of the nicotinic acetylcholine receptor subunit alpha 4 (CHRNA4) in problematic Internet use was also investigated (Montag et al., 2012). Individuals with problematic Internet use, especially females, demonstrated a significantly more frequent T- variant (CC genotype) of the rs1044396 polymorphism of the CHRNA4 gene, compared to the control group. The authors suggested that there was an interaction between the dopaminergic and cholinergic systems, which has been reported to affect cognition and anxiety; this has also been implicated in nicotine dependence.

In summary, the genetic predisposition to problematic Internet and video game use may consist of an insufficient number of dopamine receptors or insufficient amount of serotonin and dopamine, which might make individuals less able or unable to experience pleasure from activities that most people usually find rewarding. To feel normal pleasure, these individuals might engage excessively in behaviors that can stimulate the brain reward system; this mechanism may make them more vulnerable to problematic Internet and video game use (Cash et al., 2012).

CONCLUSION AND FUTURE DIRECTIONS

This chapter has discussed neuroimaging, neurophysiological, and genetic aspects of nonproblematic as well as problematic Internet and video game use. The functional and structural brain changes in response to video game use suggest that playing video games enhances visuospatial attention and visuomotor function, especially within the frontoparietal network. Additionally, problematic Internet and video game use and substance dependence seem to have abnormal reward processing in corticolimbic circuit in common. The changes in anterior cingulate cortex and posterior cingulate cortex in individuals with problematic Internet and video game use seem to be related to deficient executive functioning, impulsivity, and prominent behavioral or emotional problems. Studies of treatment-related brain changes suggest that an increase in the activity in the DLPFC and dopaminergic neurotransmission within the corticostriatal reward pathway may be associated with positive therapeutic outcomes; such changes have also been associated with effective treatments for impulse control disorders and substance dependence.

The genetic predisposition to problematic Internet and video game use may relate to a deficient number of dopamine receptors or insufficient amount of serotonin and dopamine, which may make individuals unable to derive pleasure from activities that most people find rewarding. This may make them more vulnerable to problematic Internet and video game use, just as it may increase vulnerability to frequently coexisting disorders, such as ADHD, depression, and social phobia.

Overall, the neurobiological characteristics of problematic Internet and video game use seem to be similar to those related to impulse control disorders and substance dependence in terms of the brain reward system, executive functioning, impulsivity, and behavioral or emotional problems.

Still, it would be premature to reach any firm conclusion about the brain changes in problematic Internet and video game use and the treatment-related brain changes due to the limited number of studies and the cross-sectional nature of most research. Further research using prospective and other novel designs is clearly needed to better understand the neurobiological underpinnings of problematic Internet and video game use, the relationships between brain abnormalities and problematic Internet and video game use, the role of coexisting conditions and other confounding variables, and treatment-related brain changes.

DISCLOSURE STATEMENT

This work was supported by a grant from the Korean Game Culture Foundation. The authors disclose no relationships with commercial entities and professional activities that may bias their views.

REFERENCES

American Psychiatric Association (1994). Diagnostic and Statistical Manual of Mental Disorders. Fourth Edition. American Psychiatric Association, Washington, DC.

American Psychiatric Association (2013). Diagnostic and Statistical Manual of Mental Disorders. Fifth Edition. American Psychiatric Association, Washington, DC.

Aron A, Fisher H, Mashek DJ, Strong G, Li H, Brown LL (2005). Reward, motivation, and emotion systems associated with early-stage intense romantic love. Journal of Neurophysiology 94: 327–337.

Ashburner J, Friston KJ (2000). Voxel-based morphometry—the methods. NeuroImage 11: 805–821.

Bartels A, Zeki S (2004). The neural correlates of maternal and romantic love. NeuroImage 21: 1155–1166.

Bavelier D, Achtman RL, Mani M, Focker J (2012). Neural bases of selective attention in action video game players. Vision Research 61: 132–143.

Berridge KC, Robinson TE (1998). What is the role of dopamine in reward: hedonic impact, reward learning, or incentive salience? Brain Research: Brain Research Reviews 28: 309–369.

Blanco S, Quiroga RQ, Rosso OA, Kochen S (1995). Time-frequency analysis of electro-encephalogram series. Physical Review E—Statistical Physics, Plasmas, Fluids, and Related Interdisciplinary Topics 51: 2624–2631.

Bureau M, Hirsch E, Vigevano F (2004). Epilepsy and videogames. Epilepsia 1: 24–26.

Cash H, Rae CD, Steel AH, Winkler A (2012). Internet addiction: a brief summary of research and practice. Current Psychiatry Reviews 8: 292–298.

Choi JS, Park SM, Lee J, et al (2013). Resting-state beta and gamma activity in Internet addiction. International Journal of Psychophysiology 89: 328–333.

Chuang YC (2006). Massively multiplayer online role-playing game-induced seizures: a neglected health problem in Internet addiction. Cyberpsychology and Behavior 9: 451–456.

Chuang YC, Chang WN, Lin TK, Lu CH, Chen SD, Huang CR (2006). Game-related seizures presenting with two types of clinical features. Seizure 15: 98–105.

Davidson RJ, Putnam KM, Larson CL (2000). Dysfunction in the neural circuitry of emotion regulation—a possible prelude to violence. Science 289: 591–594.

Dazzi L, Vignone V, Seu E, Ladu S, Vacca G, Biggio G (2002). Inhibition by venlafaxine of the increase in norepinephrine output in rat prefrontal cortex elicited by acute stress or by the anxiogenic drug FG 7142. Journal of Psychopharmacology 16: 125–131.

Ding WN, Sun JH, Sun YW, et al (2013). Altered default network resting-state functional connectivity in adolescents with Internet gaming addiction. PloS One 8: 26.

Donchin E (1979). Event-related brain potentials: a tool in the study of human information processing. In Begleiter H, Editor. Evoked Brain Potentials and Behavior. Plenum Press, New York, NY, pp. 13–88.

Dong G, Devito EE, Du X, Cui Z (2012). Impaired inhibitory control in "Internet addiction disorder": a functional magnetic resonance imaging study. Psychiatry Research 203: 153–158.

Dong G, Hu Y, Lin X, Lu Q (2013). What makes Internet addicts continue playing online even when faced by severe negative consequences? Possible explanations from an fMRI study. Biological Psychology 6: 182–188.

Dong G, Zhou H, Zhao X (2010). Impulse inhibition in people with Internet addiction disorder: electrophysiological evidence from a Go/NoGo study. Neuroscience Letters 485: 138–142.

Fylan F, Harding GF, Edson AS, Webb RM (1999). Mechanisms of video-game epilepsy. Epilepsia 4: 28–30.

Granek JA, Gorbet DJ, Sergio LE (2010). Extensive video-game experience alters cortical networks for complex visuomotor transformations. Cortex 46: 1165–1177.

Han DH, Bolo N, Daniels MA, Arenella L, Lyoo IK, Renshaw PF (2011). Brain activity and desire for Internet video game play. Comprehensive Psychiatry 52: 88–95.

Han DH, Hwang JW, Renshaw PF (2010a). Bupropion sustained release treatment decreases craving for video games and cue-induced brain activity in patients with Internet video game addiction. Experimental and Clinical Psychopharmacology 18: 297–304.

Han DH, Kim SM, Lee YS, Renshaw PF (2012a). The effect of family therapy on the changes in the severity of on-line game play and brain activity in adolescents with on-line game addiction. Psychiatry Research 202: 126–131.

Han DH, Kim YS, Lee YS, Min KJ, Renshaw PF (2010b). Changes in cue-induced, prefrontal cortex activity with video-game play. Cyberpsychology, Behavior, and Social Networking 13: 655–661.

Han DH, Lee YS, Yang KC, Kim EY, Lyoo IK, Renshaw PF (2007). Dopamine genes and reward dependence in adolescents with excessive Internet video game play. Journal of Addiction Medicine 1: 133–138.

Han DH, Lyoo IK, Renshaw PF (2012b). Differential regional gray matter volumes in patients with on-line game addiction and professional gamers. Journal of Psychiatric Research 46: 507–515.

Higuchi S, Motohashi Y, Liu Y, Maeda A (2005). Effects of playing a computer game using a bright display on presleep physiological variables, sleep latency, slow wave sleep and REM sleep. Journal of Sleep Research 14: 267–273.

Hoeft F, Watson CL, Kesler SR, Bettinger KE, Reiss AL (2008). Gender differences in the mesocorticolimbic system during computer game-play. Journal of Psychiatric Research 42: 253–258.

Hong SB, Kim JW, Choi EJ, et al (2013a). Reduced orbitofrontal cortical thickness in male adolescents with Internet addiction. Behavioral and Brain Functions 9: 1744–9081.

Hong SB, Zalesky A, Cocchi L, et al (2013b). Decreased functional brain connectivity in adolescents with Internet addiction. PloS One 8: 25.

Hou H, Jia S, Hu S, et al (2012). Reduced striatal dopamine transporters in people with Internet addiction disorder. Journal of Biomedicine and Biotechnology 854524: 13.

Huettel SA, Song AW, McCarthy G (2009). Functional Magnetic Resonance Imaging. Sinauer Associates, Sunderland, MA.

Hutton C, De Vita E, Ashburner J, Deichmann R, Turner R (2008). Voxel-based cortical thickness measurements in MRI. NeuroImage 40: 1701–1710.

Janes AC, Nickerson LD, Frederick B, Kaufman MJ (2012). Prefrontal and limbic resting state brain network functional connectivity differs between nicotine-dependent smokers and non-smoking controls. Drug and Alcohol Dependence 125: 252–259.

Kasteleijn-Nolst Trenite DG, da Silva AM, Ricci S, et al (1999). Video-game epilepsy: a European study. Epilepsia 4: 70–74.

Kasteleijn-Nolst Trenite DG, da Silva AM, Ricci S, et al (2002). Video games are exciting: a European study of video game-induced seizures and epilepsy. Epileptic Disorders 4: 121–128.

Kätsyri J, Hari R, Ravaja N, Nummenmaa L (2012). The opponent matters: elevated fMRI reward responses to winning against a human versus a computer opponent during interactive video game playing. Cerebral Cortex 23: 2829–2839.

Kim SH, Baik SH, Park CS, Kim SJ, Choi SW, Kim SE (2011). Reduced striatal dopamine D2 receptors in people with Internet addiction. Neuroreport 22: 407–411.

Kim SM, Han DH, Lee YS, Kim JE, Renshaw PF (2012). Changes in brain activity in response to problem solving during the abstinence from online game play. Journal of Behavioral Addictions 1: 41–49.

Ko CH, Liu GC, Hsiao S, et al (2009). Brain activities associated with gaming urge of online gaming addiction. Journal of Psychiatric Research 43: 739–747.

Ko CH, Liu GC, Yen JY, Yen CF, Chen CS, Lin WC (2013). The brain activations for both cue-induced gaming urge and smoking craving among subjects comorbid with Internet gaming addiction and nicotine dependence. Journal of Psychiatric Research 47: 486–493.

Ko CH, Yen JY, Chen CS, Chen CC, Yen CF (2008). Psychiatric comorbidity of Internet addiction in college students: an interview study. CNS Spectrums 13: 147–153.

Koepp MJ, Gunn RN, Lawrence AD, et al (1998). Evidence for striatal dopamine release during a video game. Nature 393: 266–268.

Krishnan L, Kang A, Sperling G, Srinivasan R (2013). Neural strategies for selective attention distinguish fast-action video game players. Brain Topography 26: 83–97.

Kühn S, Gallinat J (2014). Amount of lifetime video gaming is positively associated with entorhinal, hippocampal and occipital volume. Molecular Psychiatry 19: 842–847.

Kühn S, Romanowski A, Schilling C, et al (2011). The neural basis of video gaming. Translational Psychiatry 1: e53.

Lee YS, Han DH, Yang KC, et al (2008). Depression like characteristics of 5HTTLPR polymorphism and temperament in excessive Internet users. Journal of Affective Disorders 109: 165–169.

Leech R, Kamourieh S, Beckmann CF, Sharp DJ (2011). Fractionating the default mode network: distinct contributions of the ventral and dorsal posterior cingulate cortex to cognitive control. Journal of Neuroscience 31: 3217–3224.

Littel M, van den Berg I, Luijten M, van Rooij AJ, Keemink L, Franken IH (2012). Error processing and response inhibition in excessive computer game players: an event-related potential study. Addiction Biology 17: 934–947.

Lorenz RC, Kruger JK, Neumann B, et al (2013). Cue reactivity and its inhibition in pathological computer game players. Addiction Biology 18: 134–146.

Mathiak KA, Klasen M, Weber R, Ackermann H, Shergill SS, Mathiak K (2011). Reward system and temporal pole contributions to affective evaluation during a first person shooter video game. BMC Neuroscience 12: 1471–2202.

Mishra J, Zinni M, Bavelier D, Hillyard SA (2011). Neural basis of superior performance of action videogame players in an attention-demanding task. Journal of Neuroscience 31: 992–998.

Montag C, Kirsch P, Sauer C, Markett S, Reuter M (2012). The role of the CHRNA4 gene in Internet addiction: a case-control study. Journal of Addiction Medicine 6: 191–195.

Naqvi NH, Bechara A (2009). The hidden island of addiction: the insula. Trends in Neurosciences 32: 56–67.

Page ME, Lucki I (2002). Effects of acute and chronic reboxetine treatment on stress-induced monoamine efflux in the rat frontal cortex. Neuropsychopharmacology 27: 237–247.

Pearson JM, Heilbronner SR, Barack DL, Hayden BY, Platt ML (2011). Posterior cingulate cortex: adapting behavior to a changing world. Trends in Cognitive Sciences 15: 143–151.

Pope HG, Gruber AJ, Hudson JI, Huestis MA, Yurgelun-Todd D (2001). Neuropsychological performance in long-term cannabis users. Archives of General Psychiatry 58: 909–915.

Pruessner JC, Champagne F, Meaney MJ, Dagher A (2004). Dopamine release in response to a psychological stress in humans and its relationship to early life maternal care: a positron emission tomography study using [11C]raclopride. Journal of Neuroscience 24: 2825–2831.

Rahmim A, Zaidi H (2008). PET versus SPECT: strengths, limitations and challenges. Nuclear Medicine Communications 29: 193–207.

Rolls ET (2000). The orbitofrontal cortex and reward. Cerebral Cortex 10: 284–294.

Rolls ET, Grabenhorst F (2008). The orbitofrontal cortex and beyond: from affect to decision-making. Progress in Neurobiology 86: 216–244.

Rushton DN (1981). "Space invader" epilepsy. Lancet 317: 501.

Shapira NA, Goldsmith TD, Keck PE, Khosla UM, McElroy SL (2000). Psychiatric features of individuals with problematic Internet use. Journal of Affective Disorders 57: 267–272.

Sun Y, Ying H, Seetohul RM, et al (2012). Brain fMRI study of craving induced by cue pictures in online game addicts (male adolescents). Behavioural Brain Research 233: 563–576.

Sutton S, Tueting P, Zubin J, John ER (1967). Information delivery and the sensory evoked potential. Science 155: 1436–1439.

Tanabe J, Nyberg E, Martin LF, et al (2011). Nicotine effects on default mode network during resting state. Psychopharmacology 216: 287–295.

Tanaka S, Ikeda H, Kasahara K, et al (2013). Larger right posterior parietal volume in action video game experts: a behavioral and voxel-based morphometry (VBM) study. PloS One 8: e66998.

Tapert SF, Schweinsburg AD, Barlett VC, et al (2004). Blood oxygen level dependent response and spatial working memory in adolescents with alcohol use disorders. Alcoholism, Clinical and Experimental Research 28: 1577–1586.

Thalemann R, Wolfling K, Grusser SM (2007). Specific cue reactivity on computer game-related cues in excessive gamers. Behavioral Neuroscience 121: 614–618.

Weaver E, Gradisar M, Dohnt H, Lovato N, Douglas P (2010). The effect of presleep video-game playing on adolescent sleep. Journal of Clinical Sleep Medicine 6: 184–189.

Weber R, Ritterfeld U, Mathiak K (2006). Does playing violent video games induce aggression? Empirical evidence of a functional magnetic resonance imaging study. Media Psychology 8: 39–60.

Weng CB, Qian RB, Fu XM, et al (2013). Gray matter and white matter abnormalities in online game addiction. European Journal of Radiology 82: 1308–1312.

Yen JY, Ko CH, Yen CF, Wu HY, Yang MJ (2007). The comorbid psychiatric symptoms of Internet addiction: attention deficit and hyperactivity disorder (ADHD), depression, social phobia, and hostility. Journal of Adolescent Health 41: 93–98.

Yuan K, Cheng P, Dong T, et al (2013). Cortical thickness abnormalities in late adolescence with online gaming addiction. PloS One 8: e53055.

Zhang Y, Tian J, Yuan K, et al (2011). Distinct resting-state brain activities in heroin-dependent individuals. Brain Research 1402: 46–53.

Zhou Y, Lin FC, Du YS, et al (2011). Gray matter abnormalities in Internet addiction: a voxel-based morphometry study. European Journal of Radiology 79: 92–95.

5 Video Game Violence and Offline Aggression

Christopher L. Groves and
Craig A. Anderson

INTRODUCTION

Technological progress over the past several decades has revolutionized human life and interaction. Media are no longer consumed solely through the family-shared television or radio. Instead, tablets, smartphones, home computers, and video game consoles are each capable of providing an unprecedented access to television shows, movies, and video games. Indeed, the data support the notion that media use is quite high. According to Rideout et al. (2010), youth spend approximately 7 1/2 hours per day consuming some form of media. Such high consumption quickly inspires questions about what psychological effects will result from the access brought by the digital age.

Media use often allows viewers and players to engage with rich stories that contain characters, themes, lessons, and portrayals that make lasting impressions. It would be naïve to think that viewers merely observe media passively without relating to the content in meaningful ways. Viewers identify with characters and learn from their mistakes and successes. For this reason, research has often focused on major content themes within media and on their effects on subsequent behavior, beliefs, attitudes, and more. Unsurprisingly, one of the most prevalent themes in modern media is violence. No group is immune to this exposure. In a survey by Worth et al. (2008), 71% of 14-year-olds in the United States and even 35% of 10-year-olds reported viewing at least one extremely violent movie. For children living in homes without rules regarding violent content, this percentage rose to 87%. Similarly, Gentile (2008) found that more than 90% of video games rated as appropriate for children age 10 years and older contained violence.

Since Albert Bandura's (1965) classic Bobo doll study, the foundations of observation theory have provided a convincing theoretical framework through which the effects of violent media use are understood. In this study, children who observed a model aggressing toward a toy Bobo doll were found to spontaneously replicate this aggressive behavior. However, numerous theoretical advances have revealed that the relationship between viewing violence and subsequent aggressive behavior is a complex one; numerous psychological processes are at work, processes that can be well understood with the use of modern social-cognitive theories. This chapter will focus on the relationship between exposure to video game violence and aggressive behavior.

AGGRESSION AND VIOLENT MEDIA

The study of violent media often focuses on aggressive behavior as an outcome. Before proceeding, it is important to consider how researchers define aggression. Aggression is commonly defined as "any behavior directed toward another individual that is carried out with the proximate (immediate) intent to cause harm. In addition, the perpetrator must believe that the behavior will harm the target, and that the target is motivated to avoid the behavior" (Anderson and Bushman, 2002, p. 28). Violence, on the other hand, is considered an extreme form of aggression (Anderson and Bushman, 2002). In research contexts, the presence of media violence is often characterized by the presence of aggressive content—that is, characters harming others who wish to avoid such harm. Interestingly, in one experimental study by Anderson et al. (2007), individuals playing video games with lower-level aggressive content (no gory violence) demonstrated increases in aggressive behavior that were at least as large as those shown by participants who played a more graphically violent game. Because the findings of this study suggest that there is little or no difference between the effects of lower-level and higher-level aggressive media content and because most published studies have not distinguished between such types of content, this chapter will not make that distinction and will use the terms "aggression" and "violence" interchangeably.

Several content analyses have concluded that a large proportion of the contemporary mass media contains violence (e.g., Yokota and Thompson, 2000; Thompson and Haninger, 2001; Thompson et al., 2006; Linder and Gentile, 2009). Furthermore, hundreds of studies have been conducted on the effects of violent television programs and video games (e.g., Wartella and Reeves, 1985; Paik and Comstock, 1994; Bushman and Huesmann, 2006; Anderson et al., 2010). The consistent finding, accepted by a wide array of scientific societies, is that violent media use can be a risk factor for increases in aggressive behavior and a host of aggression-related variables (American Psychological Association, 2005; American Academy of Pediatrics, 2009; International Society for Research on Aggression, 2012; Society for the Psychological Study of Social Issues, 2014). This link has been observed across gender, age groups, and cultures (e.g., Anderson et al., 2003, 2010).

Importantly, the effects of violent media have been demonstrated across a variety of aggression measures. One commonly used measure of aggression is Taylor's Competitive Reaction Time Task (TCRTT). This task involves participants competing against an ostensible other participant in reaction time trials (the participant wins a trial by clicking a box faster than his or her opponent). Prior to each trial, the participants select an aversive noise volume (60–105 dB) and/or duration (0.5–5 seconds) to administer to their opponent if they beat the opponent on that trial. Several studies from different laboratories using different versions of the TCRTT have demonstrated that brief, violent video game play leads participants to administer more punitive noise blasts than those who played an equally exciting nonviolent game (e.g., Bushman and Gibson, 2011; Engelhardt et al., 2011; Anderson et al., 2004).

In another aggression measure, the "hot sauce paradigm," researchers explain to participants that they are taking part in a two-part study. The first part involves media use, and in the second part, participants select foods for another person to eat. They are informed that the person dislikes spicy food but are given the opportunity to administer an amount of hot sauce that this person must eat. In studies utilizing this paradigm, violent video game play consistently leads to increases in the amount of hot sauce administered to the other person (e.g., Barlett et al., 2009). Other studies have examined the effects of violent media on verbal aggression such as insulting another person (Parke et al., 1977; Krcmar and Farrar, 2009); on children's aggressiveness during a period of free play or at school (Silvern and Williamson, 1987; Anderson et al., 2007); and even on the frequency of committing seriously violent or delinquent behaviors as an adolescent or adult (e.g., Huesmann et al., 2003; Boxer et al., 2009; DeLisi et al., 2013).

THEORETICAL PROCESSES

As previously mentioned, the effect of violent media content is very robust and has been demonstrated across many studies. Research has therefore begun to shift to studying the psychological processes that may give rise to this effect. Currently, the General Aggression Model (GAM; Anderson and Bushman, 2002; Anderson and Carnagey, 2014) is the most comprehensive theoretical framework for understanding violent media effects. This model integrates a host of overlapping theories of human aggression, including social-cognitive, personality, and biologic factors. It has been applied to understanding the observed increases in aggression resulting from a number of stimuli, including temperature change, provocation, and pain, and ranging from relatively minor forms of aggression to major psychopathologies involving violence (Gilbert and Daffern, 2011) (Figure 5.1).

The GAM describes both short-term and long-term processes involved in the development and maintenance of aggressive behavior patterns. The single episode begins with two forms of input: the person and the situation. Contained within the person are all characteristics of the individual that carry across situations. These include biologic dispositions (e.g., testosterone levels, genetic propensities toward aggressiveness) and personality characteristics (e.g., general hostility, perceiving others' ambiguous behavior as aggressive, trait aggression, and attitudes and beliefs that support or inhibit aggressive responses). The second form of input is the situation itself. This factor includes all elements within an immediate social

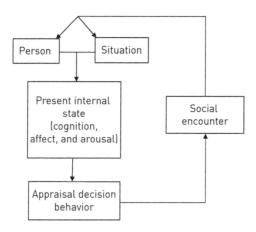

FIGURE 5.1
Short-term processes within the General Aggression Model.

encounter that can influence aggression—facilitative ones (e.g., provocation, warm temperatures, or violent media use) and inhibitory ones (e.g., being in a church or receiving a compliment). Importantly, both the person and situation variables can also include protective (or inhibiting) factors that affect aggression. For example, aggression is inhibited when individuals find themselves in a setting where aggressive responses are seen as especially inappropriate (e.g., a funeral). Similarly, person factors such as having low testosterone or being female are protective against aggression. In fact, aggression is often best understood within a risk and resilience approach in which risk and protective factors interact to produce aggressive (or non-aggressive) responses (Gentile and Bushman, 2012).

Within the GAM, the person and situation factors influence the internal states, which refer to the person's affect, cognitions, and arousal. For example, when provoked (e.g., bumped in a hallway), individuals often experience increases in aggressive affect (e.g., anger), aggressive cognitions (e.g., aggressive fantasizing), and arousal (e.g., increased heart rate). These internal states are highly interactive and may reinforce or inhibit one another. For example, following provocation, individuals may interpret the provocation as unjustified, which can then lead to increases in anger and arousal.

These internal states feed into decision-making processes whereby the individual appraises the situation. The initial appraisal is usually very fast, effortless, and automatic, and it may be made without conscious awareness. After an initial appraisal is made, the individual decides whether it is sufficient. If it is, an impulsive behavioral response occurs (e.g., a verbal insult). If the initial appraisal is deemed unsatisfying and if the individual possesses sufficient time and cognitive resources, reappraisal occurs, in which the individual considers alternative explanations of the initial harmful event and alternative behavioral options (Barlett and Anderson, 2011). When a behavioral option is considered appropriate, a thoughtful action (or inaction) occurs. It is important to note that reappraisal does not guarantee a nonaggressive response. For example, an initial appraisal may be relatively benign (e.g., harm was unintended), but reappraisal may lead to a decision that the initial harm was intended, which in turn leads to an aggressive response.

When the behavioral response is selected and enacted, the ongoing situation is influenced and feeds back into the situational input during the next episode (see Figure 5.1). In other words, the GAM presents a type of behavioral feedback loop in which the situational and individual variables interact, affecting internal states and decision-making processes before a behavior is enacted, which then affects the situation. The newly changed situation feeds back into the situational input variable and initiates a new cycle. Furthermore, with repeated cycles, long-term learning processes are also affected. For example, if an aggressive response "works," the person is rewarded for the entire decision-making process that led to the aggressive response, resulting in changes in beliefs, expectations, and so on. This is in agreement with social learning and social-cognitive theories.

This cyclical process helps people better understand the violence escalation cycle (Figure 5.2). Within this cycle, two individuals or two groups (e.g., high school cliques, political parties, or even nations) engage in increasingly aggressive responses following provocation. An initial, triggering event is perceived by the acting party as unintentional, justified, and relatively mild. However, the second party perceives this action as intentional, unjustified, and harmful and retaliates in a way that it believes is justified. The first party perceives this as an unjustified overretaliation and reacts in a way it believes is justified retaliation. Thus, the cycle begins anew, and each act of retaliation is more serious than the preceding bout of violence. These aggressive behaviors continue to escalate until one party is no longer able to retaliate or a successful intervention occurs (Anderson et al., 2008a).

Because the broad nature of the GAM allows its application across an entire range of human aggression phenomena, it serves as a solid theoretical foundation for understanding media violence effects. The text below describes some of the more specific theories within the GAM that can help explain aggressive outcomes following violent media use.

Priming Effects

A major influential theory that contributes to the explanatory power of the GAM is the cognitive neoassociation theory proposed by Berkowitz (1990, 1993). This theory posits that aggression occurs when individuals experience aversive events, which leads to negative affect, which in turn primes a host of aggression-related knowledge structures. Perhaps one of the most valuable aspects of this theory is its knowledge structure approach to an understanding of how aggression-related cues increase aggression.

According to this approach, cognitive concepts, emotions, and behavioral scripts are interconnected in memory (Collins and Loftus, 1975), forming a web of associations that are used to process information and assist in making decisions about optimal behavioral outcomes in any given situation. The theory states that activation of a given concept will automatically activate related concepts in memory. For example, the word "murder" will strongly activate concepts such

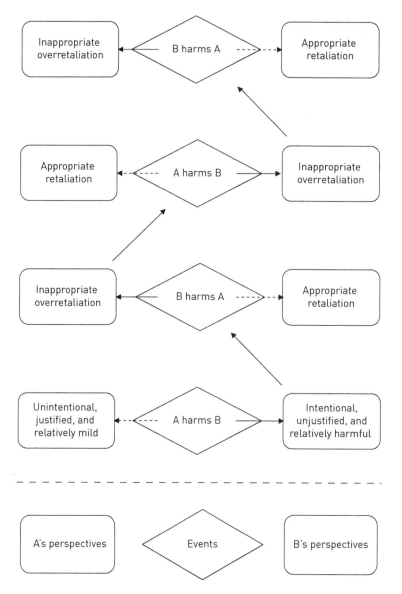

FIGURE 5.2
Violence escalation cycle.

as "kill," "attack," or "gun" but will likely not activate unrelated concepts such as "banana." When people are exposed to images of violence, violence-related concepts are subsequently activated, and this effectively primes the mind to utilize such concepts.

This theory has received empirical support from numerous psychological studies. A direct way to test it is to examine the accessibility of aggressive thoughts following violent video game play. One popular method is to offer an opportunity to complete fragmented words that produce aggression-related or aggression-unrelated words. For example, the word fragment "ki_ _" can be completed to produce the word "kill" or "kind," and individuals with greater accessibility to aggressive thoughts are more likely to complete this fragment to produce the word "kill." Several studies have demonstrated this increased accessibility following violent video game play (e.g., Carnagey and Anderson, 2005; Barlett and Rodeheffer, 2009).

In another study, participants were asked to play one of three versions of the same game. The games were identical except that one had a violent content. In one version, players shot at enemy soldiers; in another, they watered flowers; and in the final version, they clicked shapes. Following game play, participants completed an association task. The results showed that participants who had played the violent version were more likely to associate aggression-related terms with their self-concept (Bluemke et al., 2010). Other studies have measured aggressive thought accessibility using dramatically different methods but produced similar results. These include increases in amount of violent content provided in a story completion task (Anderson et al., 2003), increased speed of aggressive word recognition (Bösche, 2010), increases in rating aggressive and ambiguous word pairs as similar (Bushman and Anderson, 2002), and even increases in negative attitudes toward Arab and Muslim populations after playing a game that included terrorist themes (Saleem and Anderson, 2013).

As mentioned, these effects are thought to invoke fundamental learning processes. Therefore, the same processes that account for the harmful effects of violent games should be at play when playing video games increases positive behaviors. For example, playing video games with prosocial content seems to reduce the accessibility of aggressive thoughts (Greitemeyer and Osswald, 2009) and studies have demonstrated that playing prosocial video games increases prosocial behavior (Gentile et al., 2009; Prot et al., 2014).

The cognitive processes described above are at least partially responsible for the behavioral outcomes that have been observed (Anderson and Dill, 2000; Carnagey and Anderson, 2005; Barlett and Anderson, 2013). Indeed, a recent longitudinal study found that the aggression-enhancing effect of violent video game play was wholly mediated by changes in aggressive thinking patterns (Gentile et al., 2014). Findings such as these indicate that the positive and negative effects of video game play are two sides of the same coin (i.e., that aggressive and helping behaviors resulting from related content exposure seem to be mediated by the same underlying learning processes).

Script Theory

Related to the concept of knowledge structure development and priming, "script theory" (Huesmann, 1988) states that individuals organize much information in a way that helps guide behavior within specific social contexts, much as a theatrical script guides actors' behaviors. When in a restaurant, for example, individuals are fully aware of the socially appropriate behaviors associated with the place. Patrons enter the establishment and wait to be seated, they order drinks and then food, eat, pay, leave a tip, and leave. Script theory elucidates the ways in which seemingly disconnected knowledge structures (e.g., those related to aggressive thoughts) are organized to guide behavior.

For example, violent media often portray violent actions in ways that consistently reward aggression. Normal real-world negative consequences in such television shows and movies are underrepresented. According to such scripts, action movie heroes rarely experience, first hand, the collateral damage associated with their actions. In video games, this is extended further by rewarding players with points, in-game currency, or virtual items for killing enemies. Such portrayals make aggressive actions appear more rewarding and less damaging than in reality. A parallel that one can draw is with aggressive fantasizing, which often involves rehearsing mental imagery in which violent actions are rewarded. Indeed, television violence has been associated with aggressive fantasizing in males (Viemerö and Paajanen, 1992). In addition, individuals who imagine themselves acting as the violent characters they view are more likely to exhibit aggressive behavior (Leyens and Picus, 1973; Konijn et al., 2007). Other research indicates that for those exposed to high levels of violence, aggressive fantasizing is associated with increases in aggressive behavior (Smith et al., 2009). In line with this research, people exposed to high levels of media violence are more likely to interpret ambiguous situations in a hostile manner (Anderson et al., 2007; Möller and Krahé, 2009). For example, individuals exposed to media with a highly violent content were more likely to believe that a person in a fictional scenario who bumped someone while taking a drink was doing so intentionally (Möller and Krahé, 2009). In this case, individuals are, in a sense, filling out the missing details of a situation by utilizing the aggressive scripts developed as a result of violent media use.

Excitation Transfer

Violent media are naturally exciting (Zillmann, 1971; Anderson et al., 2004)—this is one reason why many of us enjoy such content in the first place. Unsurprisingly, increases in the severity of media violence are associated with increases in arousal. For example, research has found that seeing blood in video games is associated with increases in heart rate (Barlett et al., 2008). Similarly, auditory cues such as screaming victims also produce arousal, as measured by increases in the galvanic skin response (Jeong et al., 2012). Furthermore, more visually realistic games also produce increases in arousal, as measured by blood pressure, body temperature, and skin conductance (Ivory and Kalyanaraman, 2007; Barlett and Rodeheffer, 2009).

Individuals who become aroused do not experience an immediate return to baseline when the arousing stimulus is removed. Instead, such arousal is carried into future situations and can affect subsequent behavior. When individuals encounter a provoking situation following an arousing event, their residual arousal may be attributed to the provoking situation instead of the previously arousing event. This effectively enhances aggressive reactions in a process known as "excitation transfer" (Zillman, 1971, 1972). Therefore, when individuals consume violent media, whether passively (as in television and movies) or actively (as in video games), they may become more aggressive in situations that occur immediately afterward, because the arousal produced by such media may be transferred to these situations. For this reason, the best studies of media violence and aggressive behavior control for arousal either by including equally arousing violent and nonviolent games or by assessing and statistically controlling for arousal (e.g., Anderson et al., 2004).

Desensitization to Violence

When individuals are repeatedly exposed to an aversive stimulus, they may habituate to that stimulus; that is, they fail to be influenced to the same degree as they were on first presentation. This habituation process occurs when individuals are repeatedly exposed to violent imagery and affects emotional reactions and empathy for the victims (Funk et al., 2004). The typical anxiety-related responses to violent imagery are important in inhibiting aggression. However, when the normally aversive reactions that individuals have to images or thoughts of violence are diminished, inhibitory effects are no longer present, aggressive thoughts and behaviors increase (Bartholow et al., 2005, 2006; Engelhardt et al., 2011; Krahé et al., 2011), and helping behavior decreases (Bushman and Anderson, 2009).

Critically, this desensitization effect may lead individuals to perceive real-life violence as more acceptable following violent media use (Mullin and Linz, 1995). In other words, the desensitization toward violence is not limited to other forms of fictional violence. In a study by Carnagey et al. (2007), individuals randomly assigned to play a violent video game were less physiologically aroused by subsequent viewing of real-life violence than nonviolent game control players. Other studies found that viewing sexually violent films led individuals to experience less empathy for the victims of such violence and attribute more blame to them (Mullin and Linz, 1995; Dexter et al., 1997). Furthermore, it was reported that high exposure to media violence produced brain activity normally associated with the processing of emotional information and preparation for aggressive behavior (Kronenberger et al., 2005; Mathews et al., 2005; Weber et al., 2006; Hummer et al., 2010; Strenziok et al., 2010; Bailey et al., 2011).

The desensitization process has been found both in brief, short-term contexts, as well as in studies of long-term effects. For example, habitual violent video game players demonstrated reduced brain activity normally associated with exposure to aversive stimuli and violent imagery (Bartholow et al., 2006). Similarly, long-term violent media use has been positively associated with favorable attitudes toward violence and negatively associated with empathy with victims (e.g., Funk et al., 2004; Anderson et al., 2010; Prot et al., 2014). Both effects can be seen as resulting from the reduced emotional and physiologic responses to violence.

Aggressive Beliefs and Attitudes

Media violence may also influence propensities toward aggression through changes in the way individuals perceive behaviors of others and interpret social information (Crick and Dodge, 1994; Dodge, 2011). For example, a major determinant of whether one is to respond aggressively is his or her interpretation of ambiguous behaviors and stimuli. Thus, individuals who tend to interpret an ambiguous situation (e.g., a bump in the hallway) in hostile terms (e.g., believing that a bump in the hallway was intentional) are more likely to respond aggressively (Orobio de Castro et al., 2002). This tendency, known as the hostile attribution bias, is greater among frequent violent media users (Möller and Krahé, 2009) and has been demonstrated in the short-term experiments (Kirsh, 1998; Bushman and Anderson, 2002) as well as longitudinal studies (Anderson et al., 2007; Möller and Krahé, 2009). The longitudinal studies have found that violent media use increased hostile attribution biases which, in turn, increased aggression.

Media violence can also influence other beliefs that individuals have about people and the world around them, including beliefs about appropriate ways of reacting to others (Funk et al., 2004; Bushman and Huesmann, 2006). For example, in a longitudinal study by Möller and Krahé (2009), participants read a brief vignette in which a confrontation was described between them and another same-sex peer. Participants were provided with a list of possible reactions to this scenario and rated how appropriate each response was. Individuals who engaged with violent video games at baseline were more likely to endorse more aggressive responses subsequently, and this in turn predicted increases in aggression. This finding suggests that violent video games can produce changes in individuals' beliefs about what constitutes normal reactions to confrontation (i.e., that aggressive responses are appropriate and normal).

Attention Effects

Recent research has suggested that screen media exposure might also increase violence through its effects on attention, executive control, and impulsivity. For example, in one longitudinal study, the amount of exposure to television at ages 1 and 3 years predicted attention problems at age 7 years (Christakis et al., 2004). Indeed, research linking hours of watching television by young children to later attention disorders led the American Academy of Pediatrics to recommend that children younger than 3 years of age not view any screen media at all.

In recent years, some reports have claimed that playing fast-paced violent games can improve attention (e.g., Green and Bavelier, 2006). But what the research actually shows is that playing such games, which requires players to quickly notice and respond to visual changes throughout the screen, is associated with better visuospatial skills. That is, players of violent games practice attending and responding to rapid changes on a computer screen and become better at such visuospatial tasks. Indeed, several experimental studies suggest that as few as 10 hours of training in such games can significantly improve visuospatial skills (Subrahmanyam and Greenfield, 1994; Green and Bavelier, 2006; Achtman et al., 2008; Basak et al., 2008; Boot et al., 2008; Green et al., 2010), although some studies have failed to replicate this finding.

There is a distinction to be made between attention paid to visual stimuli that are inherently attracting attention and attention necessary to perform basic cognitive tasks. The latter is impaired in individuals with attention deficit hyperactivity disorder (ADHD), impulsivity, or executive control problems. It is possible, but remains to be proven, that the attentional sensitivity to peripheral stimuli that violent games seem to improve may be distracting and interfere with successful maintenance of focused attention on stimuli or thought processes that are not inherently attention-grabbing. For example, video game players are often required to attend to multiple peripheral stimuli, and the fidgeting child nearby may automatically draw their attention and distract them from a reading task. Indeed, several studies have reported a correlation between video game play and attention problems (e.g., Mistry et al., 2007; Bioulac et al., 2008; Gentile, 2009; Bailey et al., 2010, 2011), with some longitudinal studies providing stronger causal evidence (Swing et al., 2010; Gentile et al., 2012).

Of critical relevance to this chapter, the amount of screen media exposure—especially exposure to violent media (television and video games)—is associated with high levels of impulsive aggression through its effects on attention (Swing and Anderson, 2014). Importantly, this effect was found even after statistically controlling for increases in aggression as a result of screen media's effects on aggressive cognition and affect (Swing and Anderson, 2014. In other words, the effects of screen media on attention and the subsequent effects on aggression seem unique and independent of the other processes described above (Swing and Anderson, 2014).

DEBATE ON VIOLENT MEDIA EFFECTS

Despite the wealth of evidence in support of an effect of violent media on aggression-related outcomes, such evidence often goes underreported in news media (Bushman and Anderson, 2001). Consequently, many in the public believe that the "jury is still out" on the influence of violent media. Furthermore, a small group of researchers have been claiming that there is no effect of violent media on aggression-related outcomes (Ferguson et al., 2008; Ferguson and Kilburn, 2009, 2010; Ferguson and Savage, 2012; Ferguson, 2013; Ferguson and Dyck, 2012; Elson and Ferguson, 2014). Most of the concerns cited by these critics are methodologic in nature, and this chapter will highlight some of the more prominent criticisms mentioned in the literature and how they have been addressed.

Demand Characteristics

One criticism is that violent media research induces participants to respond desirably to please researchers. Thus, research participants presumably understand the purpose of a given study and behave aggressively following violent video game play (or violent television viewing) to provide support to the researchers' hypotheses (Ferguson and Dyck, 2012; Ferguson, 2013). Although this criticism has potential to invalidate findings, it is common practice to assess participants' understanding of the research and exclude individuals who are aware of the study hypothesis from data analyses (e.g., Bartholow and Anderson, 2002; Anderson et al., 2004; Konijn et al., 2007; Anderson and Carnagey, 2009; Gentile et al., 2009). Furthermore, there is good reason to believe that even if they know the study hypothesis, participants may be more likely to change their behavior to disprove the hypothesis, given that aggression is a socially undesirable behavior. Indeed, empirical research dedicated to addressing this possibility seems to confirm this notion, as demonstrated by a study in which aggressive behavior in video game players was reduced when the measure of aggression was too transparent (Bender et al., 2013). In other words, these individuals seemed motivated to disconfirm—not prove—the hypotheses of the researchers.

Frustration and Arousal

Another criticism is that variables such as frustration and arousal confound effects of the violent media. According to Ferguson and Savage (2012), "Studies where experimental subjects are exposed to violence, and control subjects are exposed to something calm or boring, may report statistically significant differences between groups due to the differences in excitement or arousal elicited by the material rather than the violent content itself" (p. 131). This criticism can apply only to the short-term effects of violent media. As already noted, several longitudinal studies demonstrate a long-term effect of violent media on aggressive tendencies. Direct tests also demonstrate that the effect of violent content occurs independently of frustration. For example, in one study (Williams, 2009), individuals were randomly assigned to play one of several games in which frustration and violent content were manipulated. Although frustration was found to increase aggression, so too was violent content, and thus frustration cannot solely account for aggression-related outcomes seen in other research. In still other studies, arousal is one of the most commonly controlled variables, either statistically, or through the pilot testing of video games in which equally arousing games are selected and compared (e.g., Anderson et al., 2004; Arriaga et al., 2008; Anderson and Carnagey, 2009). Indeed, starting with Anderson and Dill (2000), many experimental studies of violent video game effects have controlled for a host of potential confounds (e.g., frustration, difficulty, enjoyment, competitiveness) and still found the hypothesized effects (e.g., Arriaga et al., 2008, Barlett et al., 2008; Anderson and Carnagey, 2009; Williams, 2009).

Attraction Hypothesis

It has also been suggested that effects of exposure to violent media may be "better explained as a byproduct of 'third' variables, such as exposure to family violence and innate violence motivation" (Ferguson et al., 2008, p. 2). In other words, violent media do not increase aggression; instead, aggressive children and adults are attracted to violent media. This "attraction hypothesis" has received considerable empirical attention, but two main types of research have refuted it. First, experimental studies in which participants are randomly assigned to play a violent or a nonviolent video game control for individual differences in levels of aggressiveness. As shown in several such studies, violent game play causes significant increases in aggressive behavior, aggressive cognition, aggressive affect, and desensitization/lack of empathy (Anderson et al., 2010). Second, longitudinal studies have controlled for initial levels of aggressiveness in order to rule out attraction effects (e.g., Ostrov et al., 2006; Anderson et al., 2007, 2008b; Möller and Krahé, 2009; Gentile et al., 2011, 2014), yet their results are consistent with the hypothesis that exposure to violent media is a risk factor for aggression.

Measures of Aggression Are Invalid and Not Standardized

This criticism is targeted primarily (but not solely) at the use of the TCRTT as a measure of aggressive behavior. The measure has been described above, in the section on aggression and violent media. According to Ferguson (2013), measures such as the TCRTT "do *not* measure aggression, but vaguely approximate it in some way" and "children (and adults) wishing to be aggressive do not chase after their targets with . . . headphones with which to administer bursts of white noise" (p. 6). However, measures similar to the TCRTT have been found to demonstrate high levels of validity and to be closely associated with relevant variables, including alcohol consumption, self-reported physical aggression, and even the genetic markers linked with aggression (Giancola and Parrott, 2008).

Measures such as the TCRTT have also been criticized on the grounds that aggression can be coded in multiple ways (e.g., through the number of high blasts, consideration of intensity or duration indices only, or an average intensity and duration). Such variability and lack of standardization may allow researchers to choose the coding method that suits their particular hypothesis (Ferguson, 2013). This criticism suggests that studies using the TCRTT should produce larger effect sizes than those that do not use it; contrary to this, the largest meta-analysis (Anderson et al., 2010) found that use of the TCRTT actually produced slightly smaller effect sizes. Also, in many studies multiple coding methods derived from the TCRTT have been used, and all had a tendency to show the same effects.

Discrepant Findings

There are hundreds of empirical studies dedicated to testing the effect of violent video game play on aggression (Anderson et al., 2010). Although, as a whole, this literature reveals largely consistent effects, there are studies in which no differences in downstream effects are found between violent and nonviolent games. Some find such contrasting findings as evidence that the issue is still not settled as to whether violent video game play affects aggression. It is important, however, to note that these contrary findings are largely derived from a very small number of studies (e.g., Ferguson et al., 2008). A recent meta-analysis (Greitemeyer and Mügge, 2014) compared the effect sizes observed in studies published by major proponents of violent video game effects on aggression (Anderson and Bushman) with effect sizes reported in studies by the opponents of these effects (Ferguson) and effect sizes from all other relevant studies. It was found that the Anderson and Bushman studies produced average effect sizes of 0.19, whereas the Ferguson studies produced average effect sizes of 0.02. Critically, the effect sizes produced by the Anderson and Bushman studies were comparable to those of the studies by other "neutral" researchers (0.20).

There are many possible reasons why smaller effects are observed in some studies. For example, studies in all fields produce varying effect sizes simply based on the usual random variation in samples. Another reason involves variations in methods and measures. One particularly serious possibility in the video game domain is that some researchers may fail to identify and exclude inappropriate study participants and may use methods (e.g., transparent aggression measures) that produce null effects. As previously noted, there is also a related issue that some video game players may be strongly motivated to disconfirm (not prove) the hypothesis that violent video game play increases aggression (Bender et al., 2013).

CONCLUSION

The ways in which media, particularly violent media, influence viewers (and now players) is an old question, with a literature nearly as old as television. The theoretical accounts of how and why aggressive outcomes arise following violent media consumption are relatively solid; they are built on decades of research. Nevertheless, criticisms are frequently leveled at this literature, demanding evidence criteria beyond what is expected in other areas of psychological study. Those criticisms have been addressed, often with sound research (e.g., Bushman & Anderson, 2010; Bushman, Rothstein, and Anderson, 2010; Huesmann, 2010; Sacks et al., 2011). Although disagreement in research can fuel scientific progress, undue critical discourse has the potential to undermine the public's ability to understand the effects of violent media. Of course, dissent should not be stifled, and the only way forward is to conduct more research to further refine understanding of the issues at hand and help foster more informed consumer choices.

DISCLOSURE STATEMENT

The authors disclose no relationships with commercial entities and professional activities that may bias their views.

REFERENCES

Achtman RL, Green, CS, Bavelier D (2008). Video games as a tool to train visual skills. Restorative Neurology and Neuroscience 26: 435–446.
American Academy of Pediatrics (2009). Policy statement—media violence. Pediatrics 124: 1495–1503.
American Psychological Association (2005). APA calls for reduction of violence in interactive media used by children and adolescents. Available at http://www.apa.org/news/press/releases/2005/08/video-violence.aspx Retrieved June 20, 2013.

Anderson CA, Buckley KE, Carnagey NL (2008a). Creating your own hostile environment: a laboratory examination of trait aggression and the violence escalation cycle. Personality and Social Psychology Bulletin 34: 462–473.

Anderson CA, Bushman BJ (2002). Human aggression. Annual Review of Psychology 53: 27–51.

Anderson CA, Carnagey NL (2009). Causal effects of violent sports video games on aggression: is it competitiveness or violent content? Journal of Experimental Social Psychology 45: 731–739.

Anderson CA, Carnagey NL (2014). The role of theory in the study of media violence: the General Aggression Model. In Gentile DA, Editor. Media Violence and Children. Second Edition. Praeger, Westport, CT.

Anderson CA, Carnagey NL, Eubanks J (2003). Exposure to violent media: the effects of songs with violent lyrics on aggressive thoughts and feelings. Journal of Personality and Social Psychology 84: 960–971.

Anderson CA, Carnagey NL, Flanagan M, Benjamin AJ, Eubanks J, Valentine JC (2004). Violent video games: specific effects of violent content on aggressive thoughts and behavior. Advances in Experimental Social Psychology 36: 199–249.

Anderson CA, Dill KE (2000). Video games and aggressive thoughts, feelings, and behavior in the laboratory and in life. Journal of Personality and Social Psychology 78: 772–790.

Anderson CA, Gentile DA, Buckley K (2007). Violent Video Game Effects on Children and Adolescents. Oxford University Press, Oxford, UK.

Anderson CA, Sakamoto A, Gentile DA, et al (2008b). Longitudinal effects of violent video games on aggression in Japan and the United States. Pediatrics 122: e1067–e1072.

Anderson CA, Shibuya A, Ihori N, et al (2010). Violent video game effects on aggression, empathy, and prosocial behavior in Eastern and Western countries: a meta-analytic review. Psychological Bulletin 136: 151–173.

Arriaga P, Esteves F, Carneiro P, Monteiro MB (2008). Are the effects of unreal violent video games pronounced when playing with a virtual reality system? Aggressive Behavior 34: 521–538.

Bailey K, West R, Anderson CA (2010). A negative association between video game experience and proactive cognitive control. Psychophysiology 47: 34–42.

Bailey K, West R, Anderson CA (2011). The influence of video games on social, cognitive, and affective information processing. In Decety J, Cacioppo J, Editors. Handbook of Social Neuroscience. Oxford University Press, New York, NY, pp. 1001–1011.

Bandura A (1965). Influence of models' reinforcement contingencies on the acquisition of imitative responses. Journal of Personality and Social Psychology 1(6): 589–595.

Barlett CP, Anderson CA (2013). Examining media effects: the General Aggression and General Learning Models. In Scharrer E, Editor. Media Effects/Media Psychology. Blackwell-Wiley, Hoboken, NJ, pp. 1e–20e.

Barlett CP, Anderson CA (2011). Re-appraising the situation and its impact on aggressive behavior. Personality and Social Psychology Bulletin 37: 1564–1573.

Barlett CP, Branch O, Rodeheffer C, Harris R (2009). How long do the short-term violent video game effects last? Aggressive Behavior 35: 225–236.

Barlett CP, Harris RJ, Bruey C (2008). The effect of the amount of blood in a violent video game on aggression, hostility, and arousal. Journal of Experimental Social Psychology 44: 539–546.

Barlett CP, Rodeheffer C (2009). Effects of realism on extended violent and nonviolent video game play on aggressive thoughts, feelings and physiological arousal. Aggressive Behavior 35: 213–224.

Bartholow BD, Anderson CA (2002). Effects of violent video games on aggressive behavior: potential sex differences. Journal of Experimental Social Psychology 38: 283–290.

Bartholow BD, Bushman BJ, Sestir MA (2006). Chronic violent video game exposure and desensitization: behavioral and event-related brain potential data. Journal of Experimental Social Psychology 42: 532–539.

Bartholow, B. D., Sestir, M. A., & Davis, E. B. (2005). Correlates and consequences of exposure to video game violence: Hostile personality, empathy, and aggressive behavior. Personality and Social Psychology Bulletin 31(11): 1573–1586.

Basak C, Boot WR, Voss MW, Kramer AF (2008). Can training in a real-time strategy video game attenuate cognitive decline in older adults? Psychology and Aging 23: 765.

Bender J, Rothmund T, Gollwitzer M (2013). Biased estimation of violent video game effects on aggression: contributing factors and boundary conditions. Societies 3: 383–398.

Berkowitz L (1990). On the formation and regulation of anger and aggression: a cognitive neoassociationistic analysis. American Psychologist 45: 494–503.

Berkowitz L (1993). Pain and aggression: some findings and implications. Motivation and Emotion 17: 277–293.

Bioulac S, Arfi L, Bouvard MP (2008). Attention deficit/hyperactivity disorder and video games: a comparative study of hyperactive and control children. European Psychiatry 23: 134–141.

Bluemke M, Friedrich M, Zumbach J (2010). The influence of violent and nonviolent computer games on implicit measures of aggressiveness. Aggressive Behavior 36: 1–13.

Boot WR, Kramer AF, Simons DJ, Fabiani M, Gratton G (2008). The effects of video game playing on attention, memory, and executive control. Acta Psychologica 129: 387–398.

Bösche W (2010). Violent video games prime both aggressive and positive cognitions. Journal of Media Psychology 22: 139–246.

Boxer P, Huesmann LR, Bushman BJ, O'Brien M, Moceri D (2009). The role of violent media preference in cumulative developmental risk for violence and general aggression. Journal of Youth and Adolescence 38: 417–428.

Bushman BJ, Anderson CA (2009). Comfortably numb: desensitizing effects of violent media on helping others. Psychological Science 20: 273–277.

Bushman BJ, Anderson CA (2001). Media violence and the American public: scientific facts versus media misinformation. American Psychologist 56: 477–489.

Bushman BJ, Anderson CA (2010). Much ado about something: violent video game effects and a school of red herring. Reply to Ferguson and Kilburn. Psychological Bulletin 136: 182–187.

Bushman BJ, Anderson CA (2002). Violent video games and hostile expectations: a test of the general aggression model. Personality and Social Psychology Bulletin 28: 1679–1686.

Bushman BJ, Huesmann LR (2006). Short-term and long-term effects of violent media on aggression in children and adults. Archives of Pediatrics & Adolescent Medicine 160: 348–352.

Bushman B J, Gibson B (2011). Violent video games cause an increase in aggression long after the game has been turned off. Social Psychological and Personality Science, 2(1): 29–32.

Bushman BJ, Rothstein HR, Anderson CA (2010). Much ado about something: Violent video game effects and a school of red herring: Reply to Ferguson and Kilburn. Psychological Bulletin 136: 182–187.

Carnagey NL, Anderson CA (2005). The effects of reward and punishment in violent video games on aggressive affect, cognition, and behavior. Psychological Science 16: 882–889.

Carnagey NL, Anderson CA, Bushman BJ (2007). The effect of video game violence on physiological desensitization to real life violence. Journal of Experimental Social Psychology 43: 489–496.

Christakis DA, Zimmerman FJ, DiGiuseppe DL, McCarty CA (2004). Early television exposure and subsequent attentional problems in children. Pediatrics 113: 708–713.

Collins AM, Loftus EF (1975). A spreading activation theory of semantic processing. Psychological Review 82: 407–428.

Crick NR, Dodge KA (1994). A review and reformulation of social information-processing mechanisms in children's social adjustment. Psychological Bulletin 115: 74–101.

DeLisi M, Vaughn MG, Gentile DA, Anderson CA, Shook J (2013). Violent video games, delinquency, and youth violence: new evidence. Youth Violence and Juvenile Justice 11: 132–142.

Dexter HR, Penrod SD, Linz D, Saunders D (1997). Attributing responsibility to female victims after exposure to sexually violent films. Journal of Applied Social Psychology 27: 2149.

Dodge AK (2011). Social information processing patterns as mediators of the interaction between genetic factors and life experiences in the development of aggressive behavior. In Shaver P, Editor. Human Aggression and Violence: Causes, Manifestations, and Consequences. American Psychological Association, Washington, DC, pp. 165–185.

Elson M, Ferguson CJ (2014). Twenty-five years of research on violence in digital games and aggression: empirical evidence, perspectives, and debate gone astray. European Psychologist 19: 33–46.

Engelhardt CR, Bartholow BD, Kerr GT, Bushman BJ (2011). This is your brain on violent video games: neural desensitization to violence predicts increased aggression following violent video game exposure. Journal of Experimental Social Psychology 47: 1033–1036.

Engelhardt CR, Bartholow BD, Saults SJ (2011). Violent and nonviolent video games differentially affect physical aggression for individuals high vs. low in dispositional anger. Aggressive Behavior 37: 539–546.

Ferguson CJ (2013). Adolescents, Crime, and the Media: A Critical Analysis. Springer Science + Business Media, New York, NY.

Ferguson CJ, Dyck D (2012). Paradigm change in aggression research: the time has come to retire the General Aggression Model. Aggression and Violent Behavior 17: 220–228.

Ferguson CJ, Kilburn J (2009). The public health risks of media violence: a meta-analytic review. Journal of Pediatrics 154: 759–763.

Ferguson CJ, Kilburn J (2010). Much ado about nothing: the misestimation and over-interpretation of violent video game effects in Eastern and Western nations: comment on Anderson et al. (2010). Psychological Bulletin 136: 174–178.

Ferguson CJ, Rueda SM, Cruz AM, Ferguson DE, Fritz S, Smith SM (2008). Violent video games and aggression: causal relationship or byproduct of family violence and intrinsic violence motivation? Criminal Justice and Behavior 35: 311–332.

Ferguson CJ, Savage J (2012). Have recent studies addressed methodological issues raised by five decades of television violence research? A critical review. Aggression and Violent Behavior 17: 129–139.

Funk JB, Baldacci HB, Pasold T, Baumgardner J (2004). Violence exposure in real-life, video games, television, movies, and the internet: is there desensitization? Journal of Adolescence 27: 23–39.

Gentile DA (2009). Pathological video game use among youth 8 to 18: a national study. Psychological Science 20: 594–602.

Gentile DA (2008). The rating systems for media products. In Calvert S, Wilson B, Editors. The Handbook of Children, Media and Development. Blackwell Publishing, Hoboken, NJ, pp. 527–551.

Gentile DA, Anderson CA, Yukawa N, et al (2009). The effects of prosocial video games on prosocial behaviors: international evidence from correlational, longitudinal, and experimental studies. Personality and Social Psychology Bulletin 35: 752–763.

Gentile, D. A., & Bushman, B. J. (2012). Reassessing media violence effects using a risk and resilience approach to understanding aggression. Psychology of Popular Media Culture 1(3): 138.

Gentile DA, Coyne SM, Walsh DA (2011). Media violence, physical aggression and relational aggression in school age children: a short-term longitudinal study. Aggressive Behavior 37: 193–206.

Gentile DG, Li D, Khoo A, Prot S, Anderson CA (2014). Mediators and moderators of long-term violent video game effects on aggressive behavior: practice, thinking, and action. Journal of the American Medical Association Pediatrics 168: 450–457.

Gentile DG, Swing EL, Lim CG, Khoo A (2012). Video game playing, attention problems, and impulsiveness: evidence of bidirectional causality. Psychology of Popular Media Culture 1: 62–70.

Giancola, P. R., & Parrott, D. J. (2008). Further evidence for the validity of the Taylor aggression paradigm. Aggressive behavior 34(2): 214--229.

Gilbert F, Daffern M (2011). Illuminating the relationship between personality disorder and violence: contributions of the General Aggression Model. Psychology of Violence 1: 230–244.

Green CS, Bavelier D (2006). Effect of action video games on the spatial distribution of visuospatial attention. Journal of Experimental Psychology: Human Perception and Performance 32: 1465.

Green CS, Li R, Bavelier D (2010). Perceptual learning during action video game playing. Topics in Cognitive Science 2: 202–216.

Greitemeyer T, Mügge DO (2014). Video games do affect social outcomes: a meta-analytic review of the effects of violent and prosocial video game play. Personality and Social Psychology Bulletin 40: 578–589.

Greitemeyer T, Osswald S (2009). Prosocial video games reduce aggressive cognitions. Journal of Experimental Social Psychology 45: 896–900.

Huesmann RL (1988). An information processing model for the development of aggression. Aggressive Behavior 14: 13–24.

Huesmann RL. (2010). Nailing the coffin shut on doubts that violent video games stimulate aggression: Comment on Anderson et al. (2010). Psychological Bulletin 136(2): 179–181.

Huesmann RL, Moise-Titus J, Podolski C, Eron LD (2003). Longitudinal relations between children's exposure to TV violence and their aggressive and violent behavior in young adulthood: 1977-1992. Developmental Psychology 39: 201–221.

Hummer TA, Wang Y, Kronenberger WG, et al (2010). Short-term violent video game play by adolescents alters prefrontal activity during cognitive inhibition. Media Psychology 13: 136–154.

International Society for Research on Aggression (2012). Report of the media violence commission. Aggressive Behavior 38: 335–341.

Ivory JD, Kalyanaraman S (2007). The effects of technological advancement and violent content in video games on players' feelings of presence, involvement, physiological arousal, and aggression. Journal of Communication 57: 532–555.

Jeong EJ, Biocca FA, Bohil CJ (2012). Sensory realism and mediated aggression in video games. Computers in Human Behavior 28: 1840–1848.

Kirsh SJ (1998). Seeing the world through "Mortal Kombat" colored glasses: violent video games and the development of a short-term hostile attribution bias. Childhood 5: 177–184.

Konijn EA, Bijvank NM, Bushman BJ (2007). I wish I were a warrior: the role of wishful identification in effects of violent video games on aggression in adolescent boys. Developmental Psychology 43: 1038–1044.

Krahé B, Möller I, Huesmann LR, Kirwil L, Felber J, Berger A (2011). Desensitization to media violence: links with habitual media violence exposure, aggressive cognitions, and aggressive behavior. Journal of Personality and Social Psychology 100: 630–646.

Krcmar M, Farrar K (2009). Retaliatory aggression and the effects of point of view and blood in violent video games. Mass Communication and Society 12: 115–138.

Kronenberger WG, Mathews VP, Dunn DW, et al (2005). Media violence exposure and executive functioning in aggressive and control adolescents. Journal of Clinical Psychology 61: 725–737.

Leyens JP, Picus S (1973). Identification with the winner of a fight and name mediation: their differential effects upon subsequent aggressive behavior. British Journal of Social and Clinical Psychology 12: 374–377.

Linder JR, Gentile DA (2009). Is the television rating system valid? Indirect, verbal, and physical aggression in programs viewed. Journal of Applied Developmental Psychology 30: 286–297.

Mathews VP, Kronenberger WG, Wang Y, Lurito JT, Lowe MJ, Dunn DW (2005). Media violence exposure and frontal lobe activation measured by functional magnetic resonance imaging in aggressive and nonaggressive adolescents. Journal of Computer Assisted Tomography 29: 287–292.

Mistry KB, Minkovitz CS, Strobino DM, Borzekowski DL (2007). Children's television exposure and behavioral and social outcomes at 5.5 years: does timing of exposure matter? Pediatrics 120: 762–769.

Möller I, Krahé B (2009). Exposure to violent video games and aggression in German adolescents: a longitudinal analysis. Aggressive Behavior 35: 75–89.

Mullin CR, Linz D (1995). Desensitization and resensitization to violence against women: effects of exposure to sexually violent films on judgments of domestic violence victims. Journal of Personality and Social Psychology 69: 449–459.

Orobio de Castro B, Veerman JW, Koops W, Bosch JD, Monshouwer HJ (2002). Hostile attribution of intent and aggressive behavior: a meta-analysis. Child Development 73: 916–934.

Ostrov JM, Gentile DA, Crick NR (2006). Media exposure, aggression and prosocial behavior during early childhood: a longitudinal study. Social Development 15: 612–627.

Paik H, Comstock G (1994). The effects of television violence on antisocial behavior: A meta-analysis. Communication Research 21(4): 516–546.

Parke RD, Berkowitz L, Leyens JP, West SG, Sebastian RJ (1977). Some effects of violent and nonviolent movies on the behavior of juvenile delinquents. In Berkowitz L, Editor. Advances in Experimental Social Psychology, vol. 10. Academic Press, New York, NY, pp. 135–172.

Prot S, Gentile DG, Anderson CA, et al (2014). Long-term relations between prosocial media use, empathy and prosocial behavior. Psychological Science 25: 358–368.

Rideout VJ, Foehr UG, Roberts DF (2010). Generation M2: Media in the Lives of 8-18 Year Olds. Henry J Kaiser Foundation, Menlo Park, CA.

Sacks DP, Bushman BJ, Anderson CA (2011). Do violent video games harm children? Comparing the scientific amicus curiae "experts" in Brown V. Entertainment Merchants Association. Northwestern University Law Review Colloquy 106: 1–12.

Saleem M, Anderson CA (2013). Arabs as terrorists: effects of stereotypes within violent contexts on attitudes, perceptions and affect. Psychology of Violence 3: 84–99.

Silvern SB, Williamson PA (1987). The effects of video game play on young children's aggression, fantasy, and prosocial behavior. Journal of Applied Developmental Psychology 8: 453–462.

Smith CE, Fischer KW, Watson MW (2009). Toward a refined view of aggressive fantasy as a risk factor for aggression: interaction effects involving cognitive and situational variables. Aggressive Behavior 35: 313–323.

Society for the Psychological Study of Social Issues, Anderson CA, Bushman BJ, Donnerstein E, Hummer TA, Warburton W (2014). SPSSI research summary on media violence. Available at http://www.spssi.org/index.cfm?fuseaction=page.viewP age&pageID=1899&nodeID=1 Retrieved on April 4, 2014.

Strenziok M, Krueger F, Pulaski SJ, et al (2010). Lower lateral orbitofrontal cortex density associated with more frequent exposure to television and movie violence in male adolescents. Journal of Adolescent Health 46: 607–609.

Subrahmanyam K, Greenfield, PM (1994). Effect of video game practice on spatial skills in girls and boys. Journal of Applied Developmental Psychology 15: 13–32.

Swing EL, Anderson CA (2014). The role of attention problems and impulsiveness in media violence effects on aggression. Aggressive Behavior 40: 197–203.

Swing E, Gentile DA, Anderson CA, Walsh DA (2010). Television and video game exposure and the development of attention problems. Pediatrics 126: 214–221.

Thompson KM Haninger K (2001). Violence in E-rated video games. Journal of the American Medical Association 286: 591–598.

Thompson KM, Tepichin K Haninger K (2006). Content and ratings of mature-rated video games. Archives of Pediatric and Adolescent Medicine 160: 402–410.

Viemerö V, Paajanen S (1992). The role of fantasies and dreams in the TV viewing-aggression relationship. Aggressive Behavior 18: 109–116.

Wartella E, Reeves B (1985). Historical trends in research on children and the media: 1900-1960. Journal of Communication 35: 118–133.

Weber R, Ritterfeld U, Mathiak K (2006). Does playing violent video games induce aggression? Empirical evidence of a functional magnetic resonance imaging study. Media Psychology 8: 39–60.

Williams KD (2009). The effects of frustration, violence, and trait hostility after playing a video game. Communication and Society 12: 291–310.

Worth KA, Chambers JG, Nassau DH, Rakhra BK, Sargent JD (2008). Exposure of US adolescents to extremely violent movies. Pediatrics 122: 306–312.

Yokota F, Thompson KM (2000). Violence in G-rated animated feature films. Journal of the American Medical Association 283: 2716–2720.

Zillmann D (1971). Excitation transfer in communication-mediated aggressive behavior. Journal of Experimental Social Psychology 7: 419–434.

6 Cyberchondria

An Old Phenomenon in a New Guise?

Vladan Starcevic and David Berle

INTRODUCTION

Searching for health information online has become very common. One survey suggests that more than 75% of participants in nine countries (Russia, China, India, Mexico, Brazil, United States, Italy, Australia, and Germany) use the Internet for health-related queries (McDaid and Park, 2010). Close to 90% of adult Internet users in the United States reported looking for health information on the Internet at least once (Harris Poll, 2010). The ever-increasing number of visits to health websites (e.g., Howell, 2013) indicates that the Internet may have become the most popular, if not the most important source, of health-related information.

These trends are not surprising. The Internet costs little; online information is easy to access and quick to obtain; there are no bureaucratic hurdles, referral letters, and waiting lists; and the anonymity allows a person to make any kind of inquiry without feeling embarrassed. Such a shift from relying for health information on physicians, medical textbooks, encyclopedias, or popular health journals to using a medium as simple and ubiquitous as the Internet is likely to have a variety of consequences, both positive and negative. This chapter will focus on the latter.

The way any information obtained online is utilized depends both on how it is presented and how the Internet user responds to it. When it comes to users of online health-related information, there are large differences between them. Thus, some people handle with relative ease Internet-derived medical information, even when it is abundant and conflicting, whereas others have difficulty with it. Individuals who become alarmed when engaging in online health-related searches, yet keep on continuing with this activity, are often referred to as "cyberchondriacs" and represent the subject of this chapter.

THE CONCEPT OF CYBERCHONDRIA

The term "cyberchondria" has a brief but fascinating history (Starcevic and Berle, 2013). Not unlike other pathologies that have been attributed to the Internet (e.g., "Internet addiction"), it was introduced and promoted by the popular media, and researchers and health care professionals became interested in it only later. The term is deceptively simple, especially when one looks at its etymology. Thus, one meaning of cyberchondria is that it is the modern "version" of hypochondriasis (Koehler, 2005) and that, like its terminological predecessor, it is a mental disorder (Valley, 2001). On the other side of the spectrum of its meanings, cyberchondria has sometimes been interpreted as merely seeking health-related information on the Internet (Taylor, 2002). Neither of these extreme views has been accepted by "mainstream" mental health professionals, but they seem popular with the media. From time to time, such meanings of cyberchondria are directly or indirectly espoused, causing much terminological confusion.

Over the years, a number of more balanced definitions of cyberchondria have been proposed, as shown in Table 6.1. The common ingredients of these definitions are health anxiety and online searches for health-related information. Definitions differ in terms of how they portray the cause of cyberchondria or the sequence of occurrence of its components. Some suggest that people with cyberchondria are affected by primary, excessive health anxiety and that it motivates them to repeatedly seek relevant information online, which, however, only exacerbates their anxiety (Belling, 2006; White and Horvitz, 2009a; Recupero, 2010; Starcevic and Berle, 2013; McElroy and Shevlin, 2014). Other definitions imply that excessive

Table 6.1 Definitions of Cyberchondria

Source and Reference	Definition
Belling, 2006 (p. 385)	"Health anxiety exacerbated by exposure to Internet-based information"
Harding et al., 2008 (p. 315)	"Excessive health anxiety generated from online health searches"
White and Horvitz, 2009a (p. 1)	"Unfounded escalation of concerns about common symptomatology, based on the review of search results and literature on the Web"
Recupero, 2010 (p. 26)	"Escalation of health-related fears by consumers who use the Internet to research health and medical information"
Fergus, 2013 (p. 735)	"Searching for medical information on the Internet" [that] "is associated with an exacerbation of health anxiety"
Starcevic and Berle, 2013 (p. 206)	"Excessive or repeated search for health-related information on the Internet, driven by distress or anxiety about health, which only amplifies such distress or anxiety"
Aiken and Kirwan, 2014 (p. 158)	"Anxiety resulting from health-related search online"
McElroy and Shevlin, 2014 (p. 259)	"Increase in anxiety about one's own health status, as a result of excessive reviews of online health information"

health-related searches on the Internet are the primary cause of heightened health anxiety (Harding et al., 2008; Aiken and Kirwan, 2014). In other words, people who had never been preoccupied with health or illness could develop high levels of health anxiety solely because of online health searches. The direction of causality and the primacy in the relationship between online health-related searches and heightened health anxiety have not been a subject of any study, although it appears more plausible for excessive health anxiety, even at subclinical levels, to be chronologically primary.

The other conceptual issue is about the essence of cyberchondria: is it synonymous with health anxiety or does it primarily refer to a behavior (online health searches) that increases health anxiety? Although most definitions mention both components, only two (Fergus, 2013; Starcevic and Berle, 2013) emphasize the centrality of the behavioral aspects of cyberchondria (i.e., excessive or repeated searches for health-related information online). This distinction may seem subtle, but cyberchondria conceptualized as a behavioral component of heightened health anxiety or hypochondriasis differs importantly from cyberchondria that is meant to denote a pathological emotional state (i.e., excessive health anxiety) and may lead to different suggestions for treatment interventions. Also, the latter conceptualization might imply that cyberchondria is a distinct psychiatric disorder—a premature and misleading proposition.

A recent study describing a development and initial validation of the Cyberchondria Severity Scale reported that cyberchondria was a multidimensional construct with the following five components: compulsion, distress, excessiveness, reassurance, and mistrust of medical professionals (McElroy and Shevlin, 2014). "Compulsion" refers to an unwanted aspect of performing online health searches, which interferes with functioning in multiple ways. "Distress" denotes negative emotional states and physiological reactions associated with online health searches, such as difficulty relaxing and sleeping, worrying, anxiety, distress, tendency to panic, irritability, and loss of appetite. "Excessiveness" pertains to the time-consuming and repetitive nature of online health searches, with one or multiple sources often being consulted. "Reassurance" refers to seeking reassurance from a medical professional. "Mistrust of medical professionals" suggests an inner conflict as to whether a person should trust his or her own physician or the results of the Internet searches.

This multidimensional conceptualization reflects a broad, syndrome-like approach to cyberchondria. It almost gives cyberchondria the status of a disorder, with the possibility of transforming its various components into diagnostic criteria. For example, interference with functioning is the usual diagnostic criterion for any mental disorder. The conceptualization of some of the dimensions seems controversial (e.g., the unwanted nature of performing health-related searches on the Internet because this activity is usually described as egosyntonic), whereas it appears redundant for other aspects of cyberchondria (e.g., inclusion of seeking reassurance from physicians in addition to online health searches constituting a reassurance-seeking behavior in their own right). Also, the "distress" component encompasses emotional features such as irritability and symptoms such as loss of appetite and sleep disturbance in addition to anxiety and worry. Regardless, this study demonstrates that there is an ongoing diversity of views on cyberchondria, calling for further research.

"Cyberchondria by proxy" is a related concept that has received very little empirical research. It refers to experiencing "anxiety when conducting health-related search for others" (Aiken and Kirwan, 2014, p. 158). There is an analogy with "hypochondria by proxy," although this term has been used much less often that hypochondriasis.

RELATIONSHIP BETWEEN CYBERCHONDRIA AND HEALTH ANXIETY

As already noted, it is usually assumed that there is a strong relationship between cyberchondria and health anxiety or hypochondriasis (which usually refers to a more severe form of health anxiety). After all, the term "cyberchondria" is directly derived from hypochondriasis. However, hypochondriasis has been used reluctantly by medical practitioners, mainly because of the pejorative connotations of the term and conceptual problems, which led to its elimination from the *Diagnostic and Statistical Manual of Mental Disorders,* fifth edition (American Psychiatric Association, 2013). In contrast, cyberchondria as a term seems to be surviving and continues to be used by researchers and clinicians, perhaps to facilitate communication.

The relationship between cyberchondria and health anxiety or hypochondriasis has not been a subject of much research, but this link has generally been supported (Eastin and Guinsler, 2006; Baumgartner and Hartmann, 2011; Muse et al., 2012; Aiken and Kirwan, 2014; Singh and Brown, 2014). However, all these studies were conducted in nonclinical subjects, often university students, with sample sizes ranging from 20 to 250. Therefore, there remains a question about the representativeness of these populations and the extent to which the findings of studies apply to clinical populations. Furthermore, the paucity of research does not allow any conclusions to be made about the prevalence of cyberchondria and demographic factors associated with it (e.g., age, gender and educational level).

Studies in the United States, the Netherlands, and the United Kingdom have demonstrated that higher levels of health anxiety are associated with more Internet use to search for health-related information (Eastin and Guinsler, 2006; Baumgartner and Hartmann, 2011; Muse et al., 2012; Singh and Brown, 2014). This increased use of the Internet refers to a greater amount of time spent online looking for medical information (Muse et al., 2012; Singh and Brown, 2014), greater frequency of performing online health searches (Baumgartner and Hartmann, 2011), and a higher likelihood of searching for greater quantity (Eastin and Guinsler, 2006; Muse et al., 2012) and greater variety of medical information online (Muse et al., 2012). Comparisons of individuals with high and low levels of health anxiety showed that the former used message boards, online health support groups, and/or health forums more frequently and that they were more distressed and afraid and felt less reassured during online health searches or as a result of them

(Baumgartner and Hartmann, 2011; Muse et al., 2012). These findings suggest that people with prominent health anxiety, perhaps contrary to their expectations, do not tend to experience relief when they go online and do not feel reassured from medical information obtained on the Internet. Only one study reported a correlation between health anxiety and experience of relief after performing online health searches (Singh and Brown, 2014).

In some studies (Eastin and Guinsler, 2006; Singh and Brown, 2014), health anxiety was also associated with a greater likelihood of visiting a physician after performing online health searches. This underscores the inability of these searches to provide sufficient reassurance and is even more striking considering that individuals with high levels of health anxiety have a tendency to find interactions with medical practitioners unsatisfying or perceive physicians with mistrust (Guo et al., 2002; von Scheele et al., 2010; Singh and Brown, 2014).

It is important to note that these studies were cross-sectional and, as such, do not point to the direction of causality in the relationship between cyberchondria and health anxiety. As already mentioned, it is usually assumed that people are more likely to conduct multiple health searches on the Internet because of their preexisting high levels of health anxiety, but engaging in this activity may also cause or exacerbate health anxiety. In fact, it has been found that using the Internet for health purposes increases health anxiety in a large number of individuals (White and Horvitz, 2009b) and that it is associated with increased symptoms of depression (Bessière et al., 2010). The possibility that such use of the Internet may play some etiological role in health anxiety or even depression is intriguing and should be studied prospectively.

In one study, significant relationships were found between "Internet addiction," health anxiety, and cyberchondria (Ivanova, 2013). Another study has reported an association between health anxiety and certain characteristics of "addiction" to using the Internet for health purposes (Singh and Brown, 2014). Significant correlations were found between health anxiety and unsuccessful attempts to decrease health-related Internet use, feeling restless and irritable when not performing online searches, staying online longer than intended, increase in health-related Internet use over time, and various negative consequences of such use, including interference with multiple domains of functioning. These results led to a suggestion of possible "health-related Internet addiction" (Singh and Brown, 2014). This is an interesting proposition that calls for further research and a better understanding of cyberchondria, because it is difficult to see how an anxiety-producing or anxiety-amplifying behavior that does not seem to be enjoyable can be "addictive." Perhaps some individuals find cyberchondria pleasurable or rewarding (e.g., by "playing a doctor" or trying to resolve a diagnostic puzzle), thereby making it "addictive."

Finally, a significant positive correlation was found between anxiety resulting from online health searches for oneself and anxiety resulting from online health searches for others (Aiken and Kirwan, 2014). This implies that individuals with cyberchondria may be just as excessively concerned about the health of others (usually close family members and dependents), attempting to diagnose them online and/or taking additional measures as a consequence of such concerns.

Cyberchondria has not been a subject of much theorizing and research. This is to some extent a consequence of the lack of consensus about the very concept of cyberchondria, as noted above.

One recently proposed model of cyberchondria postulates that it is essentially a form of reassurance-seeking behavior that occurs on the Internet in response to an increased anxiety or distress and a failure of reassurance following initial online health searches (Starcevic and Berle, 2013). This is to be distinguished from online health searches that occur after reassuring and therefore reinforcing effects of initial such searches. The model is partly supported by the finding of a nonclinical study that there were different effects of seeking health information on the Internet; although about 50% of people engaged in online health searches reported less health anxiety after the searches, 40% experienced more health anxiety (White and Horvitz, 2009b). The reasons for these different effects are insufficiently understood, but it can be hypothesized that factors such as higher levels of "baseline" health anxiety might have served as a predisposition to experience more anxiety after online health searches.

This model of cyberchondria (Starcevic and Berle, 2013) also proposes several factors that may reinforce and maintain cyberchondria. These include a difficulty distinguishing between real risk and an artificial, technologically created one, with the consequent anxiety-amplifying conclusions about the unlikely probabilities; effects of the wealth of online information and a need for the "perfect" explanation; intolerance of ambiguity and uncertainty, especially during online health searches; and the questionable trustworthiness of the sources of online information. There is some support for the role of each of these factors.

White and Horvitz (2009a) demonstrated that nonclinical participants in their study had a tendency to erroneously believe that the higher ranking of search results meant a greater probability that the higher-ranking illness (e.g., a brain tumor) explained a particular symptom (e.g., a headache) that had initiated an online query. A failure to distinguish between the ranking of search results and the probability of such results explaining the initial query is more likely to escalate health anxiety than to reassure and more likely to lead to further online searches.

Perfectionist tendencies and a need for thorough explanation often characterize individuals with high levels of health anxiety or hypochondriasis (Starcevic, 1990; Starcevic et al., 1992; Sakai et al., 2010). This may fuel cyberchondria in such individuals because of the wealth of health information on the Internet and an expectation that the Internet may be the right medium to provide them with that "perfect" explanation for their health-related query.

The outcome of performing online health-related searches is often unpredictable, because the Internet is not "designed" to always provide relevant, accurate, nonconflicting, and reassuring information. Thus, information obtained online can either decrease uncertainty (Wilson et al., 2002) or increase it (Harding et al., 2008). This may depend on the way the information is presented but also on the personality characteristics of Internet users. If the effect of online health searches is a predominant increase in uncertainty, it can reinforce cyberchondria through ongoing attempts to arrive at "closure"; this may occur especially in individuals with high levels of health anxiety who have trouble tolerating uncertainty (Deacon and Abramowitz, 2008; Boelen and Carleton, 2012). Individuals with prominent difficulty tolerating uncertainty were found to be at an increased risk for anxiety disorders when exposed to online medical information (Norr et al., 2014), and they were especially likely to develop cyberchondria (Fergus, 2013). As it appears that intolerance of uncertainty is an important factor here, it should be investigated whether and to what extent its high levels also contribute to the maintenance of cyberchondria.

Findings regarding the effects of the perceived trustworthiness and reliability of the health websites on the levels of health anxiety have been conflicting. Two studies suggested that such an effect did not exist (Muse et al., 2012; Singh and Brown, 2014), whereas two other studies reported that health anxiety might be more likely to occur in response to the information obtained from the more credible online sources (Eastin and Guinsler, 2006; Baumgartner and Hartmann, 2011). If the relationship between the perceived trustworthiness and levels of health anxiety is confirmed by further research, this may support the notion that the time-consuming struggle by people with health anxiety to distinguish between trustworthy and untrustworthy health websites reinforces cyberchondria.

PREVENTIVE EFFORTS

Efforts to prevent cyberchondria or minimize its effects involve its most specific component—the fact that it is an Internet-based behavior. Consequently, the target of prevention is the interaction between humans and the Internet that might lead to anxiety-amplifying online health searches. This endeavor can succeed only with a productive collaboration between information technology professionals, search engine architects, website designers, health care providers, psychologists, researchers, public health specialists, administrators, and others.

There are a number of technical measures that may aid in preventive efforts. One such measure is the ranking of online health search results based on true probability of the link between particular symptoms and diagnoses (e.g., White and Horvitz, 2009a). The other is the construction of evidence-based diagnostic algorithms that take into account a variety of information (e.g., age, gender, smoking status, and consumption of alcohol) provided by Internet users in addition to the nature of symptoms. These algorithms have already been embedded in a number of online "symptom checkers," some of which are considered reliable and have been recommended (e.g., Loos, 2013). The purpose of these symptom checkers is not self-diagnosis but provision of a range of possible diagnoses that may be considered and discussed when visiting physicians and other health care providers.

Other approaches to preventing cyberchondria have also been proposed. They include provision of unambiguous, precise, evidence-based, and user-friendly health information on the Internet (White and Horvitz, 2009a). Also, online "health information literacy" can be improved by promoting exposure of Internet users to credible online health information resources (Ghaddar et al., 2012) and by educating them to critically appraise results of online health searches and Internet-derived health information (Berezovska et al., 2010). A categorization of health websites based on their quality is quite difficult, but it might minimize concerns about their trustworthiness. These concerns have been found to be particularly common among older adults (Miller and Bell, 2012). Addressing them adequately might not only help these people learn to distinguish between high-quality and low-quality health websites as well as decrease the likelihood of developing cyberchondria. Chapter 8 illustrates difficulties in "regulating" health-related material on the Internet even when it comes to something with self-evident negative consequences such as suicidality. Chapter 9 discusses efforts to categorize mental health websites on the basis of their quality

MANAGEMENT APPROACHES

Treatment of cyberchondria should be based on its clear and widely accepted definition and conceptualization. In the absence of that, little can be said about its management. Although no treatment has been specifically developed for cyberchondria, it is reasonable to suggest that cyberchondria should not be treated in isolation and without taking into account the context in which it appears. This context is usually that of health anxiety or hypochondriasis and, therefore, it seems that cyberchondria would best be addressed as part of a comprehensive treatment approach to those conditions. Such an approach entails psychoeducation about health anxiety, hypochondriasis, and cyberchondria, and a thorough case formulation that would identify specific precipitants of cyberchondria, reasons for this behavior, its consequences, and factors that maintain it.

Cyberchondria may be precipitated by the appearance of a new symptom or an illness in a close family member. Curiosity about an apparent scientific breakthrough in the understanding or management of a life-threatening illness or curiosity about a "new disease" discussed in mass media may also trigger cyberchondria. Of particular importance may be the precipitants that undermine the credibility of the medical profession and medical practice. These include media reports about new studies that contradict what previous research had shown or question established medical doctrine, as well as discoveries of the dangerous side effects of commonly prescribed medications, unreliable results of standard medical tests, or previously unknown risks of routine medical procedures. It is plausible that different precipitants are linked with different internal dynamics of cyberchondria; this means that a good understanding of the precipitants might help therapists focus on and address the specific aspects of cyberchondria.

The main purpose of cyberchondria is to alleviate health-related anxiety or distress, but as a safety behavior, it usually results in more anxiety or distress (e.g., Olatunji et al., 2011). This discrepancy between the purpose of cyberchondria and its consequences may seem puzzling to patients and calls for a formulation-based understanding and explanation.

The best empirically supported treatment for health anxiety and hypochondriasis is cognitive-behavioral therapy (e.g., Bouman, 2014), which targets factors considered to maintain the disorder. These include safety behaviors such as reassurance seeking and avoidance, various maladaptive assumptions and beliefs about symptoms, health and disease, misinterpretations, and selective attention to health-related and illness-related internal and external stimuli. The technique of exposure and response prevention has been most useful for addressing the behavioral aspects of health anxiety and hypochondriasis (such as reassurance seeking), whereas cognitive interventions have been effective in modifying specific health-related cognitions, misinterpretations of bodily sensations, and overestimation of risk and danger. Attentional training has been used to target selective attention.

Some of these therapeutic approaches could also be used in the management of cyberchondria. The general goals of management would be refraining from excessive and unnecessary seeking of medical information on the Internet and being able to perform online health searches without becoming overly anxious. In the course of a modified exposure and response prevention task, patients could be gradually exposed to increasingly more anxiety-provoking health information from reliable websites in order for them to habituate to this information. Following such exposure, patients would be asked to limit their online health searches by time and encouraged to only consult trustworthy and authoritative sites. They would also be instructed to make every effort not to check or seek reassurance elsewhere and not to engage in other safety behaviors as a substitute for excessive online health searches. Once patients believe that they have a degree of control over their urges to perform online health searches and feel more confident when they interact with online health material, they could be encouraged to do broader searches if necessary. The rationale for this is to convey to patients that they need to discover for themselves that online health information is not inherently threatening and they have acquired tools to manage it.

Other factors considered to reinforce cyberchondria would also need to be targeted. For example, through a series of exercises, patients would be encouraged to accept and tolerate a reasonable degree of uncertainty and abandon a futile quest for perfect explanations. This means that absolute clarity about online health information would not be pursued, as such a pursuit might lead to another cycle of cyberchondria. The issue of trust would also need to be addressed, both as it pertains to a distinction between trustworthy and untrustworthy websites and trustworthiness of information obtained online versus that received from a physician. This issue may be particularly important in cases that were precipitated by a sudden undermining of the credibility of medical professionals.

CONCLUSION

Like many other concepts that have appeared in the digital age, there is no consensus about the definition and meaning of cyberchondria. Still, its link with health anxiety is indisputable, as is the related behavior—excessive and/or repeated looking for health-related information on the Internet. Further research, especially in clinical subjects, is needed to understand whether there is something unique about seeking reassurance for health concerns on the Internet. If there is, and if such behavioral pattern is specifically associated with a set of external validating variables, perhaps cyberchondria could be considered a distinct form of psychopathology. In the absence of such evidence, cyberchondria is appropriately regarded as a behavioral manifestation of health anxiety and hypochondriasis.

Much can be done to decrease the risk of developing cyberchondria. "Technical" measures may help present online health information in a way that would increase clarity and decrease discrepancies and confusion. This would entail developing new, evidence-based algorithms linking symptoms (which are the usual point of entry for online health-related searches) and diseases, so that other relevant factors are also taken into consideration. It would be very helpful to develop a system of categorizing health websites on the basis of the quality of information they provide. Another task is to improve online health information literacy, which would enable Internet users to critically appraise this information, without escalating their health-related concerns and feeling overwhelmed.

Management of people with cyberchondria should follow its conceptual framework. At present, features of cyberchondria may be most effectively addressed by using case formulation and applying the techniques that have been successfully used in the treatment of health anxiety and hypochondriasis. This involves understanding the precipitants, purpose and consequences of cyberchondria in each particular patient and targeting factors that may maintain this behavior. In addition, any coexisting psychopathology would need to be addressed, as well as personality traits and factors such as mistrust and intolerance of uncertainty. Such an approach needs to be developed in further detail, which would then allow efficacy testing. This is an important task, considering that reliance on online sources of health information is likely to increase in the future, which may also increase the risk of cyberchondria.

DISCLOSURE STATEMENT

The authors disclose no relationships with commercial entities and professional activities that may bias their views.

REFERENCES

Aiken M, Kirwan G (2014). The psychology of cyberchondria and "cyberchondria by proxy." In Power A, Kirwan G, Editors. Cyberpsychology and New Media: A Thematic Reader. Psychology Press, East Sussex, UK, pp. 158–169.
American Psychiatric Association (2013). Diagnostic and Statistical Manual of Mental Disorders. Fifth Edition. American Psychiatric Association, Washington, DC.
Baumgartner SE, Hartmann T (2011). The role of health anxiety in online health information search. Cyberpsychology, Behavior, and Social Networking 14: 613–618.

Belling C (2006). Hypochondriac hermeneutics: medicine and the anxiety of interpretation. Literature and Medicine 25: 376–401.

Berezovska I, Buchinger K, Matsyuk O (2010). Evolving facets of cyberchondria: primum non nocere "first, do no harm." In Kalogiannakis M, Stavrou D, Mchaelidis P, Editors, Proceedings of the Seventh International Conference on Hands-on Science (HSci2010). The University of Crete, Rethymno, Greece, pp. 125–130.

Bessière K, Pressman S, Kiesler S, Kraut R (2010). Effects of Internet use on health and depression: a longitudinal study. Journal of Medical Internet Research 12: e6.

Boelen PA, Carleton RN (2012). Intolerance of uncertainty, hypochondriacal concerns, obsessive-compulsive symptoms, and worry. Journal of Nervous and Mental Disease 200: 208–213.

Bouman TK (2014). Cognitive and behavioral models and cognitive-behavioral and related therapies for health anxiety and hypochondriasis. In Starcevic V, Noyes, R, Editors. Hypochondriasis and Health Anxiety: A Guide for Clinicians. Oxford University Press, New York, NY, pp. 149–198.

Deacon B, Abramowitz JS (2008). Is hypochondriasis related to obsessive-compulsive disorder, panic disorder, or both? An empirical evaluation. Journal of Cognitive Psychotherapy 22: 115–127.

Eastin MS, Guinsler NM (2006). Worried and wired: effects of health anxiety on information-seeking and health care utilization behaviors. Cyberpsychology and Behavior 9: 494–498.

Fergus TA (2013). Cyberchondria and intolerance of uncertainty: examining when individuals experience health anxiety in response to Internet searches for medical information. Cyberpsychology, Behavior, and Social Networking 16: 735–739.

Ghaddar SF, Valerio MA, Garcia CM, Hansen L (2012). Adolescent health literacy: the importance of credible sources for online health information. Journal of School Health 82: 28–36.

Guo Y, Kuroki T, Yamashiro S, Koizumi S (2002). Illness behaviour and patient satisfaction as correlates of self-referral in Japan. Family Practice 19: 326–332.

Harding KJ, Skritskaya N, Doherty E, Fallon BA (2008). Advances in understanding illness anxiety. Current Psychiatry Reports 10: 311–317.

Harris Poll (2010). "Cyberchondriacs" on the rise? Those who go online for healthcare information continues to increase. Available at http://www.harrisinteractive.com/vault/HI-Harris-Poll-Cyberchondriacs-2010-08-04.pdf Retrieved on April 14, 2014.

Howell D (2013). Why WebMD tops stock gains with Aruba, Shutterstock. Available at http://news.investors.com/technology/022213-645435-webmd-health-aruba-shutterstock-top-stock-market-today.htm Retrieved on May 19, 2014.

Ivanova E (2013). Internet addiction and cyberchondria—their relationship with well-being. Journal of Education Culture and Society 1: 57–70.

Koehler S (2005). A look into cyberchondria: using the Internet to diagnose your health symptoms. Available at http://www.voices.yahoo.com/a-look-into-cyberchondria-using-internet-diagnose-2747.html Retrieved on May 17, 2014.

Loos A (2013). Cyberchondria: too much information for the health anxious patient? Journal of Consumer Health on the Internet 17: 439–445.

McDaid D, Park A-L (2010). Online health: untangling the web. Available at http://www.bupa.com.au/staticfiles/Bupa/HealthAndWellness/MediaFiles/PDF/LSE_Report_Online_Health.pdf Retrieved on March 6, 2014.

McElroy E, Shevlin M (2014). The development and initial validation of the Cyberchondria Severity Scale (CSS). Journal of Anxiety Disorders 28: 259–265.

Miller LMS, Bell RA (2012). Online health information seeking: the influence of age, information trustworthiness, and search challenges. Journal of Aging and Health 24: 525–541.

Muse K, McManus F, Leung C, Meghreblian B, Williams JMG (2012). Cyberchondriasis: fact or fiction? A preliminary examination of the relationship between health anxiety and searching for health information on the Internet. Journal of Anxiety Disorders 26: 189–196.

Norr AM, Capron DW, Schmidt NB (2014). Medical information seeking: impact on risk for anxiety psychopathology. Journal of Behavior Therapy and Experimental Psychiatry 45: 402–407.

Olatunji BO, Etzel EN, Tomarken AJ, Ciesielski BG, Deacon B (2011). The effects of safety behaviors on health anxiety: an experimental investigation. Behaviour Research and Therapy 49: 719–728.

Recupero PR (2010). The mental state examination in the age of the Internet. Journal of the American Academy of Psychiatry and the Law 38: 15–26.

Sakai R, Nestoriuc Y, Nolido NV, Barsky AJ (2010). The prevalence of personality disorders in hypochondriasis. Journal of Clinical Psychiatry 71: 41–47.

Singh K, Brown RJ (2014). Health-related Internet habits and health anxiety in university students. Anxiety, Stress, & Coping 27: 542–554.

Starcevic V (1990). Relationship between hypochondriasis and obsessive-compulsive personality disorder: close relatives separated by nosological schemes? American Journal of Psychotherapy 44: 340–347.

Starcevic V, Berle D (2013). Cyberchhondria: towards a better understanding of excessive health-related Internet use. Expert Review of Neurotherapeutics 13: 205–213.

Starcevic V, Kellner R, Uhlenhuth EH, Pathak D (1992). Panic disorder and hypochondriacal fears and beliefs. Journal of Affective Disorders 24: 73–85.

Taylor H (2002). Cyberchondriacs update. Available at http://www.harrisinteractive.com/vault/Harris-Interactive-Poll-Research-Cyberchondriacs-Update-2002-05.pdf Retrieved on May 22, 2014.

Valley P (2001). New disorder, cyberchondria, sweeps the Internet. Available at http://www.nzherald.co.nz/technology/news/article.cfm?c_id=5&objectid=185422 Retrieved on April 27, 2014.

von Scheele C, Nordgren L, Kempi V, Hetta J, Hallborg A (2010). A study of so-called hypochondriasis. Psychotherapy and Psychosomatics 54: 50–56.

White RW, Horvitz E (2009a). Cyberchondria: studies of the escalation of medical concerns in Web search. ACM Transactions on Information Systems 27(4), Article 23: 1–37.

White RW, Horvitz E (2009b). Experiences with Web search on medical concerns and self diagnosis. In Proceedings from the American Medical Informatics Association Annual Symposium 2009 (AMIA 2009). Curran Associates, Red Hook, NY, pp. 696–700.

Wilson T, Ford N, Ellis D, Foster A, Spink A (2002). Information seeking and medical searching. Part 2: uncertainty and its correlates. Journal of the American Society for Information Science and Technology 53: 704–715.

7 Cyberbullying
A Mental Health Perspective

Matthew W. Savage, Sarah E. Jones, and Robert S. Tokunaga

INTRODUCTION

Reports of cyberbullying have grown as technology has increasingly saturated all sectors of life. Of adolescents online, nearly one in three have experienced some form of cybervictimization (Lenhart, 2010)—enough for cyberbullying to be deemed a public health risk (David-Ferdon and Hertz, 2007) that requires attention (Li, 2007a, 2007b). The large proportion of adolescent cyberbullying victims may relate to the growing use of social networking sites in that age group; approximately 95% of American adolescents aged 12 to 17 years are regular Internet users, and 80% of them also subscribe to social networking sites (Lenhart et al., 2011). The Centers for Disease Control and Prevention (2014) recently cautioned the general public about the cyberbullying risk inherent to the use by adolescents of these new technologies. Emerging research (e.g., Walker et al., 2011), however, shows that individuals well beyond their adolescent years are also vulnerable. This chapter will review the state of knowledge of cyberbullying with a focus on its primary characteristics, including comparisons to traditional bullying, prevalence rates, and what is known about its demographic features. It will then discuss mental health considerations. Finally, it will review prevention strategies and suggest areas for future research.

DEFINITION

The term "electronic aggression" was recently put forward by the Centers for Disease Control and Prevention to refer to all types of technologically mediated hostile acts, including Internet harassment and bullying. As defined by the Centers for Disease Control and Prevention (2014), electronic aggression is "any type of harassment or bullying that occurs via e-mail, a chat room, instant messaging, a website (including blogs), or text messaging" (p. 1). In scholarly research articles, such behavior has also been variably designated "cyber harassment" (Beran and Li, 2005, 2007), "cyber victimization" (Dempsey et al., 2009), "online harassment" (Wolak et al., 2007), "Internet harassment" (Ybarra et al., 2006), "Internet bullying" (Williams and Guerra, 2007), "online aggression" (Ybarra, 2004; Ybarra and Mitchell, 2004), and "cyber stalking" (Spitzberg and Hoobler, 2002). These terms, however, have not caught on in the popular press, whereas the designation "cyberbullying" has been much more widely adopted.

Patchin and Hinduja (2006) were the first to offer a concise definition, describing cyberbullying as "willful and repeated harm inflicted through the medium of electronic text" (p. 152). Although this conceptual definition provided a good starting point, it did not address some of important characteristics of cyberbullying. Consequently, other definitions have been proposed. For example, Tokunaga (2010) presented an integrative definition of cyberbullying, describing it as "any behavior performed through electronic or digital media by individuals or groups that repeatedly communicates hostile or aggressive messages intended to inflict harm or discomfort on others" (p. 278). This definition incorporates several salient characteristics of cyberbullying: electronic or digital technology (e.g., communication across one or more digital media); harm or discomfort (e.g., messages that insult, attack, embarrass, exclude, spread rumors about, or harm the relationships of the cybervictim); and action by an individual working alone or a group working collectively.

TRADITIONAL BULLYING VERSUS CYBERBULLYING

Descriptions of cyberbullying tend to adhere closely to established characteristics of traditional bullying: aggressive acts made with harmful intent; repetition; and, increasingly, a focus on the imbalance of power between perpetrator and victim (Olweus, 1993; Smith and Brain, 2000). With regard to intent, Olweus (2003) has suggested that traditional bullying occurs when a person or group engages in any negative action intended to inflict injury, hurt, or discomfort. Researchers largely agree that such intent is a primary requisite for an act to be considered bullying (Stephenson and Smith, 1989). Traditional bullying and cyberbullying overlap in this core feature of intentional hurt. Cyberbullies wish to inflict harm on their targets and execute a series of calculated behaviors to do so. However, cyberbullying goes beyond traditional bullying in its enlistment of modern technology as a powerful tool. So, a cyberbully's intention to cause psychological distress is similar to that of the traditional bully, but it may be magnified through the combination of aggressive urges with sophisticated, modern electronic techniques (Olweus, 1993; Nansel et al., 2001).

Technology-aided bullying can be more severe and pervasive because of the cyberbully's anonymity and the ubiquitous nature of the Internet (Pratarelli et al., 1999; Patchin and Hinduja, 2006). It can also be more "creative" and can extend beyond traditional bullying to include impersonation or identity theft, hacking, rumor mongering, cyberstalking, online embarrassment, humiliation or teasing, and infected e-mails or software (Willard, 2007). Other manifestations include exhibition of unapproved photographs, videos, or other multimedia materials (Ybarra and Mitchell, 2004; von Marées and Petermann, 2012). Moreover, unlike traditional bullying, a attacks of cyberbullying are not limited to the school bus or the playground but can take place wherever the Internet or digital device goes—that is, anywhere (Patchin and Hinduja, 2006). Technology makes it so that nowhere, including the home, can feel entirely safe for the victim.

Also, with regard to the repetition component, traditional bullies must repeatedly hurt their victims for the behavior to be considered bullying. Cyberbullies often exhibit repeated acts of aggression, but it is also possible for them to repeatedly hurt their victim through a single action. For example, a cyberbully might post one embarrassing photograph of the victim on a social networking site. Although he or she has not repeatedly attacked the victim, the cyberbullying act can be replicated many times in the virtual world through endless forwarding and sharing by many people across e-mail accounts, texting platforms, or social networking sites, sometimes to the point of becoming an Internet "meme" (e.g., Roberts, 2014). In this way, it is easier for a single act of aggression to reverberate and echo in online contexts, essentially revictimizing the target every time the aggression is reproduced.

Finally, with respect to power, traditional bullies are considered more powerful due to physical strength, popularity, or intelligence (e.g., Felix et al., 2011), targeting victims who are perceived as less powerful in the physical world (Williams and Guerra, 2007). Early cyberbullying research did not focus on a power differential between perpetrators and victims, but some scholars (e.g., Wolak et al., 2007; Vandebosch and Van Cleemput, 2008) later asserted that the use of the term "bullying" could apply only if a power hierarchy existed between a strong perpetrator and a weak victim. However, in contrast to traditional bullying, power for cyberbullies can take on new attributes and draw on new sources. For example, strength can be derived from technological proficiency (Patchin and Hinduja, 2006), tipping the balance of power in favor of those who are more skilled in navigating the Internet and in using electronic devices. To that end, those who perceive themselves as disempowered offline may feel stronger online and may be empowered to take revenge in cyberspace. Anonymity also modifies the power dynamic in cyberbullying, further highlighting the divergence from traditional bullying. If victims do not know the identity of the perpetrator, they forfeit some power—the old adage "knowledge is power" seems to apply here as well. Thus, anonymity and electronic dexterity can both alter the balance of power in new ways in the cyberbullying experience.

Assessing similarities and differences between the two types of bullying helps provide a good definition of cyberbullying. As stated, many definitions have been proposed (Tokunaga, 2010), with a fair degree of overlap with regard to harmful intent and repetition. Power issues, however, were not considered an important feature in early cyberbullying research. This seems to be changing; increasingly, cyberbullying is reserved to describe technology-enabled behaviors that meet the three-part criteria of traditional bullying (i.e., intention, repetition, and power imbalance) (Wolak et al., 2007).

PREVALENCE

It is estimated that 39% of the world's population (2.7 billion people) are now online (International Telecommunication Union, 2013). As more people gain access to the Internet, there is an increased potential for cybervictimization (Belsey, 2005; Aricak et al., 2008). In addition to better access, the very nature of connectivity is changing due to mobile devices, which in turn is also changing the cyberbullying experience. Smartphones and tablets now offer mobile access to social networking sites. Those often nurture superficial "friending," which may result in shallow relationships that can be easily exploited (Srivastava, 2012). In the United States, approximately 56% of adults and 34% of teenagers own smartphones, and nearly 37% of adults and 23% of teenagers own tablets (Smith, 2013; Zickuhr, 2013). Also, high percentages of young adults continue to join social networking sites (Duggan and Brenner, 2013). Although the increased connectivity has allowed users to take advantage of the wondrous capabilities of modern technology, it has also positioned them to be dangerously vulnerable to cyberbullying attempts (Srivastava, 2012). This has helped elevate cyberbullying to a global concern, which may explain the recent rise in warnings by public service entities such as the Pew Research Center (Duggan and Brenner, 2013).

Studies of cyberbullying suggest that large proportions of adolescents report being cyberbullying perpetrators and victims. Perpetration rates reported in the cyberbullying literature range from 4% (Kowalski and Limber, 2007) to 35% (Hinduja and Patchin, 2008). However, most scholars note that self-reported perpetration measures are likely to underestimate rates of cyberbullying and suffer from social desirability bias. For that reason, victimization rates may be more accurate. Survey data indicate that 20% to 40% of youths have been victimized by a cyberbully (Li, 2006, 2007a, 2007b, 2008; Patchin and Hinduja, 2006; Aricak et al., 2008; Dehue et al., 2008; Hinduja and Patchin, 2008; Smith et al., 2008; Topcu et al., 2008; Ybarra and Mitchell, 2008). In Patchin and Hinduja's (2006) study, for example, 384 youths aged 9 to 18 years were surveyed. Among them, 29% had been victimized, 11% had been perpetrators, and more than 47% had been witnesses.

Of note, studies limit their questions about the cyberbullying experience to a time frame that differs among studies (Ybarra, 2004; Ybarra and Mitchell, 2004, 2008; Williams and Guerra, 2007; Wolak et al., 2007; Dehue et al., 2008). Common time frames used in cyberbullying prevalence studies include 1 month prior to the study (e.g., Dempsey et al., 2009); the year prior to the study (e.g., Wolak et al., 2007); the current semester or past 2 to 3 months (e.g., Wang et al., 2009); and "forever" (i.e., no time frame is specified) (e.g., Hinduja and Patchin, 2008). No research has examined whether or how the specified time frame may affect recall and the prevalence rate found in the study.

As will be discussed, the prevalence of cyberbullying among adults is unknown, but some insight can be gathered from research on cyberstalking.

AGE, GENDER, AND CYBERBULLYING

Most cyberbullying studies have focused on minors, and only a few published articles have examined cyberbullying in adults (e.g., Slonje and Smith, 2008; Walker et al., 2011). Yet, cyberbullying is not restricted to a particular age, group even if the term "bullying" generally evokes thoughts of young children and schoolyards. For instance, some scholars have argued that bullying may be a useful construct to describe some persistent hostile behavior in adults, such as workplace aggression or other forms of abuse (e.g., Tracy et al., 2006). Also, in the online world, "flaming" is a well-documented phenomenon that is comparable to cyberbullying. It refers to abusive or harsh language used against adults and children alike (Lea et al., 1992; Witmer, 1997).

Cyberstalking, which is often discussed within adult age groups, can also qualify as cyberbullying in some respects. Defined as the repeated pursuit of an individual using electronic or Internet-capable devices (Reyns et al., 2012), 26% of stalking victims' experiences in the United States included forms of cyberstalking (Baum et al., 2009). Numbers seem higher among young adults on college campuses, with 40.8% reporting that they were cyberstalked and nearly 5% reporting that they perpetrated cyberstalking (Reyns et al., 2012). Most recently, the National Cyber Security Alliance and McAfee released a report indicating that cyberstalking now affects 20% of American adults (National Cyber Security Alliance, 2013). Of note, cyberstalking studies have focused on investigating prevalence by investigating victim perspectives using self-report surveys. As a result, reports of perpetration prevalence are unknown.

However, within the samples studied in the cyberbullying scientific literature, the association between age and victimization is inconsistent. A majority of studies did not find a significant association (Ybarra, 2004; Patchin and Hinduja, 2006; Beran and Li, 2007; Wolak et al., 2007; Juvonen and Gross, 2008; Smith et al., 2008; Didden et al., 2009; Katzer et al., 2009; Varjas et al., 2009), but a minority did (Kowalski and Limber, 2007; Ybarra et al., 2007; Dehue et al., 2008; Hinduja and Patchin, 2008; Slonje and Smith, 2008; Ybarra and Mitchell, 2008). The age range and other characteristics of the samples studied may explain the conflicting findings. Studies with more restricted age ranges seem to reveal some trends: in Kowalski and Limber's (2007) study of 11- to 14-year-olds and a Ybarra et al.'s (2006, 2007) study of 10- to 15-year-olds, a positive association was found between age and victimization rate (as age increased, so did victimization prevalence). Other researchers, in contrast, uncovered a negative association in their wider age range sample of 12- to 20-year-olds (as age increased, victimization prevalence decreased) (Dehue et al., 2008; Slonje and Smith, 2008). Still, the majority of studies with wide age ranges did not yield statistically significant associations (e.g., Ybarra, 2004; Patchin and Hinduja, 2006; Wolak et al., 2007; Juvonen and Gross, 2008; Smith et al., 2008; Didden et al., 2009; Katzer et al., 2009).

In their study of 3339 American youths, Williams and Guerra (2007) found that 4.5% of fifth graders, 12.9% of eighth graders, and 9.9% of high school students reported having been victims of cyberbullying. This suggests a possible curvilinear relationship between age and victimization, where cyberbullying is low at younger ages, rises for some time, then falls as individuals become older. However, this suggestion does not answer the question of when cyberbullying may cease to be a significant problem. Therefore, research is needed to explore whether young adults such as college students remain common victims of cyberbullying; this can help inform decisions about where to target cyberbullying prevention resources (Savage and Deiss, 2010; Deiss et al., 2012).

Biological sex differences, or what some refer to as gender differences, have been reported by scholars. Studies report that girls are more likely to cyberbully than boys because of their preference for using indirect methods of aggression (Bowie, 2007; Willard, 2007). The Internet is a likely place for utilizing indirect aggressive methods due to anonymity. Findings indicate that girls are also victims more often than boys (Kowalski and Limber, 2007). However, some studies report inconsistent findings concerning sex differences in cyberbullying. For example, Williams and Guerra (2007) found no significant difference between boys' and girls' cyberbullying perpetration rates, and Li (2006) concluded that males were more likely to be cyberbullies than females. It is clear that future research in this area is warranted.

Although there has been some inquiry into age and sex as demographic factors that are important to consider with regard to cyberbullying, there has been little attention paid to race and socioeconomic status.

MENTAL HEALTH CONSIDERATIONS

Interest in the psychological underpinnings of cyberbullying was largely fueled by high-profile cases of adolescent suicide that were attributed by the media to cyber-bullying (Klomek et al., 2011). These cases underscored the need for research into psychological causes and consequences of cyberbullying and squarely identified cyberbullying as a serious health risk for children, adolescents, and young adults. Since then, empirical research has come to confirm the suspected link between cyberbullying and suicide. Hinduja and Patchin (2010) found that both cyberbul-lying perpetrators and victims had more suicide attempts and spent more time contemplating suicide than peer controls. This process has been explained on psy-chological grounds as an activation, by the cyberbullying experience in the victim or perpetrator, of a depressive state that can be accompanied by suicidal thoughts or, in more extreme cases, suicidal behavior (Schenk and Fremouw, 2012; Bauman et al., 2013).

Several studies have shown and association between victimization and negative mood states, including depressive symptoms (Ybarra, 2004; Didden et al., 2009; Erdur-Baker and Tanrikulu, 2010; Songtag et al., 2011), low self-esteem (Ybarra et al., 2006; Didden et al., 2009; Goebert et al., 2010; Patchin and Hinduja, 2010), social anxiety (Juvonen and Gross, 2008; Kowalski et al., 2008), and internalized anger (Patchin and Hinduja, 2006; Topcu et al., 2008; Carter, 2011).

Preliminary data suggest that children and youths who have been cyberbullied may develop psychiatric problems over time. In a German study of 223 middle and high school students, females with prior victimization developed clinical depression and aggression several months later (Sourander et al., 2010). Further, the duration of cyberbullying seemed to correlate with the intensity of psychological symptoms, so that prolonged victimization corresponded to the greatest degree of psychological impairment.

Currently, scholarship theorizes that being a victim of cyberbullying incidents may exacerbate already present depressive symptoms or cause new depressive symptoms in asymptomatic individuals. However, correlational designs of studies do not allow for causal arguments and so do not clarify the directionality of this association.

Victimization affects not only the state of mind but can also lead to specific behavioral responses and other adverse manifestations. For example, somatic complaints such as headaches, bodily pains, and sleeplessness, have been reported in greater proportions among victims than healthy controls (Krankenkasse, 2011). Insomnia has also been reported and may, in turn, be responsible for the higher levels of school truancy, distractibility, and declining academic performance among victims (Beran and Li, 2007; Li, 2007a, 2007b; Katzer et al., 2009). Other manifestations of victimization extend beyond school: victims were more likely than nonvictims to develop habits such as alcohol consumption and smoking (Mitchell et al., 2007). A common conclusion in the literature is that psychological problems and maladaptive behaviors accompany victimization.

Victims who retaliate against their aggressors also exhibit psychological problems. Due to the more fluid power dynamic, retaliation may be easier to achieve, perhaps facilitating a transition from victim to perpetrator (Songtag et al., 2011). Researchers explain how those who are victimized can become angry and seek selective exposure to antisocial media content, making it more likely for them to become cyberbullies against other targets as well, beyond the aggressor (den Hamer et al. [2014]). Referred to as "bully-victims," these individuals who are simultaneously an aggressor and a victim, are nearly six times more likely as those who are only cybervictims to experience emotional distress due to harassment online, and they also tend to have poorer relationships with their caregivers (Barnow et al., 2001; Ybarra and Mitchell, 2004; Schenk and Fremouw, 2012).

These behaviors may be explained by the moderate but reliable association between perpetration and victimization (e.g., Erdur-Baker and Tanrikulu, 2010; Werner et al., 2010). In other words, it may be that cyberbullies become targets of victimization, and that those victimized are compelled to aggress against others. Scholars hypothesize that cyberbullying incidents may both exacerbate already existing depressive symptoms or cause new depressive symptoms to emerge in asymptomatic individuals. However, correlational designs do not clarify the directionality of this association.

Perpetration of cyberbullying has also been linked to psychiatric conditions, including depression and anxiety, although exact rates are difficult to find (Perren et al., 2010). Compared to controls, cyberbullies experience increased levels of aggression and social anxiety, have more primitive social skills (Harman et al., 2005), and exhibit problematic behaviors such as alcohol abuse and smoking more intensely (Katzer et al., 2009; Sourander et al., 2010). A need to redirect negative feelings has been cited as a primary cyberbullying motivator (Varjas et al., 2010). For the cyberbully, a negative internal state can also give moral "permission" to engage in planned aggression (Calvete et al., 2010).

Wright and Li (2012) provide further explanation of how anger and frustration, from which individuals try to escape, may stem from their own previous victimization. In their study of 130 college students, they found that offline and online victimization at baseline predicted "cyber-displaced aggression," or aggression against others meant to alleviate negative affective states, 6 months later. These authors reason that victimization precipitates stress with which the victim must cope. For some, the failure to cope adaptively leads to future perpetration of aggression. Other longitudinal studies, however, did not find such an association with previous victimization, when the investigation controlled for the frequency of online communication and antisocial behavior (Sticca et al., 2013).

The implications of these findings in both victims and perpetrators can be alarming. However, it is important to note that except for a few, relatively small longitudinal studies, the large majority of studies are cross-sectional, which limits the ability to draw strong conclusions or establish causality between cyberbullying and psychological problems. Therefore, a number of scenarios remain possible: (1) cyberbullying predicts psychological problems; (2) existing psychological problems make youths vulnerable to cyberbullying; (3) there is reciprocity of the variables (both cyberbullying and psychological problems are occurring concurrently); and (4) there is a spurious relationship between cyberbullying and psychological problems, which might be explained by a third variable. All four explanations are tenable, prompting calls for large, sufficiently powered longitudinal studies (e.g., Smith et al., 2006; Tokunaga, 2010).

A few longitudinal studies have explored the psychological outcomes of cyberbullying less than its risk factors. As discussed above, victimization may be one risk factor for perpetration. Another risk factor is stress stemming from general life circumstances (Dumont and Provost, 1999; Wadsworth and Compas, 2002). According to the "buffering hypothesis" (Cohen and Wills, 1985), individuals who lack support face the greatest level of stress and are the most susceptible to cyberbullying perpetration. The buffering hypothesis postulates that life stressors can be attenuated or "buffered" against with help from a person's support system, including family and friends. Indeed, a longitudinal study of 1416 adolescents randomly selected from middle schools in Cyprus found that perceived support from the family at the initial data collection point was associated with fewer cyberbullying perpetrations 1 year later (Fanti et al., 2012). Thus, it is likely that for youths and adolescents, social support may prevent cyberbullying by reducing stress that might otherwise be channeled into outward aggression.

PREVENTION

Few scientifically based strategies exist to prevent cyberbullying perpetration or help cyberbullying victims. However, three interventions aimed at prevention have received recent attention: the *Social Networking Safety Promotion and Cyberbullying Prevention* program (Arizona Attorney General's Office, 2011), the *Cyber Bullying: A Prevention Curriculum* program (Limber et al., 2008), and the *Media Heroes* program (Wölfer et al., 2013).

The *Social Networking Safety Promotion and Cyberbullying Prevention* program and accompanying Internet safety guide were developed by former Arizona Attorney General Terry Goddard (Arizona Attorney General's Office, 2011). The presentation was delivered to middle and high school students in the Phoenix metropolitan area. The greater part of the presentation focused on social network safety promotion, and a smaller segment addressed strategies to prevent cyberbullying. At the end of the presentation, an Internet safety guide was distributed to students, with the goal of promoting discussions with their parents. A recent outcome evaluation of more than 300 sixth, seventh, and eighth graders found that the group that received the presentation outperformed the control group on reports of their intention to not retaliate and intention to tell a trusted adult if cyberbullied (Roberto et al., 2014). Behavioral intention is a commonly measured outcome in prevention studies; it is not a measure of behavior change but is strongly related to future behavior. In the study by Roberto et al. (2014), there was a positive effect on other prevention variables that the intervention targeted. For example, exposure to the intervention worked to increase perceptions of susceptibility and severity in sixth and eighth graders (i.e., the intervention made them feel like cyberbullying was something that they should be prepared to handle in the future).

Arizona's *Social Networking Safety Promotion and Cyberbullying Prevention* program follows the extended parallel process model (Witte, 1993). The materials seek to change students' attitudes, intentions, and behaviors by persuading them that serious threats exist and that performing certain actions can reduce those threats. This is an example of fear appeal of the extended parallel process model with both threat and efficacy components. In the context of cyberbullying prevention campaigns, the extended parallel process model is easy to apply due to its relative simplicity. It requires manipulating only two determinants of behavior change—perceived threat and perceived efficacy. However, it would seem easier to address perceived threat and efficacy when trying to prevent future victimization but not necessarily for preventing perpetration. For example, persuasive messages can attest that one is at risk of being victimized (susceptibility) and that there are harsh consequences (severity), which can be avoided through successful strategies (response efficacy) that can easily be learned (self-efficacy). But campaign messages suggesting that cyberbullying is an act many people have tried (susceptibility) with serious consequences (severity) but that can easily be stopped (self-efficacy) by thinking before clicking (response efficacy) are weaker in terms of targeting the threat component better than the efficacy one. That is true because these efforts may cause the unintended effect of suggesting that too many people cyberbully others and because it is difficult to be convincing about the ease and effectiveness of stopping oneself from being a cyberbully. More work is needed to determine how this model might be used to prevent cyberbullying perpetration.

Cyber Bullying: A Prevention Curriculum (Limber et al., 2008) includes lessons intended for students in grades 6 to 12 and can be implemented in a civic, community or educational environment. The program has three aims: (1) to raise students' and parents' awareness of cyberbullying, (2) to equip students with the skills and resources to treat each other respectfully when using technology, and (3) to students with the skills to use technology in positive ways. It has components for parents and teachers. Eight class sessions highlight peer education. For students in middle school, the first five sessions discuss journal entries from fictional students learning about cyberbullying in a peer-led small group setting. The journals teach students how to react to cyberbullying situations. At the high school level, the stories are based on actual news events with altered details. Sessions six and seven are the same for students at both levels, and they consist of students working in groups to create a safety plan for their own social network interactions. Parents are provided with a letter explaining the curriculum. Homework assignments involve students speaking to their parents about cyberbullying. Teachers are also provided with a lesson that can be used for self-education or as part of their professional development activities.

To our knowledge, no studies have formally tested the efficacy of this program, but the approach is based on the *Olweus Bullying Prevention Program* developed for traditional bullying (Olweus, 1991). Outcome studies of the latter program have yielded good long-term success rates in Norwegian and other European samples and some short-term success in the United States (Olweus and Limber, 2010). The *Olweus Bullying Prevention Program* is based on the ecological model of behavior change, which focuses on the need to implement interventions at several levels of influence (e.g., the individual, classroom, school, home, and community). *Cyber Bullying: A Prevention Curriculum* takes a similar approach but is less comprehensive in its scope at the community level. For example, both campaigns educate students and involve parents and teachers, but the *Olweus Bullying Prevention Program* calls for more systemic requirements such as community-school partnerships.

Media Heroes (Wölfer et al., 2013) is a school-based cyberbullying prevention program used in Germany for middle school students and designed for implementation by trained teachers. The program draws on the theory of planned behavior (Ajzen, 1991) to reduce cyberbullying through increasing knowledge and competencies. This includes education on definitions, legal rights and online security options, as well as training in social skills such as empathy. The program focuses on three determinants of behavior change. First, it addresses attitudes toward the target behavior by emphasizing the consequences and legal risks. Second, it bolsters social responsibility within the classroom to foster appropriate subjective norms (i.e., the program aims to change what behavior is considered acceptable by those in the classroom). Third, it increases students' behavioral control by encouraging online protective strategies for self and others (i.e., it promotes control over perpetration behavior and knowledge of what to do if cyberbullied). In accordance with the principles of the theory of planned behavior and models of behavior change, this focus on changing attitudes, subjective norms, and behavioral control can persuade students to avoid the targeted behavior and lead to reduced cyberbullying perpetration. A recent longitudinal evaluation of the program conducted in Germany over 9 months with approximately 600 students demonstrated its effectiveness in reducing cyberbullying behavior (Wölfer et al., 2013). More research, including studies in other countries, is needed to further test this model.

In addition to the interventions described so far, a plethora of intervention materials regarding Internet safety are available online from nonprofit organizations, civic groups, and governmental agencies. Using the search term "cyberbullying" in popular online search engines easily leads one to these websites. However, content of the information presented there needs to be analyzed. Mason (2008) discussed three online resources that schools should consider using: *i-SAFE*, *NetSmartz*, and *CyberSmart*. It appears that these sites have different strengths and some areas of agreement. The *i-SAFE* program incorporates community outreach with a classroom curriculum designed to protect adolescents' online experiences. *NetSmartz*, sponsored by the National Center for Missing and Exploited Children and by Boys and Girls Clubs of America, is more tailored to adolescents through the use of online interactive activities. *CyberSmart*, developed with support from Macmillan/McGraw-Hill, is geared toward the classroom, and its online curriculum does not need to be followed in any particular order. Although these online resources have varied strengths and take different approaches, there is considerable agreement on the unique characteristics of individuals who perpetrate and are victimized and individual factors as determinants of behavior.

CONCLUSION

This examination of cyberbullying, including discussions of cyberbullying characteristics, prevalence rates, demographic features, mental health correlates, and prevention efforts, makes clear the need for further research. Some important areas that have received particularly little attention deserve special focus. For example, the changing role of power within the cyberbullying experience is not empirically understood and warrants investigation. Also, relatively little is known about prevalence across the age spectrum, and even less about other demographic features such as gender, race, and socioeconomic status. Yet better characterizing the perpetrator and the victim would have important public policy implications. Moreover, the psychiatric symptomatology that accompanies cyberbullying makes this phenomenon one of great mental health relevance, but more work is needed to elucidate any cause-and-effect relationship between victimization, perpetration, and psychological problems. And on the prevention front, various strategies drawing on a number of theoretical constructs have been recommended, including mass media, interpersonal, and curriculum-based tools. Researchers must work to make stronger connections to theory or engage in the task of theory development, all the while endeavoring to test their interventions in well-designed, "real life" efficacy studies.

Finally, much cyberbullying research focuses on specific, isolated encounters—the dyadic interaction between cyberbully and victim—and rarely attends to the "big picture" (i.e., the surrounding peer audience in cyberspace). Literature on witnesses of traditional bullying notes the relevance of bystanders to the experience and the degree to which bystanders' reactions can differ (e.g., Salmivalli et al., 1996; Olweus, 2001; Twemlow et al., 2004). Moreover, bystanders are known to play an integral role in the establishment of power structures and to have significant influence as a result of group dynamics and rules (Salmivalli et al., 1996; Salmivalli and Voeten, 2004). Cyberbullying research, however, has largely disregarded bystander behavior (Twemlow et al., 2004). Future research should address this big gap because a framework for cyberbullying cannot be fully outlined and prevention strategies cannot be effective without an appropriate, nuanced understanding of the bystander role. Such an approach would appropriately place cyberbullying within its "ecological framework of interactional influence" (Craig and Pepler, 1997, p. 54), yielding richer, more inclusive results.

DISCLOSURE STATEMENT

The authors disclose no relationships with commercial entities and professional activities that may bias their views.

REFERENCES

Ajzen I (1991). The theory of planned behavior. Organizational Behavior and Human Decision Process 50: 179–211.

Aricak T, Siyahhan S, Uzunhasanoglu A, et al (2008). Cyberbullying among Turkish adolescents. Cyberpsychology & Behavior 11: 253–261.

Arizona Attorney General's Office (2011). Internet safety. Available at http://www.azag.gov/internet-safety. Retrieved on January 15, 2014.

Barnow S, Lucht M, Freyberger HJ (2001). Influence of punishment, emotional rejection, child abuse, and broken home on aggression in adolescence: an examination of aggressive adolescents in Germany. Psychopathology 34: 167–173.

Baum K, Catalano S, Rand M, Rose K (2009). Stalking victimization in the United States. Available at http://www.ovw.usdoj.gov/docs/stalking-victimization.pdf Retrieved on February 21, 2014.

Bauman S, Toomey RB, Walker JL (2013). Associations among bullying, cyberbullying and suicide in high school students. Journal of Adolescence 36: 341–350.

Belsey B (2005). Cyberbullying: an emerging threat to the "always on" generation. Available at http://www.cyberbullying.ca/pdf/Cyberbullying_Article_by_Bill_Belsey.pdf.Retrieved on August 1, 2013.

Beran T, Li Q (2005). Cyber-harassment: a study of a new method for an old behavior. Journal of Educational Computing Research 32: 265–277.

Beran T, Li Q (2007). The relationship between cyberbullying and school bullying. Journal of Student Wellbeing 1: 15–33.

Bowie BH (2007). Relational aggression, gender and the developmental process. Journal of Child and Adolescent Psychiatric Nursing 20: 107–115.

Calvete E, Orue I, Estévez A, Villardón, Padilla P (2010). Cyberbullying in adolescents: modalities and aggressors' profile. Computers in Human Behavior 26: 1128–1135.

Carter JM (2011). Examining the relationship among physical and psychological health, parent and peer attachment, and cyberbullying in adolescents in urban and suburban environments. Doctoral dissertation. Available at http://digitalcommons.wayne.edu/ oa_dissertations/368/. Retrieved on January 30, 2014.

Centers for Disease Control and Prevention (2014). Youth violence: technology and youth—protecting your child from electronic aggression. Available at http://www. cdc.gov/violenceprevention/pdf/ea-tipsheet-a.pdf. Retrieved on January 30, 2014.

Cohen S, Wills TA (1985). Stress, social support, and the buffering hypothesis. Psychological Bulletin 98: 310–357.

Craig WM, Pepler DJ (1997). Observations of bullying and victimization in the school yard. Canadian Journal of School Psychology 13: 41–60.

David-Ferdon C, Hertz MF (2007). Electronic media, violence, and adolescents: an emerging public health problem. Journal of Adolescent Health 41(Suppl 6): S1–S5.

Dehue F, Bolman C, Vollink T (2008). Cyberbullying: youngsters' experiences and parental perception. Cyberpsychology & Behavior 11: 217–223.

Deiss DM, Savage MW, Tokunaga RS (2012). Antecedents and outcomes associated with deviant online behavior: testing a model of cyberbullying perpetration. Paper presented at the 62nd Annual International Communication Association Conference, Phoenix, AZ. Available at http://citation.allacademic.com/meta/p550275_index. html. Retrieved on January 8, 2014.

Dempsey AG, Sulkowski ML, Nichols R, Storch EA (2009). Differences between peer victimization in cyber and physical settings and associated psychosocial adjustment in early adolescence. Psychology in the Schools 46: 962–972.

den Hamer A, Konijn EA, Keijer MG (2014). Cyberbullying behavior and adolescents' use of media with antisocial content: a cyclic process model. Cyberpsychology, Behavior, and Social Networking 17: 74–81.

Didden R, Scholte RHJ, Korzilius H, et al (2009). Cyberbullying among students with intellectual and developmental disability in special education settings. Developmental Neurorehabilitation 12: 146–151.

Duggan M, Brenner J (2013). The demographics of social media users—2012. Available at http://pewinternet.org/~/media//Files/Reports/2013/PIP_SocialMediaUsers.pdf. Retrieved on September 1, 2013.

Dumont M, Provost MA (1999). Resilience in adolescents: protective role of social support, coping strategies, self-esteem, and social activities on experience of stress and depression. Journal of Youth and Adolescence 28: 343–363.

Erdur-Baker Ö, Tanrikulu İ (2010). Psychological consequences of cyber bullying experiences among Turkish secondary school children. Procedia—Social and Behavioral Sciences 2: 2771–2776.

Fanti KA, Demetriou AG, Hawa VV (2012). A longitudinal study of cyberbullying: examining risk and protective factors. European Journal of Developmental Psychology 9: 168–181.

Felix ED, Sharkey JD, Green JG, Furlong MJ, Tanigawa D (2011). Getting precise and pragmatic about the assessment of bullying: the development of the California Bullying Victimization Scale. Aggressive Behavior 37: 234–247.

Goebert D, Else I, Matsu C, Chung-Do J, Chang JY (2010). The impact of cyberbullying on substance use and mental health in a multiethnic sample. Maternal and Child Health Journal 15: 1282–1286.

Harman JP, Hansen CE, Cochran ME, Lindsey CR (2005). Liar, liar: Internet faking out but not frequency of use affects social skills, self-esteem, social anxiety, and aggression. Cyberpsychology & Behavior 8: 1–6.

Hinduja S, Patchin JW (2010). Bullying, cyberbullying, and suicide. Archives of Suicide Research 14: 206–221.

Hinduja S, Patchin JW (2008). Cyberbullying: an exploratory analysis of factors related to offending and victimization. Deviant Behavior 29: 129–156.

International Telecommunication Union (2013). The world in 2013: ICT facts and figures. Available at http://www.itu.int/en/ITU-D/Statistics/Documents/facts/ICTFactsFigures2013.pdf. Retrieved on October 1, 2013.

Juvonen J, Gross EF (2008). Extending the school grounds? Bullying experiences in cyberspace. Journal of School Health 78: 496–505.

Katzer C, Fetchenhauer D, Belschak F (2009). Cyberbullying: who are the victims? A comparison of victimization in Internet chatrooms and victimization in school. Journal of Media Psychology 21: 25–36.

Klomek AB, Sourander A, Gould MS (2011). Bullying and suicide: detection and intervention. Psychiatric Times 28: 27–31.

Kowalski RM, Limber P (2007). Electronic bullying among middle school students. Journal of Adolescent Health 41(Suppl 6): S22–S30.

Kowalski RM, Limber SP, Agatston PW (2008). Cyberbullying: Bullying in the Digital Age. Blackwell, Oxford, UK.

Krankenkasse T (2011). Cybermobbing-Gewalt unter Jugendlichen. Ergebnisse einer repräsentativen Forsa-Umfrage für Deutschland.

Lea M, O'Shea T, Fung P, Spears R (1992). "Flaming" in computer-mediated communication: observations, explanations and implications. In Lea M, Editor. Contexts of Computer-Mediated Communication. Harvester-Wheatsheaf, London, UK, pp. 89–112.

Lenhart A (2010). Cyberbullying 2010: What the research tells us. Available at http://www.slideshare.net/PewInternet/cyberbullying-2010-what-the-research-tells-us4009451. Retrieved on October 1, 2013.

Lenhart A, Madden M, Smith A, Purcell K, Zickuhr K, Rainie L (2011). Teens, kindness and cruelty on social networking sites: how American teens navigate the new world of "digital citizenship." Available at http://pewinternet.org/~/media//Files/Reports/2011/PIP_Teens_Kindness_Cruelty_sns_Report_Nov_2011_FIAL_110711.pdf. Retrieved on January 30, 2014.

Li Q (2008). A cross-cultural comparison of adolescents' experience related to cyberbullying. Educational Research 50: 223–234.

Li Q (2007a). Bullying in the new playground: research into cyberbullying and cyber victimization. Australasian Journal of Educational Technology 23: 435–454.

Li Q (2006). Cyberbullying in schools: a research of gender differences. School Psychology International 27: 157–170.

Li Q (2007b). New bottle but old wine: a research of cyberbullying in schools. Computers in Human Behavior 23: 1777–1791.

Limber SP, Kowalski RM, Agatston PW (2008). Cyber Bullying: A Prevention Curriculum for Grades 6-12. Hazelden Publishing, Center City, MN.

Mason KL (2008). Cyberbullying: a preliminary assessment for school personnel. Psychology in the Schools 45: 323–348.

Mitchell KJ, Ybarra M, Finkelhor D (2007). The relative importance of online victimization in understanding depression, delinquency, and substance use. Child Maltreatment 12: 314–324.

Nansel TR, Overpeck M, Pilla RS, Ruan WJ, Simons-Morton B, Scheidt P (2001). Aggression behaviors among US youth: prevalence and association with psychosocial adjustment. Journal of the American Medical Association 285: 2094–2100.

National Cyber Security Alliance (2013). Cyberstalking is a real crime: one in five Americans affected by unwanted contact. Available at http://www.staysafeonline.

org/about-us/news/cyberstalking-is-a-real-crime-one-in-five-americansaffected-by-unwanted-contact. Retrieved on February 21, 2014.

Olweus D (2003). A profile of bullying at school. Educational Leadership 60: 12–19.

Olweus D (1991). Bully/victim problems among schoolchildren: basic facts and effects of a school based intervention program. In Pepler DJ, Rubin KH, Editors. The Development and Treatment of Childhood Aggression. Erlbaum, Hillsdale, NJ, pp. 411–448.

Olweus D (1993). Bullying at School: What We Know and What We Can Do. Blackwell, Oxford, UK.

Olweus D (2001). Peer harassment: a critical analysis and some important issues. In Juvonen J, Graham S, Editors, Peer Harassment in School: The Plight of the Vulnerable and Victimized. Guilford Press, New York, NY, pp. 3–20.

Olweus D, Limber SP (2010). Bullying in school: evaluation and dissemination of the Olweus Bullying Prevention Program. American Journal of Orthopsychiatry 80: 124–134.

Patchin JW, Hinduja S (2006). Bullies move beyond the schoolyard: a preliminary look at cyberbullying. Youth Violence and Juvenile Justice 4: 148–169.

Patchin JW, Hinduja S (2010). Traditional and nontraditional bullying among youth: a test of general strain theory. Youth Society 43: 727–251.

Perren A, Dooley J, Shaw T, Cross D (2010). Bullying in school and cyberspace: associations with depressive symptoms in Swiss and Australian adolescents. Child and Adolescent Psychiatry and Mental Health 4: 1–10.

Pratarelli M, Browne BL, Johnson K (1999). The bits and bytes of computer/Internet addiction: a factor analytic approach. Behavior Research Methods, Instruments, and Computers 31: 305–314.

Reyns BW, Hensen B, Fisher BS (2012). Stalking in the twilight zone: extent of cyberstalking victimization and offending among college students. Deviant Behavior 33: 1–25.

Roberto AJ, Eden J, Savage MW, Ramos-Salazar L, Deiss DM (2014). Outcome evaluation results of school-based cybersafety promotion and cyberbullying prevention intervention for middle school students. Health Communication 29: 1029–1042.

Roberts C (2014). Slut shaming trend sweeping Internet, adds meme form to adolescent cyberbullying. Available at http://www.nydailynews.com/news/national/adolescents-memes-cyber-bully-article-1.1235246. Retrieved on February 11, 2014.

Salmivalli C, Lagerspetz K, Björkqvist K, Österman K, Kaukiainen A (1996). Bullying as a group process: participant roles and their relations to social status within the group. Aggressive Behavior 22: 1–15.

Salmivalli C, Voeten M (2004). Connections between attitudes, group norms and behavior associated with bullying in schools. International Journal of Behavioral Development 28: 246–258.

Savage MW, Deiss DM (2010). Sticks and stones might break my bones, but typed words will really hurt me: testing a cyberbullying victimization intervention. Paper presented at the 96th annual National Communication Association Conference, San Francisco, CA. Available at http://citation.allacademic.com/meta/p425740_index.html. Retrieved on January 8, 2014.

Schenk AM, Fremouw WJ (2012). Prevalence, psychological impact, and coping of cyberbully victims among college students. Journal of School Violence 11: 21–37.

Slonje R, Smith PK (2008). Cyberbullying: another main type of bullying? Scandinavian Journal of Psychology 49: 147–154.

Smith A (2013). Smartphone ownership—2013 update. Available at http://www.pewinternet.org/2013/06/05/smartphone-ownership-2013/. Retrieved on March 1, 2014.

Smith P, Mahdavi J, Carvalho M, Tippett N (2006). An investigation into cyber-bullying, its forms, awareness and impact, and the relationship between age and gender in cyberbullying. Report presented to the Anti-Bullying Alliance, London, UK. Available at http://www.anti-bullyingalliance.org. Retrieved on January 30, 2014.

Smith PK, Brain P (2000). Bullying in schools: lessons from two decades of research. Aggressive Behavior 26: 1–9.

Smith PK, Mahdavi J, Carvalho M, Fisher S, Russell S, Tippett N (2008). Cyberbullying: its nature and impact in secondary school pupils. Journal of Child Psychology and Psychiatry 49: 376–385.

Songtag LM, Clemans KH, Graber JA, Lyndon ST (2011). Traditional and cyber aggres-sors and victims: a comparison of psychosocial characteristics. Journal of Youth and Adolescence 40: 392–404.

Sourander A, Klomek AB, Ikonen M, et al (2010). Psychosocial risk factors associated with cyberbullying among adolescents: a population-based study. Archives of General Psychiatry 67: 720–728.

Spitzberg BH, Hoobler G (2002). Cyberstalking and the technologies of interpersonal ter-rorism. New Media and Society 4: 71–92.

Srivastava S (2012). Pessimistic side of information & communication technology: cyber bullying & legislature laws. International Journal of Advances in Computer Science and Technology 1: 14–20.

Stephenson P, Smith D (1989). Bullying in the junior school. In Tatum DP, Lane DA, Editors. Bullying in Schools. Trentham Books, Stoke-on-Trent, UK, pp. 45–58.

Sticca F, Ruggieri S, Alsaker F, Perren S (2013). Longitudinal risk factors for cyberbully-ing in adolescence. Journal of Community & Applied Social Psychology 23: 52–67.

Tokunaga RS (2010). Following you home from school: a critical review and synthe-sis of research on cyberbullying victimization. Computers in Human Behavior 26: 277–287.

Topcu C, Erdur-Baker Ö, Capa-Aydin Y (2008). Examination of cyberbullying experi-ences among Turkish students from different school types. Cyberpsychology & Behavior 11: 643–648.

Tracy SJ, Lutgen-Sandvik P, Alberts JK (2006). Nightmares, demons, and slaves: explor-ing the painful metaphors of workplace bullying. Management Communication Quarterly 20: 148–185.

Twemlow SW, Fonagy P, Sacco FC (2004). The role of the bystander in the social archi-tecture of bullying and violence in schools and communities. Annals of the New York Academy of Sciences 1036: 215–232.

Vandebosch H, Van Cleemput K (2008). Defining cyberbullying: a qualitative research into the perceptions of youngsters. Cyberpsychology & Behavior 11: 499–503.

Varjas K, Henrich CC, Meyers J (2009). Urban middle school student's perceptions of bullying, cyberbullying, and school safety. Journal of School Violence 8: 159–176.

Varjas K, Talley J, Meyers J, Parris L, Cutts H (2010). High school students' perceptions of motivations for cyberbullying: an exploratory study. Western Journal of Emergency Medicine 11: 269–273.

von Marées N, Petermann F (2012). Cyberbullying: an increasing challenge for schools. School Psychology International 33: 467–476.

Wadsworth ME, Compas BE (2002). Coping with family conflict and economic strain: the adolescent perspective. Journal of Research on Adolescence 12: 243–274.

Walker CM, Sockman BR, Koehn S (2011). An exploratory study of cyberbullying with undergraduate university students. TechTrends 55: 31–38.

Wang J, Iannotti RJ, Nansel TR (2009). School bullying among adolescents in the Unites States: physical, verbal, relational, and cyber. Journal of Adolescent Health 45: 368–375.

Werner NE, Bumpus MF, Rock D (2010). Involvement in Internet aggression during early adolescence. Journal of Youth and Adolescence 36: 607–619.

Willard N (2007). Cyberbullying and Cyberthreats: Responding to the Challenge of Online Social Aggression, Threats, and Distress. Research Press, Champagne, IL.

Williams K, Guerra N (2007). Prevalence and predictors of Internet bullying. Journal of Adolescent Health 41(Suppl 6): S14–S21.

Witmer DF (1997). Risky business: why people feel safe in sexually explicit on-line communication. Journal of Computer-Mediated Communication 2: 0.

Witte K (1993). Putting the fear back into fear appeals: the extended parallel process model. Communication Monographs 59: 329–349.

Wolak J, Mitchell K, Finkelhor D (2007). Does online harassment constitute bullying? An exploration of online harassment by known peers and online-only contacts. Journal of Adolescent Health 41(Suppl 6): S51–S58.

Wölfer R, Schultze-Krumbholz A, Zagorscak P, Jäkel A, Göbel K, Scheithauer H (2013). Prevention 2.0: targeting cyberbullying @ school. Prevention Science. E-pub.

Wright MF, Li Y (2012). Kicking the digital dog: a longitudinal investigation of young adults' victimization and cyber-displaced aggression. Cyberpsychology, Behavior, and Social Networking 15: 448–454.

Ybarra ML (2004). Linkages between depressive symptomatology and Internet harassment among young regular Internet users. Cyberpsychology & Behavior 7: 247–257.

Ybarra ML, Diener-West M, Leaf PJ (2007). Examining the overlap in Internet harassment and school bullying: implications for school intervention. Journal of Adolescent Health 41(Suppl 6): S42–S50.

Ybarra ML, Mitchell KJ (2008). How risky are social networking sites? A comparison of places online where youth sexual solicitation and harassment occurs. Pediatrics 121: e350–e357.

Ybarra ML, Mitchell KJ (2004). Online aggressor/targets, aggressors, and targets: a comparison of associated youth characteristics. Journal of Child Psychology and Psychiatry 45: 1308–1316.

Ybarra ML, Mitchell KJ, Wolak J, Finkelhor D (2006). Examining characteristics and associated distress related to Internet harassment: findings from the second Youth Internet Safety Survey. Pediatrics 118: 1169–1177.

Zickuhr K (2013). Tablet ownership 2013. Available at http://www.pewinternet.org/2013/06/10/tablet-ownership-2013/ Retrieved on March 1, 2014.

8 Life Versus Death
The Suicidal Mind, Online

Keith M. Harris

INTRODUCTION

Uttering the word "suicide" can darken any conversation, but utter a combination of "Internet" and "suicide" in the same sentence, and, beyond the expected darkness, other disturbing elements spring to mind—suicide pacts, prosuicide forums, cyberbullying, and webcam suicides. These are some of the new ways in which the ancient problem of suicide is being radically transformed, giving rise to the new reality of cybersuicide. This chapter covers research into cybersuicidology, as this new field has been called, including the epidemiology of cybersuicide, the psychosocial theories and models that have attempted to explain it, and the various variables that determine the interaction between information technology and the suicidal mind. Throughout, a rather ambitious goal will serve as guide: we will attempt to answer the increasingly common question of whether, when it comes to suicide, the Internet has been good, bad, or a "mixed bag."

Globally, suicide is one of the leading preventable causes of death, responsible for about 1 million deaths each year (World Health Organization, 2008). It is a particularly important cause of death in younger people, with those aged 20 to 24 years deemed to be at especially high risk (Patton et al., 2009). Adolescents and young adults are also an important focus of Internet suicide studies because they use the Internet extensively and their online habits are likely to continue for most of their lives (Duggan and Brenner, 2013).

Population studies have estimated the lifetime prevalence of suicidal ideation at about 10% of adults (Bromet et al., 2007; Nock et al., 2008). Suicidal ideation is important, because it can be a serious symptom of personal distress and because it is an important predictor of completed suicide (Maris et al., 1992; Beck et al., 1999). In 2013, an estimated 2.7 billion people, or 39% of the world's population, were online (International Telecommunication Union, 2013). That would mean potentially 270 million Internet users with suicidal ideation over the course of their lifetimes and perhaps at risk for suicide.

The information on risk factors for suicidal behaviors is quite robust although far from complete. Many factors have been shown to greatly increase the risk of suicidal ideation, attempts, and deaths. Foremost among them is mental illness. However, it is important to note that psychosocial risk factors, including mental illness, interact with demographic factors, making for a complex etiology. As an example, in a large multinational study on suicide risk factors, mood disorders (e.g., major depressive disorder) ranked as the most common risk factor in wealthier nations, whereas impulse control disorders (e.g., intermittent explosive disorder) were comparatively more important in lower income countries (Nock et al., 2008). Other common risk factors include substance abuse, sexual or physical abuse, unemployment, younger age, and lack of social support (eg, Carter et al., 2007; Li et al., 2011). When people think of suicidal individuals online, it is important to remember the unique factors that are at play, which might drive their thoughts and actions around suicide—physical, social, psychological, or, most likely, a combination thereof.

The earliest awareness of cybersuicide can be traced back to reports of online suicide pacts among Japanese youths. Covering one such story, the *New York Times* quoted Japanese psychologist Mafumi Usui saying "depressed young people and the Internet, it's a very dangerous mix" (New York Times, 2006). In fact, at past suicidology conferences, it was not unusual to hear calls for keeping potentially suicidal patients away from the Internet. Possibly as a sign of acceptance of the world people live in, the discourse has shifted in recent years as experts have become more likely to advocate taking advantage of new opportunities afforded by Internet-related technologies. In reacting to reports of Japanese online suicides, for example, Fred Takahashi, professor of behavioral sciences at Japan's National Defense Medical College, turned attention to solutions. "The problem in Japan is that there are more sites where people are exchanging suicide methods, looking for partners, than there are sites devoted to prevention" (Associated Press, 2003). His words echoed those of Robert Goldney, professor of psychiatry at the University of Adelaide in Australia, who stated that rather than focus attention on how the media should report suicide in a way that does not encourage copycat suicides, people should work at making best use of the media for positive results (Goldney, 2001).

Such views seem more conscious of other historic scares that are now assessed more objectively. After all, before the Internet, similar concerns were discussed about the negative psychological effects of myriad media outlets. Television, for example, dominated discussion for decades, along with theories to explain how it might influence health behaviors. The "cultivation theory" stressed that repeated television exposure to problematic or outright deviant behaviors could legitimize and normalize them (Gerbner, 2008). That seems to be at play online as well, with some individuals advocating nonsuicidal self-harm (e.g., superficial cutting, burning), anorexic starvation or purging, or, indeed, taking one's life, and other vulnerable individuals adopting these behaviors as a way to find camaraderie, validation, and a sense of belonging. But the Internet is not television. It is dynamic, interpersonal, and constantly evolving, which may justify heightened public health anxiety, even if too little research has been conducted to fully understand similarities and differences vis-à-vis older media platforms.

THE SUICIDAL MIND, ONLINE

What is often missing from the cybersuicide discussion is how information technology (IT) environments interact with the suicidal mind. Psychosocial models may not be perfect, but they help bring pertinent factors into perspective. Social cognitive theory (Bandura, 1998) can explain some of the online experiences of suicidal individuals. For example, based on this theory, we can extrapolate that suicidal individuals may model their behaviors on peers at prosuicide sites or in therapeutic forums. Their self-efficacy can influence their perceived ability to carry out a suicidal act or to seek help and reduce their suicidal feelings. Social persuasion, whether from prosuicide forums or prevention sites, is also an important determinant for how individuals at risk for suicide can be influenced online (Bandura, 1998). In addition, the theory of planned behavior has been shown to explain health-related behaviors (e.g., alcohol abuse) and how attitudes toward behaviors, rather than basic knowledge of the facts of the topic, determine positive or negative outcomes (e.g., Ajzen et al., 2011). However, despite the light that the various theories can shed on the problem, researchers rarely use them to guide their understanding of cybersuicide.

Other, more suicide-specific theories and models are also useful. The most relevant probably still comes from the father of suicidology, Edwin Shneidman. To understand suicidal individuals and their actions, Shneidman (1996) emphasized ten commonalities: the seeking of a solution, cessation of consciousness, unendurable psychological pain, frustrated psychological needs, helplessness–hopelessness, ambivalence, constrictive cognitive state, escape, communication of intention, and a consistency in lifelong coping patterns. Preliminary cybersuicide research suggests a possible role for all, but some deserve more elaboration.

Tunnel Vision

A particularly relevant commonality may be cognitive constriction. Baumeister (1990), Shneidman (1996) and others have elaborated on the tendency for suicidal people to have tunnel vision (failing to see the full spectrum of options to resolve their dilemmas) or black-and-white thinking (e.g., seeing only two options; "I will feel this anguish the rest of my life, or I can end it now and feel peace through death"). That temporary mental limitation, when experiencing suicidal thoughts, has been called cognitive constriction. The restricted aspect of the suicidal mind should be considered when evaluating the online behaviors of suicidal individuals and when designing interventions that confront the narrowed-down cognitive spectrum that they are able to consider.

Self-Disclosure

Shneidman's suicide factors also include frustrated psychological needs and communication of intention, which can be demonstrated through the suicidal individual's need for self-disclosure. The latter is important for forming new interpersonal relationships and fostering intimacy (e.g., Sprecher et al., 2013). Thompson (1999) hypothesized that self-disclosure was becoming more common online, and that it might be beneficial in identifying those at risk of suicide. Joinson pioneered the study of online self-disclosure and established an evidence base demonstrating how self-disclosure is often faciliated through online platforms (Joinson, 2001; Joinson et al., 2007). Examples of suicide-related self-disclosure are found in forums and social networking sites (e.g., Cash et al., 2013). More specifically and of relevance for suicide prevention efforts, suicidal individuals appear more likely to disclose suicide plans in an asynchronous forum (where messages may be read and responded to at varying time intervals) compared with immediate communications through either telephone help lines or personal chats (Gilat and Shahar, 2007). This might allow a better understanding of the nature of suicidality, as well as reveal warning signs that could be important for prevention efforts.

Escape

Escape is another feature of suicide highlighted by Shneidman and relevant to cybersuicide. Baumeister (1990), too, described suicide as an escape from oneself. His theory conceptualizes suicidal individuals as self-focused, self-hating and, as described above, cognitively constricted. Indeed, a small study found that suicidal people were more likely to post messages showing self-focus and unbearable pain (Barak and Miron, 2005). They desire escape from their painful world, and, as has been shown with other Internet users (e.g., Demetrovics et al., 2011), suicidal people take advantage of escapist activities. Evidence of potentially escapist activities was shown in comparisons of suicidal and nonsuicidal Internet users, with suicidal people reporting more random surfing, more time spent online, and more time spent on pornography/sex (males) and gaming (females) (Harris et al., 2014).

However, it is important to underscore that not all games offer escape in the negative pain-postponing or pain-evading sense; some may have positive social or other attributes. For example, a large Korean study examined daily behaviors as coping strategies and found that mobile or online gaming was negatively associated with suicidal ideation in both adolescent females and males (Kim et al., 2014). What is missing from the gaming analyses of these studies, however, is the type of games played. It is possible that some games, such as massively multiplayer online role-playing games, may have different effects than single-player games, due to the many social motivations for playing them (Yee, 2006). Perhaps suicidal individuals are more likely to play games for escape, whereas nonsuicidal players have other motivations.

Life-Death Ambivalence

Insufficient attention has been paid to one of Shneidman's key aspects of suicide—ambivalence. There is growing evidence of the importance of life-death ambivalence in suicide, including cybersuicide (e.g., Kovacs and Beck, 1977; Jobes and Mann, 1999; Corona et al., 2013). Thus, suicidal people have posted ambivalent forum messages (e.g., Baume et al., 1997). More directly, an anonymous online survey of 1000 adult Internet users found that about 95% of participants who were at high risk for suicide (defined as scoring above a cutoff score on a popular suicide risk assessment measure, the Suicide Behaviors Questionnaire–Revised) had debated whether to live or die and more than 33% had done so frequently (Harris et al., 2010). Behavioral evidence of their life-death debate was shown through reports that more than 50% of the high-risk participants went online to look for or confirm their reasons for living and dying but were somewhat more death-oriented. These findings demonstrate the complexity of the suicidal mind as it weighs life versus death. They also show a need to address that complexity when assessing the relationship between suicide and IT. Those in crisis are likely to be simultaneously engaged in both helpful and harmful online behaviors (e.g., Eichenberg, 2008). It is crucial to keep that in mind when designing or interpreting cybersuicide research or contemplating interventions.

IS INFORMATION TECHNOLOGY BAD FOR SUICIDAL INDIVIDUALS?

Probably no other online content generates the kind of consensus one sees around the essential "badness" of online services that encourage or facilitate self-harm. Chief among those are suicide pacts and prosuicide websites, although search engines have also been on the receiving end of some critics' wrath because doing an online search for "suicide" is often the first step toward taking one's life.

Suicide Pacts

Although relatively rare, online suicide pacts are an important example of how Internet use can lead to deadly consequences in some vulnerable individuals. Online suicide pacts seem to have originated in Japan in 2000, but it was not until 2003 that media reports exploded and a host of expert commentary emerged (Ueno, 2005). The Japanese media popularized the term "netto shinju" (ネット心中) in referring to this type of suicide. The phrase combines "net" (Internet) and "lovers' suicide pact," and it borrows from an older term romanticizing a suicide pact between lovers escaping intolerable situations. Unfortunately, such terms help glamorize and normalize suicide, which can lead to increases in suicide rates, particularly among females (e.g., Stack, 2005). Although accurate statistics are impossible to come by, Japan appears to be the leader in this phenomenon.

Rajagopal (2004) mentioned folie à deux, a shared psychosis, as one theory for suicide pacts, although empirical evidence is lacking. Many Internet suicide pacts appear to fit this model; folie à deux can occur when those involved are socially isolated and where one is more dominant (the one who initiates the plan and solicits others). Rajagopal has also warned that the epidemiology of Internet suicide pacts is likely to change over time (such as the ages of pact victims becoming younger). Other theories have also been proposed, but a sound prevention method is still lacking. Online suicide pacts are usually formed in obscure and anonymous forums, and most of the individuals involved seem to feel socially isolated and ambivalent toward life (Ikunaga et al., 2013). Research is needed to help predict who will visit those forums, how to reach out to them, and what interventions are likely to succeed.

Prosuicide Sites

What makes a website, forum, bulletin board system, or similar online location prosuicide is a matter of debate. Actively encouraging others to commit suicide is certainly one aspect. Other criteria may include presenting or allowing users to present detailed descriptions of suicide methods and allowing users to express their belief that suicide is a personal choice. There is good reason to find the above behaviors and environments unacceptable, and there have been many calls to ban prosuicide sites. However, creating a clear and specific piece of legislation to do so is fraught with difficulty, particularly if free speech laws are strong in the host country. In 2006, Australia became the first nation to make prosuicide sites illegal (Pirkis et al., 2009), although there are no known prosecutions of any website administrators to date. But, does making prosuicide sites illegal really matter given the international connectivity of the Internet? Some experts believe that the answer is "yes" regardless of any prosecutions, because such laws can do much good by raising awareness and promoting prevention efforts (Pirkis et al., 2009).

Those aligned against prosuicide sites include more than politicians and mental health professionals. Technology blog and leading IT news source *The Next Web* listed suicide and self-harm communities as the second most disturbing type of online community, just after pro–anorexia nervosa and ahead of child pornography (Falconer, 2012). The article rightly mentions the provision of how-to methods of suicide as a particularly harmful feature. However, the claim that "hundreds of teen suicides have been connected with involvement in prosuicide communities" is difficult to prove, if not difficult to imagine. Still, the theme of the suicidal person's perception of being misunderstood and his or her need to communicate with others seems to have been accurately identified in the blog (Harris et al., 2009). A *Washington Post* article, for example, quoted a young blogger of the Tumblr microblogging and social networking site who wrote about her depression and self-harm saying, "I know they're not going to judge me for self-harming. It's nice to know that you can tell your story without being judged" (Dewey, 2013).

The most infamous prosuicide site is likely alt.suicide.holiday, or ASH, which began as an unmoderated online newsgroup. The name came from the observation that suicides tend to increase around the holidays. A closer analysis showed that suicides tended to drop before holidays and spike just after, which Gabennesch

(1988) interpreted as a reflection of the "broken-promise theory." ASH has been banned in some places and by some Internet providers because it promotes suicide as a personal choice, and some members even encourage it. Overall, however, most members seem to offer support and discourage suicide. What concerns suicide prevention experts the most, however, is the suicide methods list that some sites maintain, because many suicidal people type "best suicide methods" or "how to kill yourself" in online search engines (Harris et al., 2009). Also, access to effective methods is considered one of the greatest risks for completed suicide among vulnerable individuals (Hawton, 2005; Mann et al., 2005; Wu et al., 2012).

Exit International and Church of Euthanasia are examples of other sites that might be regarded as prosuicide. Both are voluntary euthanasia sites, although Church of Euthanasia also advocates "save the planet, kill yourself," as part of what might be regarded as an ill-considered "green" philosophy for saving the Earth by reducing one's carbon footprint.

Empirical study of prosuicide sites (loosely defined) has produced some important, if incomplete, information. Niezen (2013) has discussed the wide variety of communication styles and information types that exist in suicide forums. An analysis of motivations and perceived impact of using a German suicide forum revealed mostly positive suicide prevention effects (Eichenberg, 2008). The content analysis of Japanese suicide bulletin board systems showed themes related to life-death ambivalence, psychological pain, and belongingness (Ikunaga et al., 2013). Administration of open-ended questions to 290 multinational suicidal online users, aged 18 to 71 years, revealed that visitors found prosuicide sites both supportive and negative but were more likely to have negative opinions of sites with suicide pacts (Harris et al., 2009). The latter study also confirmed the ambivalent nature of suicidality as suicide-risk survey participants reported searching for both suicide methods and professional support. In general, suicidal Internet users came away with somewhat more positive perceptions of prosuicide sites than of professionally run support sites, pointing toward a need for professionals to better adapt their online environments to fit with preferences of their target population.

Overall, however, an insufficient number of methodologically sound studies have explored prosuicide sites. That may be in part because prosuicide sites are rather rare and poorly connected via hyperlinks with other sites, which can make them difficult to access and study (Kemp and Collings, 2011). Still, one should remain objective about the magnitude of the problem; the negative effects of posting suicide methods online do not seem to have caught up with printed versions of similar material, such as Tsurumi's *The Complete Manual of Suicide* (1993) or Humphry's *Final Exit* (1991). To date, these printed books are likely to be responsible for more suicides than prosuicide sites, although that could change in coming years.

Webcam Suicides

Webcam broadcasts of "live" suicides are another area of concern. It is possible that the suicide victims are making a cry for help by performing their suicidal acts in public view. Evidence for the desire for rescue has been found repeatedly in ambivalent or low-lethality suicide attempts (e.g., Linehan et al., 2006; Wasserman and Stack, 2008). Cyberbullying (see Chapter 7) should also be a focus of research, and studies have implicated bullying in webcam suicides, prosuicide forums, and social networks where suicides have been reported (Bauman et al., 2013).

Beyond considering banning prosuicide sites, it might serve prevention efforts well to take action against bullying behaviors. It is also important to keep in mind that, although somewhat less likely than their victims, bullies also seem to be at an increased suicide risk (Hinduja and Patchin, 2010). Many people are exposed to bullying communications each day, often resulting in a passive bystander effect where the observer does nothing to help. A recent study produced preliminary indicators of how and when university students might provide help in such cases (Aldrich et al., 2014). More research is needed to understand bystander effect factors (a situation where, as mentioned, people do not offer help to someone in need when other observers are present), the role of good Samaritans (those who contrary to passive bystanders, offer assistance), and the difficult question of how and why people watch others killing themselves (Polder-Verkiel, 2012).

Searching for Suicide on the Internet

Because it is believed that the online quest for suicide starts with a search box, a common practice in cybersuicide research involves typing in suicide-related search terms and then analyzing the results (e.g., Biddle et al., 2008; Recupero et al., 2008; Westerlund et al., 2012; Ayers et al., 2013; Gunn and Lester, 2013; Song et al., 2014). Search terms have included "suicide," "suicide methods," and the more academic "deliberate self-harm" (Prasad and Owens, 2001).

Cybersuicide research, like other Internet-related research, requires a basic understanding of the technologies involved. Unfortunately, some studies do not indicate methodology, such as clearing the browser's search history and cache. Such stored information can lead to "filter bubbles"—search results unique to the individual user. It is necessary to take advantage of appropriate IT tools. For example, there are several analysis tools, including free applications such as PageRank, SimilarWeb, and Up-rank, all of which provide indicators of a page's importance (Liu and Li, 2011). Although site popularity is important because it relates to its impact on the population of interest, the quality of a site's information and features is of greater concern.

Another research method utilizes archived search engine data. Suicide-related search terms can be analyzed by frequency over time and compared with national suicide rates to observe any trends. Results from a simple correlational study of searches (e.g., "commit suicide") done at the state level in the United States showed positive associations with state suicide rates (Gunn and Lester, 2013). A more elaborate study, also using Google Trends data, compared 2006 to 2010 mental health searches in the United States and Australia (Ayers et al., 2013). It found that all assessed mental health problems, including suicide, showed seasonal patterns with winter peaks and summer troughs. Another more recent study went a step further, analyzing search terms in connection with the destination users ultimately clicked on among the search's results (Wong et al., 2013). That study used archived (2006) suicide-related searches of the America Online subscribers and found that only 2 out of 1314 sites users visited could be categorized as prosuicide. The advantage of the Wong et al. (2013) study is that actual search terms and ultimate website destinations were analyzed.

One of the more advanced cybersuicidology studies used empirically derived suicide search terms (e.g., "suicide methods") and then-state-of-the-art software (e.g., *Virtual Observatory for the Study of Online Networks*) to conduct a hyperlinked network analysis of more than 1000 suicide-related sites (Kemp and Collings, 2011). The researchers classified sites according to their primary purpose (e.g., providing information or support) and mapped out how they were linked to other sites. Results showed suicide prevention sites to be centralized and focused on support networks, whereas suicide method sites had few links to other sites, making it difficult for users to find additional sites of the same type.

Overall, the limitations of these studies are notable. It is not possible to know the true level of suicide risk of the searchers in any of the studies—some searches may have been done by researchers conducting the above studies. In addition, it is not known how Internet users responded to or behaved at the destination sites, or if they followed links to other sites. More research is clearly needed to understand whether and when search behaviors translate into self-harm or finding support and help.

IS INFORMATION TECHNOLOGY GOOD FOR SUICIDAL INDIVIDUALS?
Help Seeking

An important finding is that suicidal people are less likely than nonsuicidal people to seek help from any type of help source (e.g., Wilson et al., 2005). Of course, some suicidal people do seek help, including assistance from general health professionals or mental health professionals shortly before their suicide (Draper et al., 2008). Various theories explain help-seeking behaviors. The theory of planned behavior is useful for predicting many help-seeking actions. It states that beliefs, norms, and behavioral control predict behavioral intentions and behaviors (Ajzen, 1991). However, the prototype/willingness model goes further by including subjective norms, such as stigma (Hammer and Vogel, 2013). That is an important point because studies have consistently found people to be less likely to seek help for stigmatized problems, including suicidal thoughts (Wilson et al., 2005; Perkins et al., 2013).

Help-seeking research has shown important differences between online and offline help seeking for suicidal ideation. For example, a recent study (Seward and Harris, n.d.) confirmed that, overall, suicidal people were less likely to seek help from face-to-face sources than nonsuicidal people (controlling for age, sex, and ethnicity). However, suicidal young adults (aged 18 to 29 years) were about equally likely to seek help from online help sources as nonsuicidal young adults.

In addition, suicidal participants were statistically more likely to choose social networking sites for support, compared with their nonsuicidal counterparts. Seward and Harris (n.d.) also found suicidal young adults to be split between those who prefer professional support (i.e., online help sites with access to online mental health professionals) and those who prefer informal support (i.e., social networking and anonymous forums), with nearly all expressing at least modest likelihood of trying to access various sources of help. That fits well with previous research (Harris et al., 2009) and demonstrates the importance of looking at a range of online options, such as provision of help through more than one source type.

Social Support

Social support is related to help seeking, in part because friends and family make up important sources of personal assistance. A study of callers to Australia's crisis hotline Lifeline revealed that most callers were primarily seeking social support (Watson et al., 2006). There is little doubt that many of those in crisis are doing the same online. One of the advantages of the Internet is the potential for expanding and improving on social support. The Online Relationship Building Scale (ORBS; Harris et al., 2009) was developed from the perspective that interpersonal relationships are a fundamental aspect of human nature and that interpersonal voids demand to be filled (Baumeister and Leary, 1995). The ORBS assesses frequency of using the Internet to find and make new interpersonal relationships. It has been shown that suicide-risk individuals are more likely to score higher on the ORBS, as are sexual minorities (Harris, 2013). Accordingly, stigmatized individuals may be more likely to make use of IT platforms to improve their social lives. The message they seem to be sending is that one of the solutions to their problems is enhanced social support, which some help sites are beginning to address.

Online Mental Health Professionals and Online Support

Suicide prevention and support groups have been online almost since the beginning of the Internet. In 2000 to 2002, Barak and colleagues began a pioneering suicide support site, the Hebrew language SAHAR (Barak, 2007). Online support groups are believed to promote self-efficacy, interpersonal communications, and reductions in psychological distress (Barak et al., 2008). However, quality can vary, and many suicidal users express disdain for what they interpret as the condescending attitude of some sites, or an unhelpful format (Harris et al., 2009). Quality of suicide support sites is of vital importance if the sites are going to be helpful in reducing suicidality. There are several means for rating site quality, including Health on the Net (HON) and Brief DISCERN, which evaluate factors such as the qualifications of authors and identity of any funding sources. However, a consistent measure and evaluation body are still lacking. Rating of mental health websites is discussed in more detail in Chapter 9.

Volunteer helpers and other nonprofessionals are also instrumental in saving and improving lives online. Private organizations, such as the US-based QPR

Institute, have begun empirically derived online training of lay people (QPR Institute, 2011). It is crucial to train and use these informal helpers; online mental health professionals are far too few and suicidal individuals often avoid professional help. A systematic analysis of suicide-related sites found a strong need for both private and government sites to improve their provision of evidence-based information and care and other features to better help those in crisis (Szumilas and Kutcher, 2009). Quality is, once again, of vital importance because some help organizations have been shown to possibly lead to harming vulnerable individuals or produce no positive results (Freedenthal, 2010).

In addition to recommending offline treatment if appropriate, formal online therapy can be offered to the suicidal person who is already online. Recent studies have found promising, if mixed, evidence that online therapies can reduce suicide risk factors, such as depressive symptoms and suicidal ideation (Proudfoot, 2004; Van Spijker et al., 2012) (see also Chapters 9 and 10). Conducting rigorous evaluations of online treatment is necessary for the development of this field.

Another promising direction is treatment through mobile phone apps (see Chapter 13). Luxton et al. (2011) discussed developments in support of suicidal individuals through texting and gaming. As anonymous, asynchronous, and gaming activities all appear to be pertinent to suicidal people, treatment approaches and support using those features have the potential to be beneficial. Aguirre et al. (2013) located hundreds of mobile phone apps aimed at suicide, with 27 that were formally dedicated to suicide prevention. Their overall results were mixed, but a positive direction in developing these applications could be discerned. Similarly, an evaluation of a suicide prevention app for Aboriginal Australians found mixed, but promising results (Shand et al., 2013). Clearly, more work is required on designing and testing these applications.

A newer development is intelligent real-time therapy, which utilizes machine learning to provide suicide prevention treatment (Kelly et al., 2012). Just as software can distinguish reasonably well between genuine email and spam, it could also "learn" to distinguish genuine cries for help from other online postings. A similar approach utilizes information retrieval, affect analysis, and machine learning to identify suicidal individuals who are posting on public forums, so that appropriate help can be delivered in a timely manner (Li et al., 2013). Naturally, this raises privacy concerns and the possibility of false-positives, but these types of real-time responses to online cries for help could forge new roads in mental health triage and suicide prevention.

CONCLUSION

Many researchers would probably say that suicide-related sites are neither good nor bad, arguing, instead, that most are a little of both, even if they may lean one way or another (e.g., Niezen, 2013). For example, a suicide support site may not offer much support, and it may do nothing more than state an opinion on suicide, provide a crisis phone number (that may not work in the country where the search is being conducted), or give a link to a better site. At the dawn of cybersuicide research, two sites were at the top of many suicide-related searches—SuicideGirls (an adult site) and a "quiz" on suicide, which turned out to be a quiz on Christianity where the only "correct" answers supported that faith. How many people in a personal crisis ended up accessing irrelevant sites, became frustrated by not finding what they needed, and then gave up on locating help may never be known.

The Internet is a better place than it once was, which justifies optimism about the future. When one makes an online search for "suicide" today, no pornographic or proselytizing sites feature prominently in the results. Google and other search engines now routinely list crisis support sites at the top of the "suicide" search yield. Facebook also has an evolving means for reporting the cries for help of friends and others and for removing inappropriate content (e.g., graphic images of suicides, encouragement of suicidal acts). Behind the scenes, much work has been done to assist those in need. It is difficult to document the number of lives saved or improved by those actions, but their impact is likely significant.

Cybersuicidology is still young and working through some growing pains. However, 15 years of research on Internet behaviors have produced valuable information about suicide and its prevention. It is no longer possible to give an "all bad" or "all good" assessment about the interplay between suicide and IT; a more nuanced reaction is in order. That is why this statement from Vaughan Bell, a psychologist and writer on online mental health at King's College in London, resonates: "The Internet is typically discussed as if it were a set of activities when it is actually a medium upon which various activities can occur. It is, therefore, neither "good" nor "bad" for mental health, although specific activities may have an influence" (Bell, 2007, p. 445). Over the next several years, it is likely that a deeper understanding of the influence of those activities will be developed. IT-based treatments and outreach will likely expand well beyond what there is today. At the forefront will be researchers conducting randomized controlled trials and program evaluations, more professionals expanding their therapy offerings to IT platforms, and many concerned lay people pioneering unique approaches to suicide prevention. Prosuicide sites, cyberbullying, and other negative factors are unlikely to be eradicated and will continue to elicit anger and condemnation. Most in the field of cybersuicidology, however, believe that the Internet, or mobile, environment will ultimately offer more advantages than disadvantages.

DISCLOSURE STATEMENT

The author discloses no relationships with commercial entities and professional activities that may bias his views.

REFERENCES

Aguirre RTP, McCoy MK, Roan M (2013). Development guidelines from a study of suicide prevention mobile applications (apps). Journal of Technology in Human Services 31: 269–293.

Ajzen I (1991). The theory of planned behavior. Organizational Behavior and Human Decision Processes 50: 179–211.

Ajzen I, Joyce N, Sheikh S, Cote NG (2011). Knowledge and the prediction of behavior: the role of information accuracy in the theory of planned behavior. Basic and Applied Social Psychology 33: 101–117.

Aldrich RS, Harrington NG, Cerel J (2014). The Willingness to Intervene Against Suicide Questionnaire. Death Studies 38: 100–108.

Associated Press (2003). Japan worried about spurt of Internet suicide pacts. Available at http://www.smh.com.au/articles/2003/07/04/1057179108308.html. Retrieved on January 7, 2014.

Ayers JW, Althouse BM, Allem JP, Rosenquist JN, Ford DE (2013). Seasonality in seeking mental health information on Google. American Journal of Preventive Medicine 44: 520–525.

Bandura A (1998). Health promotion from the perspective of social cognitive theory. Psychology and Health 13: 623–649.

Barak A (2007). Emotional support and suicide prevention through the Internet: a field project report. Computers in Human Behavior 23: 971–984.

Barak A, Boniel-Nissim M, Suler J (2008). Fostering empowerment in online support groups. Computers in Human Behavior 24: 1867–1883.

Barak A, Miron O (2005). Writing characteristics of suicidal people on the Internet: a psychological investigation of emerging social environments. Suicide and Life-Threatening Behavior 35: 507–524.

Bauman S, Toomey RB, Walker JL (2013). Associations among bullying, cyberbullying, and suicide in high school students. Journal of Adolescence 36: 341–350.

Baume P, Cantor CH, Rolfe, A (1997). Cybersuicide: the role of interactive suicide notes on the Internet. Crisis 18: 73–79.

Baumeister RF (1990). Suicide as escape from self. Psychological Review 97: 90–113.

Baumeister RF, Leary MR (1995). The need to belong: desire for interpersonal attachments as a fundamental human motivation. Psychological Bulletin 117: 497–529.

Beck AT, Brown GK, Steer RA, Dahlsgaard KK, Grisham JR (1999). Suicide ideation at its worst point: a predictor of eventual suicide in psychiatric outpatients. Suicide and Life-Threatening Behavior 29: 1–9.

Bell V (2007). Online information, extreme communities and Internet therapy: is the Internet good for our mental health? Journal of Mental Health 16: 445–457.

Biddle L, Donovan J, Hawton K, Kapur N, Gunnell D (2008). Suicide and the Internet. British Medical Journal 336: 800–802.

Bromet EJ, Havenaar JM, Tintle N, Kostyuchenko S, Kotov R, Gluzman S (2007). Suicide ideation, plans and attempts in Ukraine: findings from the Ukraine World Mental Health Survey. Psychological Medicine 37: 807–819.

Carter GL, Page A, Clover K, Taylor R (2007). Modifiable risk factors for attempted suicide in Australian clinical and community samples. Suicide and Life-Threatening Behavior 37: 671–680.

Cash SJ, Thelwall M, Peck SN, Ferrell JZ, Bridge JA (2013). Adolescent suicide statements on MySpace. Cyberpsychology, Behavior, and Social Networking 16: 166–174.

Corona CD, Jobes DA, Nielsen AC, et al (2013). Assessing and treating different suicidal states in a Danish outpatient sample. Archives of Suicide Research 17: 302–312.

Demetrovics Z, Urbán R, Nagygyörgy K, et al (2011). Why do you play? The development of the Motives for Online Gaming Questionnaire (MOGQ). Behavior Research Methods 43: 814–825.

Dewey C (2013). Self-harm blogs pose problems and opportunities. Available at http://articles.washingtonpost.com/2013-09-09/national/41898796_1_blogs-razor-blades-self-harm. Retrieved on February 10, 2014.

Draper B, Snowdon J, Wyder M (2008). A pilot study of the suicide victim's last contact with a health professional. Crisis 29: 96–101.

Duggan M, Brenner J (2013). The demographics of social media users: 2012 Pew Internet and American Life Project. Available at http://pewInternet.org/Reports/2013/Social-media-users.aspx. Retrieved on February 24, 2014.

Eichenberg C (2008). Internet message boards for suicidal people: a typology of users. Cyberpsychology and Behavior 11: 107–113.

Falconer J (2012). 10 of the most disturbing communities on the Web. Available at http://thenextweb.com/media/2012/08/04/10-of-the-most-disturbing-communities-on-the-web/#!tkygA. Retrieved on January 31, 2014.

Freedenthal S (2010). Adolescent help-seeking and the Yellow Ribbon suicide prevention program: an evaluation. Suicide and Life-Threatening Behavior 40: 628–639.

Gabennesch H (1988). When promises fail: a theory of temporal fluctuations in suicide. Social Forces 67: 129–145.

Gerbner G (2008). Mass media and dissent. In Kurtz, LR, Editor. Encyclopedia of Violence, Peace, and Conflict. Elsevier, New York, NY, pp. 1182–1183.

Gilat I, Shahar G (2007). Emotional first aid for a suicide crisis: comparison between telephonic hotline and Internet. Psychiatry 70: 12–18.

Goldney RD (2001). The media and suicide: a cautionary view. Crisis 22: 173–175.

Gunn JF, Lester D (2013). Using Google searches on the Internet to monitor suicidal behavior. Journal of Affective Disorders 148: 411–412.

Hammer JH, Vogel DL (2013). Assessing the utility of the willingness/prototype model in predicting help-seeking decisions. Journal of Counseling Psychology 60: 83–97.

Harris KM (2013). Sexuality and suicidality: matched-pairs analyses reveal unique characteristics in non-heterosexual suicidal behaviors. Archives of Sexual Behavior 42: 729–737.

Harris KM, McLean JP, Sheffield J (2009). Examining suicide-risk individuals who go online for suicide-related purposes. Archives of Suicide Research 13: 264–276.

Harris KM, McLean JP, Sheffield J (2014). Suicidal and online: how do online behaviors inform us of this high-risk population? Death Studies 38: 387–394.

Harris KM, McLean JP, Sheffield J, Jobes D (2010). The internal suicide debate hypothesis: exploring the life versus death struggle. Suicide and Life-Threatening Behavior 40: 191–192.

Hawton K (2005). Restriction of access to methods of suicide as a means of suicide prevention. In Hawton K, Editor. Prevention and Treatment of Suicidal Behaviour: From Science to Practice. Oxford University Press, Oxford, UK, pp. 1182–1183.

Hinduja S, Patchin JW (2010). Bullying, cyberbullying, and suicide. Archives of Suicide Research 14: 206–221.

Humphry D (1991). Final Exit: The Practicalities of Self-deliverance and Assisted Suicide for the Dying. The Hemlock Society, Eugene, OR.

Ikunaga A, Nath SR, Skinner KA (2013). Internet suicide in Japan: a qualitative content analysis of a suicide bulletin board. Transcultural Psychiatry 50: 280–302.

International Telecommunication Union (2013). ITU releases latest global technology development figures. Available at http://www.itu.int/net/pressoffice/press_releases/2013/05.aspx#.Uu4MWbT54_Z. Retrieved on February 24, 2014.

Jobes DA, Mann RE (1999). Reasons for living versus reasons for dying: examining the internal debate of suicide. Suicide and Life-Threatening Behavior 29: 97–104.

Joinson AN (2001). Self-disclosure in computer-mediated communication: the role of self-awareness and visual anonymity. European Journal of Social Psychology 31: 177–192.

Joinson AN, Woodley A, Reips UD (2007). Personalization, authentication and self-disclosure in self-administered Internet surveys. Computers in Human Behavior 23: 275–285.

Kelly J, Gooding P, Pratt D, Ainsworth J, Welford M, Tarrier N (2012). Intelligent real-time therapy: harnessing the power of machine learning to optimise the delivery of momentary cognitive behavioural interventions. Journal of Mental Health 21: 404–414.

Kemp CG, Collings SC (2011). Hyperlinked suicide: assessing the prominence and accessibility of suicide websites. Crisis 32: 143–151.

Kim SM, Han DH, Trksak GH, Lee YS (2014). Gender differences in adolescent coping behaviors and suicidal ideation: findings from a sample of 73,238 adolescents. Anxiety, Stress and Coping 27: 439–454.

Kovacs M, Beck AT (1977). The wish to die and the wish to live in attempted suicides. Journal of Clinical Psychology 33: 361–365.

Li TMH, Ng BCM, Chau M, Wong PWC, Yip PSF (2013). Collective intelligence for suicide surveillance in web forums. In Pacific Asia Workshop on Intelligence and Security Informatics, PAISI 2013, Vol. 8039. LNCS, Beijing, China, pp. 29–37.

Li Z, Page A, Martin G, Taylor R (2011). Attributable risk of psychiatric and socio-economic factors for suicide from individual-level, population-based studies: a systematic review. Social Science and Medicine 72: 608–616.

Linehan MM, Comtois KA, Brown MZ, Heard HL, Wagner A (2006). Suicide Attempt Self-Injury Interview (SASII): development, reliability, and validity of a scale to assess suicide attempts and intentional self-injury. Psychological Assessment 18: 303–312.

Liu YF, Li RF (2011). Up-rank: a method for ranking web pages based on user behaviors and hyperlink. International Journal of Advancements in Computing Technology 3: 322–328.

Luxton DD, June JD, Kinn JT (2011). Technology-based suicide prevention: current applications and future directions. Telemedicine and e-Health 17: 50–54.

Mann JJ, Apter A, Bertolote J, et al (2005). Suicide prevention strategies: a systematic review. Journal of the American Medical Association 294: 2064–2074.

Maris RW, Berman AL, Maltsberger JT, Yufit RI, Editors (1992). Assessment and Prediction of Suicide. Guilford Press, New York, NY.

New York Times (2006). World briefing: Asia: Japan: Internet suicide pact takes six lives. Available at http://query.nytimes.com/gst/fullpage.html?res=9904E4D71331F932A2 5750C0A9609C8B63. Retrieved on February 17, 2014.

Niezen R (2013). Internet suicide: communities of affirmation and the lethality of communication. Transcultural Psychiatry 50: 303–322.

Nock MK, Borges G, Bromet EJ, et al (2008). Cross-national prevalence and risk factors for suicidal ideation, plans and attempts. British Journal of Psychiatry 192: 98–105.

Patton GC, Coffey C, Sawyer SM, et al (2009). Global patterns of mortality in young people: a systematic analysis of population health data. Lancet 374: 881–892.

Perkins D, Fuller J, Kelly BJ, et al (2013). Factors associated with reported service use for mental health problems by residents of rural and remote communities: cross-sectional findings from a baseline survey. BMC Health Services Research 13: 157.

Pirkis J, Neal L, Dare A, Blood RW, Studdert D (2009). Legal bans on pro-suicide web sites: an early retrospective from Australia. Suicide and Life-Threatening Behavior 39: 190–193.

Polder-Verkiel SE (2012). Online responsibility: bad Samaritanism and the influence of Internet mediation. Science and Engineering Ethics 18: 117–141.

Prasad V, Owens D (2001). Using the Internet as a source of self-help for people who self-harm. Psychiatric Bulletin 25: 222–225.

Proudfoot JG (2004). Computer-based treatment for anxiety and depression. Is it feasible? Is it effective? Neuroscience and Biobehavioral Reviews 28: 353–363.

QPR Institute (2011). QPR gatekeeper training for suicide prevention. Available at https://www.qprinstitute.com/index.html. Retrieved on March 5, 2014.

Rajagopal S (2004). Suicide pacts and the Internet: complete strangers may make cyber-space pacts. British Medical Journal 329: 1298–1299.

Recupero PR, Harms SE, Noble JM (2008). Googling suicide: surfing for suicide information on the Internet. Journal of Clinical Psychiatry 69: 878–888.

Seward AL, Harris KM (n.d.). Psychological characteristics of suicidal emerging adults seeking help online. The Suicide Study Group.

Shand FL, Ridani R, Tighe J, Christensen H (2013). The effectiveness of a suicide prevention app for indigenous Australian youths: study protocol for a randomized controlled trial. Trials 14: 396.

Shneidman ES (1996). The Suicidal Mind. Oxford University Press, New York, NY.

Song TM, Song J, An JY, Hayman LL, Woo JM (2014). Psychological and social factors affecting Internet searches on suicide in Korea: a big data analysis of Google search trends. Yonsei Medical Journal 55: 254–263.

Sprecher S, Treger S, Wondra JD, Hilaire N, Wallpe K (2013). Taking turns: reciprocal self-disclosure promotes liking in initial interactions. Journal of Experimental Social Psychology 49: 860–866.

Stack S (2005). Suicide in the media: a quantitative review of studies based on nonfictional stories. Suicide and Life-Threatening Behavior 35: 121–133.

Szumilas M, Kutcher S (2009). Teen suicide information on the Internet: a systematic analysis of quality. Canadian Journal of Psychiatry 54: 596–604.

Thompson S (1999). The Internet and its potential influence on suicide. Psychiatric Bulletin 23: 449–451.

Tsurumi W (1993). The Complete Manual of Suicide. Ohta, Tokyo, Japan.

Ueno K (2005). Suicide as Japan's major export? A note on Japanese suicide culture. Revista Espaco Academico 44. Available at http://www.espacoacademico.com.br/044/44eueno_ing.htm. Retrieved on March 4, 2014.

Van Spijker BAJ, Cristina Majo M, Smit F, Van Straten A, Kerkhof AJFM (2012). Reducing suicidal ideation: cost-effectiveness analysis of a randomized controlled trial of unguided web-based self-help. Journal of Medical Internet Research 14: e141.

Wasserman IM, Stack S (2008). Lethal locations: an application of opportunity theory to motel suicide, a research note. Death Studies 32: 757–767.

Watson RJ, McDonald J, Pearce DC (2006). An exploration of national calls to Lifeline Australia: social support or urgent suicide intervention? British Journal of Guidance and Counselling 34: 471–482.

Westerlund M, Hadlaczky G, Wasserman D (2012). The representation of suicide on the Internet: implications for clinicians. Journal of Medical Internet Research 14: e122.

Wilson CJ, Deane FP, Ciarrochi J, Rickwood D (2005). Measuring help-seeking intentions: properties of the General Help-Seeking Questionnaire. Canadian Journal of Counselling 39: 15–28.

Wong PWC, Fu KW, Yau RSP (2013). Accessing suicide-related information on the Internet: a retrospective observational study of search behavior. Journal of Medical Internet Research 15: e3.

World Health Organization (2008). Suicide prevention (SUPRE). Available at http://www.who.int/mental_health/prevention/suicide/suicideprevent/en/print.html.   Retrieved on March 6, 2014.

Wu KCC, Chen YY, Yip PSF (2012). Suicide methods in Asia: implications in suicide prevention. International Journal of Environmental Research and Public Health 9: 1135–1158.

Yee N (2006). Motivations for play in online games. Cyberpsychology and Behavior 9: 772–775.

SECTION II
OPPORTUNITIES

9 Psychoeducation and the Internet

Nicola J. Reavley and Anthony F. Jorm

INTRODUCTION

Current estimates suggest that more than 2.7 billion people have access to more than 860 million sites on the Internet (International Telecommunications Union, 2013; Netcraft, 2014). As many as 80% of Internet users in developed countries use the Internet to search for health information, typically seeking information on conditions, symptoms, diseases, and treatments (Shuyler and Knight, 2003; Pew Internet & American Life Project, 2011). Web-based information on psychiatric disorders is provided by governments, nonprofit organizations, corporations, and private individuals, and it is commonly accessed by those with a psychiatric diagnosis or their caregivers (Powell and Clarke, 2006; Ybarra and Suman, 2006; Khazaal et al., 2008a). Such information can typically be provided at little to no cost and for anyone with an Internet connection, the information is easily accessible and can be viewed anonymously, which may be important for those concerned about the stigma surrounding psychiatric disorders.

The relatively rapid increase in the amount of health information on the Internet has been closely followed by discussions about its quality and the impact that poor quality information might have on the health of those who access it. In the area of psychiatric disorders, poor quality information may increase the risk that someone who needs treatment might delay or avoid it, use inappropriate or ineffective treatments, or not adhere to treatment.

This chapter aims to outline the role of the Internet in the provision of psychoeducation in mental health. It seeks to explore the following questions:

- Is web-based information on psychiatric disorders of good quality?
- How can consumers be guided to better quality sites?
- Do quality information websites change knowledge, attitudes, and behavior?

The chapter is largely based on reviews of studies of web-based information on a range of psychiatric disorders, mainly those published in English (Reavley and Jorm, 2010). It also draws on studies that have attempted to assess the effectiveness of web-based psychoeducation interventions that typically cover information on signs and symptoms of mental illness, treatments, self-help behaviors, and where to seek help. These interventions may also incorporate skills training designed to reduce symptoms and promote healthy behaviors. This chapter focuses on the effectiveness of psychoeducation interventions in improving knowledge about mental health problems and behaviors that affect mental health, with a particular emphasis on interventions aimed at members of the general community, either because they are experiencing mental health problems themselves or are in contact with someone who is. It does not address interventions that aim to have a direct impact on symptoms of psychiatric disorders, such as Internet therapy (see Chapter 10); interventions accessed via clinical services; or universal prevention interventions, such as those carried out in schools and colleges.

IS WEB-BASED INFORMATION ON PSYCHIATRIC DISORDERS OF GOOD QUALITY? REVIEW OF RESEARCH
Methods of Assessing Quality

Since the late 1990s, researchers have conducted studies to assess the quality of web-based information on a wide range of health topics. Eysenbach et al. (2002) reviewed these studies and reported that 70% considered quality a problem. However, there is evidence that accuracy varies between health domains, with these authors noting that up to 90% of diet and nutrition information was unreliable compared to only 5% of the information on cancer.

There have been various methods of assessing information quality, with the early focus on accountability defined by Silberg et al. (1997) as including the following: authorship (authors, affiliations, and credentials clearly identified), attribution (sources and references mentioned), disclosure (ownership of the site and sponsorship disclosed), and currency (whether the site has been modified in the past month and year and whether the date the site was created or modified was specified). Since then, other assessment measures have been developed and, although these vary, most cover one or more of the following: accuracy, completeness, readability, accountability, and design and technical criteria (Jadad and Gagliardi, 1998; Eysenbach et al., 2002). The methods can be broadly divided into rating instruments to be used by experts, checklists that can be used by consumers (e.g., the DISCERN, a 16-item checklist designed to assist consumers in assessing the quality of health information; Charnock et al., 1999), codes of conduct or badges of quality that can be displayed on sites (e-Health Code of Ethics and the Health on the Net [HON] Foundation; Internet Healthcare Coalition, 2000; Health on the Net Foundation, 2010), and automated ratings (e.g., Google PageRank). Table 9.1 provides a description of rating methods.

A review of studies of the quality of web-based information on a range of psychiatric disorders found that there were variations in the methods used to assess website quality in terms of site selection and rating methods (Reavley and Jorm, 2010). Some studies assessed all available websites that met their criteria, which varied according to the study, whereas others limited their assessment to the top 10, 20, or 50 results given by common search engines.

A number of website quality studies also incorporate the development of rating instruments. In the studies described below, rating was most commonly done through expert assessment (with rating by two or more experts) or with the use of rating instruments. However, such instruments are rarely validated and many are used only once. Jadad and Gagliardi (1998) reviewed 47 Internet health information rating instruments, none of which provided information on the interobserver reliability and construct validity of the measurements. In a follow-up study, 98 instruments were identified; of 51 newly identified rating instruments, only 5 provided some information by which they could be evaluated and none were validated (Gagliardi and Jadad, 2002). This limits the ability to draw conclusions from such studies.

General Mental Health Information

Three studies assessed the overall quality of mental health information on the Internet. Nemoto et al. (2007) assessed the quality of Japanese language websites covering psychiatric disorders in 2005. They used the DISCERN and also assigned a global score. Their results showed that information on mood disorder, panic disorder, and schizophrenia was most common and concluded that the quality of information was mostly inadequate, especially regarding treatment.

In a study comparing user-contributed information about depression and schizophrenia on Wikipedia with centrally controlled online information sources, Encyclopaedia Britannica, and a psychiatry textbook, Reavley et al. (2012) assessed online content on 10 relevant topics from 14 frequently accessed websites (including Wikipedia). The content was rated by experts according to the following criteria: accuracy, up-to-dateness, breadth of coverage, referencing, and readability. The authors concluded that the quality of information on depression and schizophrenia on Wikipedia was generally as good as, or better than, that provided by centrally controlled websites, Encyclopaedia Britannica, and a psychiatry textbook.

In the most recent study, Grohol et al. (2014) reviewed the overall quality of mental health information searched for online. They used 11 common mental health terms and identified the first 20 search results of the search engines Google and Bing. The analysis included 440 web pages using the DISCERN instrument, an adaptation of the Depression Website Content Checklist, Flesch Reading Ease and Flesch-Kincaid Grade Level readability measures, HON Code badge display, and commercial status. Results showed that the information quality was higher for schizophrenia, bipolar disorder, and dysthymia, and lower for phobia, anxiety, and panic disorder websites. These researchers concluded that 67.5% of websites had

Table 9.1 Methods for Assessing Quality of Web-Based Information on Psychiatric Disorders

Rating Method	Description	Studies Using This Method
A. Validated checklists for use by nonexperts/consumers		
DISCERN	16-item checklist designed to assist consumers to assess the quality of health information (Charnock et al., 1999)	Griffiths et al. (2002); Griffiths and Christensen (2005); Serdobbel et al. (2006); Ipser et al. (2007); Nemoto et al. (2007); Akram et al. (2008); Khazaal et al. (2008b,c); Morel et al. (2008); Barnes et al. (2009); Zermatten et al. (2010); Thakor et al. (2011); Prusti et al. (2012); (Klila et al. 2013); Grohol et al. (2014)
Silberg score	9-item measure of accountability (Silberg et al., 1997)	Griffiths and Christensen (2000); Kisely et al. (2003); Murphy et al. (2004); Khazaal et al. (2008b,c,d,e); Morel et al. (2008); Zermatten et al. (2010); Klila et al. (2013)
Interactivity score	4-item measure of interactivity (including interactivity, audio or video support, supporting bodies, and the ability to send queries (Abbott, 2000)	Khazaal et al. (2008b,c,d,e); Morel et al. (2008); Zermatten et al. (2010); Klila et al. (2013)
Abbot esthetic criteria	4-item measure of esthetics (subheadings, diagrams, hyperlinks (Abbott, 2000)	Khazaal et al. (2008b,c.d,e); Morel et al. (2008); Zermatten et al. (2010); Klila et al. (2013)
Flesch reading ease score	Measure of readability (available through Microsoft Word)	Akram et al. (2008); Khazaal et al. (2008b,c.d.,e); Morel et al. (2008); Zermatten et al. (2010); Klila et al. (2013); Grohol et al. (2014)
Flesch-Kincaid reading grade education scores	Rates text based on US school years or grade levels (available through Microsoft Word)	Berland et al. (2001); Kisely et al. (2003); Khazaal et al. (2008b,c,d,e); Morel et al. (2008); Zermatten et al. (2010); Reavley et al. (2012); Klila et al. (2013); Grohol et al. (2014)
DARTS tool	5-item quality assessment tool (Narhi et al., 2008)	Prusti et al. (2012)

B. Rating instruments used by content experts

Global score

Standardized pro forma

Content quality scores

Bipolar Website Quality Checklist (BWQC)

Grounded theory methodology

Strathclyde Website Evaluation Form

Depression Website Content Checklist

Scoring form for the quality of websites about eating disorders

Christensen et al. (2000); Griffiths and Christensen (2000, 2005); Berland et al. (2001); Lissman and Boenhlein (2001); Griffiths et al. (2002); Murphy et al. (2004); Seomun et al. (2005); Bremner et al. (2006); Schrank et al. (2006); Ipser et al. (2007); Nemoto et al. (2007); Seyringer et al. (2007); Stjernsward and Ostman (2007); Touchet et al. (2007); Coquard et al. (2008); Ferreira-Lay and Miller (2008); Khazaal et al. (2008c, d); Faden et al. (2009); Barnes et al. (2009); Jorm et al. (2010); Zermatten et al. (2010); Moore and Ayers (2011); Perdaens and Pieters (2011); Smith et al. (2011); Reavley et al. (2012); Reichow et al. (2012b); Klila et al. (2013); Grohol et al. (2014)

C. Codes of conduct

HON Code

Health on the Net Foundation (2010)

Martin-Facklam et al. (2002); Khazaal et al. (2008b,c,d,e); Morel et al. (2008); Zermatten et al. (2010); Guardiola-Wanden-Berghe et al. (2011); Morgan and Montagne (2011); Klila et al. (2013); Grohol et al. (2014)

D. Automated assessment

Computer algorithm for the automated assessment of quality of evidence-based treatment information

Google page rank

Griffiths et al. (2005)

Griffiths and Christensen (2002, 2005); Serdobbel et al. (2006)

good or better quality content but that additional work needs to be done to make many of the sites more readable.

Depression

The largest number of studies—10—assessing the quality of online mental health information focused on depression (Christensen et al., 2000; Griffiths and Christensen, 2000, 2002, 2005; Berland et al., 2001; Lissman and Boehnlein, 2001; Griffiths et al., 2005; Stjernsward and Ostman, 2007; Ferreira-Lay and Miller, 2008; Zermatten et al., 2010). Methods of assessing quality varied, with the Silberg scale, which assesses accountability (Silberg et al., 1997), and the DISCERN (Charnock et al., 1999) being the most commonly used tools. The most recent study concluded that overall information quality was good (Zermatten et al., 2010), whereas studies conducted in earlier years were more likely to report overall poor quality (Griffiths and Christensen, 2000, 2002, 2005; Berland et al., 2001; Lissman and Boehnlein, 2001). There was some evidence of higher quality information from websites of government, professional, and charitable organizations (Lissman and Boehnlein, 2001; Ferreira-Lay and Miller, 2008).

Two studies assessed the quality of English and Finnish information on antidepressant drugs. Prusti et al. (2012) reported that no website provided information about all aspects of antidepressant treatment, but few provided incorrect information. The other study found that the sites WebMD and FamilyDoctor.org were of the highest quality, whereas pharmaceutical company sites were of lower quality (Morgan and Montagne, 2011).

Substance Use Disorders

Four studies assessed the quality of information on substance use disorders. They included studies of the French language information on alcohol dependence (Coquard et al., 2008, 2011), information on cannabis addiction (Khazaal et al., 2008c), and information on cocaine addiction (Khazaal et al., 2008d). All studies concluded that information quality was poor. Another study of the US college online alcohol policy information concluded that information accessibility had improved between 2002 and 2007 (Faden et al., 2009).

Bipolar Disorder

Three studies assessed quality of information on bipolar disorder, with two studies assessing English language information and concluding that the overall quality of information was good (Morel et al., 2008; Barnes et al., 2009). A study of German language information concluded that comprehensive information on the nature of the illness was more frequent in sites resulting from the search term "manic-depressive disorder," whereas the term "bipolar disorder" produced more results offering information on evidence-based therapeutic strategies (Seyringer et al., 2007).

Anxiety Disorders/Trauma

Five studies assessed information on anxiety disorders or trauma. These included information on a range of anxiety disorders (Ipser et al., 2007), social phobia (Khazaal et al., 2008e), and Dutch language information on obsessive-compulsive disorder (OCD) (Serdobbel et al., 2006). All studies concluded that quality was poor. In a more recent study, Klila et al. (2013) assessed the quality of information on OCD and concluded that this was relatively good.

Bremner et al. (2006) assessed the quality of websites related to the topic of psychological trauma. They concluded that such sites were often not useful and sometimes provided inaccurate and potentially harmful information.

Schizophrenia/Psychosis

Two studies assessed the quality of information on schizophrenia/psychosis. One assessed German websites and found that evidence-based medical information was provided by more than one-half of the sites resulting from the search term "schizophrenia" and by less than one-third of "psychosis" hits (Schrank et al., 2006). The other study, which assessed the quality of information on schizophrenia treatment, concluded that accountability, presentation, and readability were poor (Kisely et al., 2003).

Eating Disorders

Four studies assessed the quality of websites giving information on diet or eating disorders, with all reporting that the overall quality of information was of poor or variable quality and that websites did not adequately address diagnostic criteria or treatment options (Murphy et al., 2004; Guardiola-Wanden-Berghe et al., 2011; Perdaens and Pieters, 2011; Smith et al., 2011). Guardiola-Wanden-Berghe et al. (2010) assessed content quality and the relationship with authorship and/or affiliation in blogs covering the topic of eating disorders. Their results showed that indication of authorship (as opposed to anonymity) and affiliation to an institution were associated with higher quality.

Attention Deficit Hyperactivity Disorder

Two studies assessed the quality of information on attention deficit hyperactivity disorder (ADHD). Akram et al. (2008) concluded that the information was basic and incomplete and that websites by government and professional bodies were better than those in other categories. Kisely et al. (2003) reported that accountability, presentation, and readability were poor and that agreement with evidence-based practice was low. Sites scoring in the top 10% for quality were significantly more likely to be owned by an organization or have an editorial board than those in the bottom 10%.

Other Disorders and Treatments

Other studies have assessed the quality of information on pathological gambling (Khazaal et al., 2008b), female hypoactive sexual desire (Touchet et al., 2007), St. John's wort (Martin-Facklam et al., 2002; Thakor et al., 2011), postpartum mental health (Moore and Ayers, 2011), and dementia (Seomun et al., 2005). All studies reported that quality was generally poor. Reichow et al. (2012a) assessed the quality of information on autism, concluding that government websites were of higher quality than those offering a product or service.

Variation in Quality Across Mental Health Topics

Quality of information appears to be somewhat related to the topic. The highest quality information appears to be that relating to bipolar disorder, with two studies concluding that information was generally of good quality (Morel et al., 2008; Barnes et al., 2009). The most recent study of the quality of online depression information concluded that this was relatively good (Zermatten et al., 2010). However, information on other mental health topics was generally considered to be of poor quality.

Is Quality Improving?

Studies reviewing the quality of affective disorder information were carried out between 2000 and 2010. Although earlier studies generally concluded that information quality was poor, the four most recent studies, two of which assessed information on bipolar disorder, reported that the overall quality of website information was good (Ferreira-Lay and Miller, 2008; Morel et al., 2008; Barnes et al., 2009; Zermatten et al., 2010). Study methodology and quality indicators differed across the studies, but there is some evidence that information quality has been improving over time, particularly in the case of more frequently assessed topics.

Methods of Improving Quality

Despite the concerns about the quality of health information on the Internet, there is no clear agreement about the best way to improve this. Quality improvement methods include labeling and filtering information and the development of codes of conduct and seals of approval (Eysenbach and Diepgen, 1998; Wilson, 2002). Although some codes of conduct have been developed and graphic images denoting an award or approval seal appear on some websites, enforcement of breaches and the lack of consistent, universal, and well-recognized manner of indicating high-quality websites present barriers to implementation (Wilson, 2002). A number of other technological solutions have been proposed (e.g., the use of web browser encryption icons and automated quality assessments), but these also face significant barriers (Risk and Petersen, 2002; O'Grady, 2006).

In an attempt to assess the effect of feedback on website quality improvement, Jorm et al. (2010) assigned a score to 52 suicide prevention websites based on expert consensus guidelines. Administrators of half of the websites received feedback on how to improve the sites, and the other half did not receive such feedback. The feedback took the form of a letter headed "University of Melbourne Project to Evaluate and Improve Suicide Prevention Websites" and included a large university logo at the top to add authority. Websites were evaluated again 6 months later, and it was found that feedback did not lead to improvement.

HOW CAN CONSUMERS BE GUIDED TO BETTER QUALITY SITES?

As already noted, the Silberg scale (Silberg et al., 1997) and the DISCERN (Charnock et al., 1999) were the most commonly used quality assessment tools in the studies discussed above. However, evidence for links between scores on these instruments and overall site quality is mixed. In their assessments of depression sites, Griffiths and Christensen (2000) and Khazaal et al. (2008d) did not find significant associations between Silberg scores and site quality. In a recent study, Khazaal et al. (2012) concluded that the DISCERN was a good indicator of website quality. However, the DISCERN is designed to be used by consumers without content expertise and therefore does not assess scientific quality or accuracy of evidence.

Several studies investigated the links between site owner characteristics and content quality. Eight studies found that higher quality information came from websites of government, professional, or charitable organizations (Lissman and Boehnlein, 2001; Ipser et al., 2007; Akram et al., 2008; Ferreira-Lay and Miller, 2008; Barnes et al., 2009; Morgan and Montagne, 2011; Reichow et al., 2012a; Grohol et al., 2014), whereas six others found that site ownership did not predict quality (Khazaal et al., 2008b, 2008c, 2008d, 2008e; Morel et al., 2008; Klila et al., 2013). In general, characteristics associated with higher quality included government ownership, editorial boards, having information on a variety of mental health issues, having internal search engines, mentioning scientific evidence or citation of references, and an absence of financial interest. Sites by professional organizations tended to recommend one type of mental health care provider, thus limiting their quality scores to some extent. Khazaal et al. (2012) analyzed data from a number of studies and concluded that the HON label failed to predict website quality. Evidence of links between search engine page ranks and quality scores is mixed. Griffiths and Christensen (2005) assessed the links between evidence-based quality of content as measured by evidence-based depression guidelines and Google PageRank and concluded that these were correlated. Ipser et al. (2007) failed to find an association between Google PageRank and website quality, whereas Grohol et al. (2014) concluded that search engines' algorithms largely returned relevant, good quality mental health information.

A number of the studies listed the highest quality websites by topic area. Based on studies carried out since 2005, these websites are shown in Table 9.2. They can be used as a guide for consumers searching for high-quality information.

Table 9.2 Top-Rated Currently Available Websites for Psychiatric Disorders

General mental health information

Grohol et al., 2014

Help Guide.org	www.helpguide.org
Mayo Clinic	www.mayoclinic.org
National Institute of Mental Health	www.nimh.nih.gov
Psych Central	www.psychcentral.com
Wikipedia	www.wikipedia.org
WebMD	www.webmd.com
eMedicineHealth	www.eMedicineHealth.com
MedicineNet	www.medicinenet.com
WebMD	www.webmd.com

Reavley et al., 2012

Wikipedia	www.wikipedia.org
National Institute of Mental Health	www.nimh.nih.gov
WebMD	www.webmd.com

Depression

Morgan and Montagne, 2011

WebMD	www.webmd.com
FamilyDoctor.org	www.familydoctor.org

Zermatten et al., 2010

Medicinenet.com	http://www.medicinenet.com/depression/article.htm
Netdoctor.co.uk	http://www.netdoctor.co.uk/depression/index.shtml
The Royal College of Psychiatrists	http://www.rcpsych.ac.uk/default.aspx?page50

Ferreira-Lay and Miller, 2008

National Health Service (NHS)	www.nhs.uk/depression
National Institutes of Mental Health (NIMH)	www.nimh.nih.gov/health/publications/depression/complete-publication.shtml N2 10 71 www.nimh.nih.gov/publicat/depressionmenu.cfm www.nimh.nih.gov/medlineplus/depression.html
SANE	www.sane.org.uk/About___Mental___Illness/Depression.htm N3 10 66 www.sane.org.uk

Antidepressants

Morgan and Montagne, 2011

WebMD	www.WebMd.com
FamilyDoctor.org	www.FamilyDoctor.org

Bipolar disorder

Barnes et al., 2009

Black Dog Institute	www.blackdoginstitute.org.au
National Institutes of Mental Health (NIMH)	www.nimh.nih.gov
bipolar.about.com	www.bipolar.about.com

(continued)

Table 9.2 Continued

165

Psychoeducation and the Internet

Attention deficit hyperactivity disorder (ADHD)

Akram et al., 2008 (UK)

British Medical Journal Publishing Group Best Treatments	www.besttreatments.co.uk/btuk/conditions/10235.jsp
NHS Direct Health Encyclopaedia ADHD	www.nhsdirect.nhs.uk/articles/article. aspx?articleId=40 &sectionId=27010
Pharmaceutical company Janssen–Cilag Products	www.janssen-cilag.co.uk/bgdisplay. jhtml?itemname=parents_background_adhd&_ requestid=1343815&s=1

Suicide prevention

Jorm et al., 2010

Suicide.org	www.suicide.org
Suicideline	www.suicideline.org.au

Postpartum mental health

Sites for professionals (Moore and Ayers, 2011)

Postpartum.net	www.postpartum.net
Postpartum Health Alliance	www.postpartumhealthalliance.org
BabyBlues Connection	www.babybluesconnection.org
Postpartum Support	www.postpartumsupport.com
Postpartum Education and Support	www.postpartumeducationandsupport.com

Sites for mothers with postpartum mental illness (Moore and Ayers, 2011)

Post and Antenatal Depression Association	www.panda.org.au
Highland Antenatal and Postnatal Illness Support	www.hapis.org.uk
Postpartum Health Alliance	www.postpartumhealthalliance.org
Postpartum.net	www.postpartum.net
Post Natal Depression Support Association	www.pndsa.co.za

Autism

Reichow et al., 2012a

Wikipedia	www.wikipedia.org
Association for Science in Autism Treatment	www.asatonline.org
Johns Hopkins School of Public Health	www.jhsph.edu

DO QUALITY INFORMATION WEBSITES CHANGE KNOWLEDGE, ATTITUDES, AND BEHAVIOR?

Despite the considerable amount of mental health information on the Internet, relatively little is known about the links between information quality and health behaviors. It is largely unknown whether checklists such as DISCERN are useful to consumers and whether better quality information leads to better health outcomes

(Bernstam et al., 2005). Many of the studies discussed in this chapter use expert rating, and there is evidence that consumers are influenced by criteria that are different from those used by experts when evaluating information (Sillence et al., 2007; Harris et al., 2009). Thus, design features appear to play a significant part in assessment and consumers have been shown to reject clinically credible sites because of poor design (Harris et al., 2009). It is likely that readability is also important to consumers and, because many of the studies reviewed here found reading levels (based on US years of schooling or grade levels) to be relatively high, it is likely that mental health websites need to put a greater emphasis on simplicity and intelligibility. Perceived expertise and absence of bias are also relevant; for example, a consumer may mistrust a pharmaceutical company website that an expert may rate highly against evidence-based criteria (Sillence et al., 2007; Broom and Tovey, 2008). In a study of mental health-related Internet use, Lam-Po-Tang and McKay (2010) found that perceived reliability was not associated with perceived influence on health-related decision making.

Assessments of the effects of Internet information quality are further complicated by the fact that consumers typically use many sources of health information and effects may take a long time to develop. Evidence suggests that many of those who obtain information on the Internet discuss this with their health practitioners (Sillence et al., 2007; Lam-Po-Tang and McKay, 2010).

A growing number of studies have attempted to assess the impact of web-based psychoeducation interventions on knowledge and beliefs about psychiatric disorders and treatments. Web-based psychoeducation interventions typically cover information on signs and symptoms of mental illness, treatments, self-help behaviors, and where to seek help. They may also incorporate skills training designed to reduce symptoms and promote healthy behaviors. There is evidence that web-based psychoeducation interventions can improve mental health literacy, which has been defined as "knowledge and beliefs about mental disorders which aid their recognition, management, or prevention" (Jorm et al., 1997); a relatively small number of studies have shown impact on user behavior. However, longer term effects are unknown. A key issue to consider when assessing the impact of web-based interventions is whether these are supported by a clinician or appropriately trained nonprofessional or whether they are entirely automated; there is evidence that the addition of support leads to better outcomes (Richards and Richardson, 2012).

Depression and Anxiety Disorders

In one of the first randomized controlled trials to test the efficacy of web-based depression treatment, Christensen et al. (2004) assessed the impact of the mental health information website BluePages (www.bluepages.anu.edu.au) and the cognitive-behavioral therapy (CBT) skills training website MoodGYM (www.moodgym.anu.edu.au). Both users of BluePages and MoodGYM were contacted weekly by lay people to direct their use of the websites, including which sections to visit. They found that both sites improved knowledge of evidence-based treatments, including CBT. The effectiveness of MoodGYM in improving mental health literacy has been assessed in other studies, including a randomized controlled trial involving Norwegian university students with elevated psychological distress (Lintvedt et al., 2013). MoodGYM was effective in increasing depression literacy at the 2-month follow up. However, no benefits were seen in studies involving teenage males (O'Kearney et al., 2006) and teenage females (O'Kearney et al., 2009).

In a more recent study, 155 callers to Lifeline (a telephone counseling service) who met the criteria for moderate to high psychological distress, were randomly assigned to one of four conditions: (1) web CBT (MoodGYM and BluePages) plus weekly telephone tracking, (2) web CBT only, (3) weekly telephone tracking only, and (4) neither website nor telephone tracking (Farrer et al., 2012). Participants were assessed at preintervention, postintervention, and 6 and 12 months postintervention. Results showed that those in the web-only and web-plus–tracking conditions had significantly higher depression literacy at postintervention, and this was maintained in the Web-only condition at the 6-month follow-up point. No significant differences were found in depression literacy among all four conditions at 12 months.

In the context of the low rates of help seeking for mental health problems, an aim of some websites is to promote evidence-based treatments, many of which involve seeking professional help. In an attempt to assess the impact of web-based interventions on help seeking, 414 people with elevated scores on a depression assessment scale were randomly allocated to BluePages, MoodGYM, or an attention control condition (Christensen et al., 2006). Interviewers maintained weekly telephone contact with participants in all conditions over the period of the intervention (a total of six contacts of approximately 10 minutes each). Use of BluePages was associated with behavioral changes such as decreases in seeking support from friends and family and using everyday therapeutic measures (spending time with family and friends, exercising, eating chocolate, listening to music, being with pets, and doing more enjoyable things) but no increase in seeking evidence-based interventions. MoodGYM was associated with reports of help seeking for CBT, massage, and exercise. A follow-up study found these changes to be maintained over 12 months (Mackinnon et al., 2008).

A number of studies suggest that unsupported website use can have beneficial effects on mental health literacy. These include a web-based intervention (MIDonline: www.midonline.com.au), which has also been shown to improve mental health literacy relating to depression in Greek- and Italian-born immigrants (Kiropoulos et al., 2011). Deitz et al. (2009) assessed the effects of a web-based program (http://ymhonline.com/loginpage.asp) providing working parents with the knowledge and skills necessary for prevention and early intervention of mental health problems in young people. Those in the intervention group showed significantly greater knowledge about anxiety, depression, and treatment options.

Eating Disorders

StudentBodies is a program that targets women at risk for eating disorders by helping them improve their dietary practices, attitudes to the body, and body image satisfaction. It consists of eight structured weeks of readings and homework tasks (http://www.beyondblackboards.com/StudentBodies.aspx?). This program has been assessed in a number of trials, four of which involved women at high risk for eating disorders, and it has been shown to reduce eating disorder-related attitudes, especially negative body image and the desire to be thin (Beintner et al. 2012). There is some evidence that *StudentBodies* can also reduce disordered eating behaviors (Jacobi et al., 2012).

Mental Health First Aid and Caregiving Behaviors

Hart et al. (2012) conducted a study in which web users who downloaded mental health first aid guidelines from a website were invited to respond to an initial questionnaire and then, one month later, a follow-up questionnaire assessing their views on the usefulness of the documents and whether they had influenced behavior. Results showed that of 154 people who responded to the second questionnaire, 63 had provided first aid and 23 had sought care themselves. In another study, Berk et al. (2013) used the Delphi consensus method to develop a set of guidelines for caregivers of adults with bipolar disorder and then conducted an evaluation of the acceptability and usefulness of the online version of these guidelines. These authors found that at least 80% of users found the various sections of the website useful. Moreover, two-thirds of the caregivers reported using the information 1 month later.

Help Seeking for Mental Health Problems

Santor et al. (2007) examined the use and impact of a school-based health information website on high school students. Their results showed that female students, students wanting professional help, those scoring higher on depressive vulnerability measures, and students reporting more severe mood problems logged on frequently over longer periods of time, viewed information sheets, posted and viewed questions and answers, and completed the symptom screen. Visits to the website were positively associated with visits to school health centers and guidance counselors and referrals to a health professional.

Mental Health Game Websites

The popularity of computer games has led to the development of game websites that aim to improve mental health literacy. These are often targeted toward young people. *Reach Out Central* (http://roc.reachout.com.au/flash/index.html), an online gaming program designed to support the mental health of people aged 16 to 25 years, has been evaluated using a pre-post study design involving 266 young people (Shandley et al., 2010). Improvements in mental health literacy were seen postintervention. Li et al. (2013) evaluated the effectiveness of a fully automated, web-based, social network electronic game designed according to cognitive-behavioral approaches (https://apps.facebook.com/mentalhealthgame/)

in enhancing mental health knowledge. A pre-/post-test design was used, with 73 undergraduates self-assessing their mental health literacy before and after completing the game within a 3-week period. The study showed that the gaming approach was effective in enhancing young people's mental health literacy.

Summary

Research studies suggest that quality information websites can change knowledge, attitudes, and behavior to some extent, particularly for depression, which is one of the most frequently studied mental health problems. Studies have also shown benefits in eating disorder–related attitudes and behaviors, help seeking for mental health problems in school-age children, and mental health first aid behaviors. However, most studies have only assessed short-term effects and the longer term impact is unknown.

FUTURE RESEARCH DIRECTIONS

Although the speed of technology and program development means that there will be technologies and devices available in the future that we have difficulty predicting, it is likely that the area of electronic mental health as a whole will grow in importance. The recent move toward mobile phone–based interventions may have implications for web-based interventions, which may be superseded or may become adapted to particular functions (Jorm et al., 2013). Tailoring to an individual's needs is likely to increase the effectiveness of web-based interventions; this may be enhanced by further research on identifying consumers of mental health information on the Internet and on effects of this information on health behaviors such as help seeking and use of evidence-based treatments. The move toward greater interactivity, information sharing, and collaboration on the Internet (Web 2.0) may offer such opportunities.

There is also a need for greater evaluation of web-based psychoeducation interventions, because much of what is currently available has not been evaluated. One of the main goals of health education is behavioral change; therefore, it can be argued that the extent to which a web-based intervention applies recognized behavior change theories is an indicator of quality. Mental health website quality assessment can be extended to cover the extent to which sites meet the evaluation criteria arising out of such a framework and may include naturalistic reports of user behavior (Sillence et al., 2007; Frost et al., 2008). This may involve the development of innovative ways of assessing health-related behaviors and outcomes, which new technologies can support and enable.

CONCLUSION

In conclusion, the evidence suggests that the quality of mental disorder information on the Internet is variable and can depend on the topic in question, with information on bipolar disorder and depression generally being of higher quality. Information quality appears to be improving over time, particularly for more frequently assessed topics such as depression. However, despite the concerns about the quality of health information on the Internet, there is no clear agreement on the best way to improve this; the methods that have been tried, including labeling and codes of conduct, have shown mixed results.

A number of studies have assessed the characteristics of higher quality sites. These studies suggest that, in general, consumers wishing to find better quality sites should look for those that are government owned, have editorial boards, have information on a variety of mental health issues, have internal search engines, mention scientific evidence or citation of references, and have an absence of financial interest.

There is some evidence that quality information websites can change knowledge, attitudes, and behavior to some extent, particularly for depression. Studies have also shown benefits in eating disorder–related attitudes and behaviors, help seeking for mental health problems in school-age children, and mental health first aid and caregiving behaviors. However, there is a need for greater evaluation of web-based psychoeducation interventions, because much of what is currently available has not been formally assessed, particularly over the longer term. Given the rapid pace of technological change, such evaluation is likely to involve new technologies and those that are yet to be invented.

DISCLOSURE STATEMENT

The authors disclose no relationships with commercial entities and professional activities that may bias their views.

REFERENCES

Abbott VP (2000). Web page quality: can we measure it and what do we find? A report of exploratory findings. Journal of Public Health Medicine 22: 191–197.

Akram G, Thomson AH, Boyter AC, Morton MJ (2008). Characterisation and evaluation of UK websites on attention deficit hyperactivity disorder. Archives of Disease in Childhood 93: 695–700.

Barnes C, Harvey R, Wilde A, et al (2009). Review of the quality of information on bipolar disorder on the Internet. Australian and New Zealand Journal of Psychiatry 43: 934–945.

Beintner I, Jacobi C, Taylor CB (2012). Effects of an Internet-based prevention programme for eating disorders in the USA and Germany—a meta-analytic review. European Eating Disorders Revew 20: 1–8.

Berk L, Berk M, Dodd S, et al (2013). Evaluation of the acceptability and usefulness of an information website for caregivers of people with bipolar disorder. BMC Medicine 11: 162.

Berland GK, Elliott MN, Morales LS, et al (2001). Health information on the Internet: accessibility, quality, and readability in English and Spanish. Journal of the American Medical Association 285: 2612–2621.

Bernstam EV, Shelton DM, Walji M, Meric-Bernstam F (2005). Instruments to assess the quality of health information on the World Wide Web: what can our patients actually use? International Journal of Medical Informatics 74: 13–19.

Bremner JD, Quinn J, Quinn W, Veledar E (2006). Surfing the net for medical information about psychological trauma: an empirical study of the quality and accuracy of trauma-related websites. Medical Informatics and the Internet in Medicine 31: 227–236.

Broom A, Tovey P (2008). The role of the Internet in cancer patients' engagement with complementary and alternative treatments. Health (London) 12: 139–155.

Charnock D, Shepperd S, Needham G, Gann R (1999). DISCERN: an instrument for judging the quality of written consumer health information on treatment choices. Journal of Epidemiology and Community Health 53: 105–111.

Christensen H, Griffiths KM, Jorm AF (2004). Delivering interventions for depression by using the Internet: randomised controlled trial. British Medical Journal 328: 265.

Christensen H, Griffiths KM, Medway J (2000). Sites for depression on the web: a comparison of consumer, professional and commercial sites. Australian and New Zealand Journal of Public Health 24: 396–400.

Christensen H, Leach LS, Barney L, Mackinnon AJ, Griffiths KM (2006). The effect of web based depression interventions on self reported help seeking: randomised controlled trial. BMC Psychiatry 6: 13.

Coquard O, Fernandez S, Khazaal Y (2008). Assessing the quality of French language web sites pertaining to alcohol dependency. Sante Mentale au Quebec 33: 207–224.

Coquard O, Fernandez S, Zullino D, Khazaal Y (2011). A follow-up study on the quality of alcohol dependence-related information on the web. Substance Abuse Treatment, Prevention and Policy 6: 13.

Deitz DK, Cook RF, Billings DW, Hendrickson A (2009). A web-based mental health program: reaching parents at work. Journal of Pediatric Psychology 34: 488–494.

Eysenbach G, Diepgen TL (1998). Towards quality management of medical information on the Internet: evaluation, labelling, and filtering of information. British Medical Journal 317: 1496–1500.

Eysenbach G, Powell J, Kuss O, Sa ER (2002). Empirical studies assessing the quality of health information for consumers on the world wide web: a systematic review. Journal of the American Medical Association 287: 2691–2700.

Faden VB, Corey K, Baskin M (2009). An evaluation of college online alcohol-policy information: 2007 compared with 2002. Journal of Studies on Alcohol and Drugs Suppl: 28–33.

Farrer L, Christensen H, Griffiths KM, Mackinnon A (2012). Web-based cognitive behavior therapy for depression with and without telephone tracking in a national helpline: secondary outcomes from a randomized controlled trial. Journal of Medical Internet Research 14: e68.

Ferreira-Lay P, Miller S (2008). The quality of Internet information on depression for lay people. Psychiatric Bulletin 32: 170–173.

Frost JH, Massagli MP, Wicks P, Heywood J (2008). How the social web supports patient experimentation with a new therapy: the demand for patient-controlled and patient-centered informatics. AMIA Annual Symposium Proceedings: 217–221.

Gagliardi A, Jadad AR (2002). Examination of instruments used to rate quality of health information on the Internet: chronicle of a voyage with an unclear destination. British Medical Journal 324: 569–573.

Griffiths KM, Christensen H (2000). Quality of web based information on treatment of depression: cross sectional survey. British Medical Journal 321: 1511–1515.

Griffiths KM, Christensen H (2002). The quality and accessibility of Australian depression sites on the World Wide Web. Medical Journal of Australia 176(Suppl): S97–S104.

Griffiths KM, Christensen H (2005). Website quality indicators for consumers. Journal of Medical Internet Research 7: e55.

Griffiths KM, Tang TT, Hawking D, Christensen H (2005). Automated assessment of the quality of depression websites. Journal of Medical Internet Research 7: e59.

Grohol JM, Slimowicz J, Granda R (2014). The quality of mental health information commonly searched for on the Internet. Cyberpsychology, Behavior, and Social Networking 17: 216–221.

Guardiola-Wanden-Berghe R, Gil-Perez JD, Sanz-Valero J, Wanden-Berghe C (2011). Evaluating the quality of websites relating to diet and eating disorders. Health Information & Libraries Journal 28: 294–301.

Guardiola-Wanden-Berghe R, Sanz-Valero J, Wanden-Berghe C (2010). Eating disorders blogs: testing the quality of information on the Internet. Eating Disorders 18: 148–152.

Harris PR, Sillence E, Briggs P (2009). The effect of credibility-related design cues on responses to a web-based message about the breast cancer risks from alcohol: randomized controlled trial. Journal of Medical Internet Research 11: e37.

Hart LM, Jorm AF, Paxton SJ, Cvetkovski S (2012). Mental health first aid guidelines: an evaluation of impact following download from the World Wide Web. Early Intervention in Psychiatry 6: 399–406.

Health on the Net Foundation (2010). Health on the Net Foundation code of conduct (HONcode). Available at http://www.hon.ch/HONcode/Pro/intro.html. Retrieved on April 10, 2010.

International Telecommunications Union (2013). The world in 2013: ICT facts and figures. Available at http://www.itu.int/en/ITU-D/Statistics/Pages/stat/default.aspx. Retrieved on March 7, 2014.

Internet Healthcare Coalition (2000). e-Health code of ethics (May 24). Journal of Medical Internet Research 2: e9.

Ipser JC, Dewing S, Stein DJ (2007). A systematic review of the quality of information on the treatment of anxiety disorders on the Internet. Current Psychiatry Reports 9: 303–309.

Jacobi C, Volker U, Trockel MT, Taylor CB (2012). Effects of an Internet-based intervention for subthreshold eating disorders: a randomized controlled trial. Behaviour Research and Therapy 50: 93–99.

Jadad AR, Gagliardi A (1998). Rating health information on the Internet. Navigating to knowledge or to Babel? Journal of the American Medical Association 279: 611–614.

Jorm AF, Fischer JA, Oh E (2010). Effect of feedback on the quality of suicide prevention websites: randomised controlled trial. British Journal of Psychiatry 197: 73–74.

Jorm AF, Korten AE, Jacomb PA, et al (1997). "Mental health literacy": a survey of the public's ability to recognise mental disorders and their beliefs about the effectiveness of treatment. Medical Journal of Australia 166: 182–186.

Jorm AF, Morgan AJ, Malhi GS (2013). The future of e-mental health. Australian and New Zealand Journal of Psychiatry 47: 104–106.

Khazaal Y, Chatton A, Cochand S, et al (2008a). Internet use by patients with psychiatric disorders in search for general and medical information. Psychiatric Quarterly 79: 301–309.

Khazaal Y, Chatton A, Cochand S, et al (2008b). Quality of web-based information on pathological gambling. Journal of Gambling Studies 24: 357–366.

Khazaal Y, Chatton A, Cochand S, Zullino D (2008c). Quality of web-based information on cannabis addiction. Journal of Drug Education 38: 97–107.

Khazaal Y, Chatton A, Cochand S, Zullino D (2008d). Quality of web-based information on cocaine addiction. Patient Education and Counseling 72: 336–341.

Khazaal Y, Chatton A, Zullino D, Khan R (2012). HON label and DISCERN as content quality indicators of health-related websites. Psychiatric Quarterly 83: 15–27.

Khazaal Y, Fernandez S, Cochand S, Reboh I, Zullino D (2008e). Quality of web-based information on social phobia: a cross-sectional study. Depression and Anxiety 25: 461–465.

Kiropoulos LA, Griffiths KM, Blashki G (2011). Effects of a multilingual information website intervention on the levels of depression literacy and depression-related stigma in Greek-born and Italian-born immigrants living in Australia: a randomized controlled trial. Journal of Medical Internet Research 13: e34.

Kisely S, Ong G, Takyar A (2003). A survey of the quality of web based information on the treatment of schizophrenia and attention deficit hyperactivity disorder. Australian and New Zealand Journal of Psychiatry 37: 85–91.

Klila H, Chatton A, Zermatten A, et al (2013). Quality of web-based information on obsessive compulsive disorder. Neuropsychiatric Disease and Treatment 9: 1717–1723.

Lam-Po-Tang J, McKay D (2010). Dr Google, MD: a survey of mental health-related Internet use in a private practice sample. Australasian Psychiatry 18: 130–133.

Li TM, Chau M, Wong PW, Lai ES, Yip PS (2013). Evaluation of a web-based social network electronic game in enhancing mental health literacy for young people. Journal of Medical Internet Research 15: e80.

Lintvedt OK, Griffiths KM, Sorensen K, et al (2013). Evaluating the effectiveness and efficacy of unguided Internet-based self-help intervention for the prevention of depression: a randomized controlled trial. Clinical Psychology and Psychotherapy 20: 10–27.

Lissman TL, Boehnlein JK (2001). A critical review of Internet information about depression. Psychiatric Services 52: 1046–1050.

Mackinnon A, Griffiths KM, Christensen H (2008). Comparative randomised trial of online cognitive-behavioural therapy and an information website for depression: 12-month outcomes. British Journal of Psychiatry 192: 130–134.

Martin-Facklam M, Kostrzewa M, Schubert F, Gasse C, Haefeli WE (2002). Quality markers of drug information on the Internet: an evaluation of sites about St. John's wort. American Journal of Medicine 113: 740–745.

Moore D, Ayers S (2011). A review of postnatal mental health websites: help for healthcare professionals and patients. Archives of Women's Mental Health 14: 443–452.

Morel V, Chatton A, Cochand S, Zullino D, Khazaal Y (2008). Quality of web-based information on bipolar disorder. Journal of Affective Disorders 110: 265–269.

Morgan M, Montagne M (2011). Drugs on the Internet, part II: antidepressant medication web sites. Substance Use and Misuse 46: 1628–1641.

Murphy R, Frost S, Webster P, Schmidt U (2004). An evaluation of web-based information. International Journal of Eating Disorders 35: 145–154.

Narhi U, Pohjanoksa-Mantyla M, Karjalainen A, et al (2008). The DARTS tool for assessing online medicines information. Pharmacy World and Science 30: 898–906.

Nemoto K, Tachikawa H, Sodeyama N, et al (2007). Quality of Internet information referring to mental health and mental disorders in Japan. Psychiatry and Clinical Neurosciences 61: 243–248.

Netcraft (2014). December 2013 web server survey. Available at www.netcraft.com. Retrieved on January 6, 2014.

O'Grady L (2006). Future directions for depicting credibility in health care web sites. International Journal of Medical Informatics 75: 58–65.

O'Kearney R, Gibson M, Christensen H, Griffiths KM (2006). Effects of a cognitive-behavioural Internet program on depression, vulnerability to depression and stigma in adolescent males: a school-based controlled trial. Cognitive Behaviour Therapy 35: 43–54.

O'Kearney R, Kang K, Christensen H, Griffiths K (2009). A controlled trial of a school-based Internet program for reducing depressive symptoms in adolescent girls. Depression and Anxiety 26: 65–72.

Perdaens S, Pieters G (2011). Eating disorders on the Internet. A review of the quality of Dutch websites. Tijdschrift voor Psychiatrie 53: 695–703.

Pew Internet & American Life Project (2011). Health topics. Pew Internet, Washington, DC. Available at http://www.pewinternet.org/Reports/2011/HealthTopics.aspx. Retrieved on February 5, 2014.

Powell J, Clarke A (2006). Internet information-seeking in mental health: population survey. British Journal of Psychiatry 189: 273–277.

Prusti M, Lehtineva S, Pohjanoksa-Mantyla M, Bell JS (2012). The quality of online antidepressant drug information: an evaluation of English and Finnish language web sites. Research in Social and Administrative Pharmacy 8: 263–268.

Reavley NJ, Jorm AF (2010). The quality of mental disorder information websites: a review. Patient Education and Counseling 85: e16–25.

Reavley NJ, Mackinnon AJ, Morgan AJ, et al (2012). Quality of information sources about mental disorders: a comparison of Wikipedia with centrally controlled web and printed sources. Psychological Medicine 42: 1753–1762.

Reichow B, Halpern JI, Steinhoff TB, et al (2012a). Characteristics and quality of autism websites. Journal of Autism and Developmental Disorders 42: 1263–1274.

Reichow B, Naples A, Steinhoff T, Halpern J, Volkmar FR (2012b). Brief report: consistency of search engine rankings for autism websites. Journal of Autism and Developmental Disorders 42: 1275–1279.

Richards D, Richardson T (2012). Computer-based psychological treatments for depression: a systematic review and meta-analysis. Clinical Psychology Review 32: 329–342.

Risk A, Petersen C (2002). Health information on the Internet: quality issues and international initiatives. Journal of the American Medical Association 287: 2713–2715.

Santor DA, Poulin C, LeBlanc JC, Kusumakar V (2007). Online health promotion, early identification of difficulties, and help seeking in young people. Journal of the American Academy of Child and Adolescent Psychiatry 46: 50–59.

Schrank B, Seyringer ME, Berger P, Katschnig H, Amering M (2006). Schizophrenia and psychosis on the Internet. Psychiatrische Praxis 33: 277–281.

Seomun GA, Lee SJ, Chang SO, Lee SJ (2005). An evaluation study of dementia information providing websites in Korea [in Korean]. Taehan Kanho Hakhoe Chi 35: 631–640.

Serdobbel Y, Pieters G, Joos S (2006). Obsessive compulsive disorder and the Internet. An evaluation of Dutch-language websites and quality indicators. Tijdschrift voor Psychiatrie 48: 763–773.

Seyringer ME, Schrank B, Berger P, Katschnig H, Amering M (2007). Bipolar disorder and manic-depressive disorder on the Internet. Neuropsychiatrie 21: 172–178.

Shandley K, Austin D, Klein B, Kyrios M (2010). An evaluation of "Reach Out Central": an online gaming program for supporting the mental health of young people. Health Education Research 25: 563–574.

Shuyler KS, Knight KM (2003). What are patients seeking when they turn to the Internet? Qualitative content analysis of questions asked by visitors to an orthopaedics Web site. Journal of Medical Internet Research 5: e24.

Silberg WM, Lundberg GD, Musacchio RA (1997). Assessing, controlling, and assuring the quality of medical information on the Internet: Caveant lector et viewor—Let the reader and viewer beware. Journal of the American Medical Association 277: 1244–1245.

Sillence E, Briggs P, Harris PR, Fishwick L (2007). How do patients evaluate and make use of online health information? Social Science and Medicine 64: 1853–1862.

Smith AT, Kelly-Weeder S, Engel J, et al (2011). Quality of eating disorders websites: what adolescents and their families need to know. Journal of Child and Adolescent Psychiatric Nursing 24: 33–37.

Stjernsward S, Ostman M (2007). Depression, e-health and family support. What the Internet offers the relatives of depressed persons. Nordic Journal of Psychiatry 61: 12–18.

Thakor V, Leach MJ, Gillham D, Esterman A (2011). The quality of information on websites selling St. John's wort. Complementary Therapies in Medicine 19: 155–160.

Touchet BK, Warnock JK, Yates WR, Wilkins KM (2007). Evaluating the quality of websites offering information on female hypoactive sexual desire disorder. Journal of Sex and Marital Therapy 33: 329–342.

Wilson P (2002). How to find the good and avoid the bad or ugly: a short guide to tools for rating quality of health information on the Internet. British Medical Journal 324: 598–602.

Ybarra ML, Suman M (2006). Help seeking behavior and the Internet: a national survey. International Journal of Medical Informatics 75: 29–41.

Zermatten A, Khazaal Y, Coquard O, Chatton A, Bondolfi G (2010). Quality of web-based information on depression. Depression and Anxiety 27: 852–858.

10 Internet-Based Psychotherapy

Gerhard Andersson

INTRODUCTION

Modern technology is being incorporated in health care contexts—from the increasingly popular electronic medical records to more recent experimental applications, such as remote monitoring of medication adherence via smartphone (Warmerdam et al., 2012). Although some of these developments are noticeable to all who deliver mental health care, it is probably less well known that a parallel development has occurred when it comes to the delivery of psychological treatment itself, particularly the delivery of psychotherapy via the Internet (Andersson, 2014a). Clinicians may have used text messaging or e-mail with their clients or perhaps even conducted a web conference over Skype, but it is less likely that they have used structured online treatment programs or are knowledgeable about them. This chapter introduces this new and growing research and treatment platform.

To set the scope of the discussion, it helps to distinguish Internet-based psychotherapy from other online treatments or information pursuit activities. A first distinction is between Internet-based psychotherapy and the provision of information in the form of psychoeducation (see Chapter 9). There are countless websites that passively offer visitors information and advice. Those cannot be regarded as psychotherapy even if they are used as adjuncts to other treatments, including psychotherapy, and even if they lead to some benefits in some individuals at little or no cost (Donker et al., 2009).

A second distinction relates to differences in technological complexity, interactivity, and adaptability among platforms. Online therapy programs vary greatly in technological complexity. A particularly technology-heavy therapy format is virtual reality (see Chapter 12), which for long was too expensive for broad Internet delivery but whose costs are gradually decreasing (Emmelkamp, 2005). On the opposite end of the technology and cost continuum are the old text-based interventions (i.e., self-help books), which are commonly referred to as bibliotherapy (Watkins, 2008). The Internet can be used to present those books online in a rather linear format, sometimes with relatively minor additions, such as interactive elements, pictures, or film and audio files. This form of online therapy has been the most investigated (Andersson and Titov, 2014) and constitutes the bulk of the studies presented here.

The definition of Internet-delivered therapy in this chapter includes the role of the guiding therapist and describes the treatment as "a therapy that is based on self-help books, guided by an identified therapist who gives feedback and answers to questions, with a scheduling that mirrors face-to-face treatment, and which also can include interactive online features such as queries to obtain passwords in order to get access to treatment modules" (Andersson et al., 2008a, p. 164). This definition underscores the role of the therapist, whereas the technology platform is somewhat deemphasized, because programs vary widely in their technology features and level of interactivity. The amount of treatment information provided may also vary, ranging from short one-chapter texts (Christensen et al., 2006) to complete books of nearly 200 pages (Andersson et al., 2006). The information, however, can be adaptable and tailored to the patient's needs, expanding or shrinking as clinically indicated and as broadband access permits, and with possible inclusion of pictures, online lectures, or film and audio clips.

A third distinction from other treatment delivery reflects a long-standing question in the Internet-delivered psychotherapy literature about the amount of contact between clinician and patient during assessment and treatment. Computerized cognitive-behavioral therapy (CBT) programs were available even before the arrival of the Internet (e.g., Marks et al., 1998), often in the form of CD-ROMs. Those often required patients to arrive at the clinic at set times to participate in the computerized program. More sophisticated fully automated versions exist today (see Chapter 11); they require no clinician contact and can be administered remotely, either via CD or Internet. These programs, however, tend to be less effective than guided Internet therapy programs (Titov et al., 2008; Berger et al., 2011; Johansson and Andersson, 2012) that incorporate interactions with a therapist, and they usually generate higher dropout rates (Melville et al., 2010). As this chapter will show, even minimal weekly clinician contact to provide encouragement and feedback on homework assignments seems to boost results and promote program adherence (Palmqvist et al., 2007).

There is another form of Internet-based psychotherapy in which the contact is provided in the form of a live chat unfolding in real time with full therapist involvement (Kessler et al., 2009) and with or without face-to-face communication via webcam (Storch et al., 2011). Thus, Internet-based psychotherapy can be either nonguided, guided with minimal therapist contact, or provided in real time with full therapist involvement as it would be in traditional or telephone-based psychotherapy. This chapter focuses mainly on guided, Internet-based psychotherapy (in particular, Internet-guided CBT or ICBT) in which limited therapist support is offered. Unguided programs are addressed elsewhere (see Chapter 11). Real-time treatments are only briefly discussed because they do not require a standardized treatment program per se and can be very close to regular face-to-face therapy. There is also much less research on real-time delivery of Internet treatments, but a literature on other forms of online counseling does exist (Richards and Vigano, 2013). The following sections will (1) introduce guided Internet-based psychotherapy; (2) review the role of the guiding clinician; (3) describe efficacy and effectiveness; (4) highlight what is known about outcome mediators; and (5) discuss future trends in the field, including blended treatments.

HOW IS THE INTERNET USED IN GUIDED INTERNET-BASED PSYCHOTHERAPY?

The first component of Internet-based psychotherapy is the assessment. Patients and research participants who think they may benefit can register for treatment or a research study online, and self-report measures need to be complemented by a structured diagnostic interview (e.g., Sheehan et al., 1998). In clinical implementations of Internet treatment, the initial diagnostic interview is often conducted face-to-face in the therapist's office (Andersson and Hedman, 2013). However, in research studies, diagnostic interviews have typically been conducted via telephone so as not to require the subjects to travel (Cacciola et al., 1999). It is important to emphasize that questionnaire-derived diagnoses do not replace the need for a comprehensive diagnostic interview (Carlbring et al., 2002). As for online administration of self-report questionnaires, it is now well established that it performs equally well or better than paper-and-pencil administration (primarily because the problem of missing items can be avoided in Internet administration) (Carlbring et al., 2007; Hedman et al., 2010; Holländare et al., 2010). However, some "offline" questionnaires may require new validation and psychometric testing for reliable administration online (Buchanan, 2003). Whether questionnaires are administered online or in a paper-and-pencil format, it is important to adhere to the same format throughout the intervention (Carlbring et al., 2007). An advantage of online administration of outcome measures is that weekly administration can be linked to obtaining access to the next treatment step, which is good for research in which the therapy process is investigated (Ljótsson et al., 2013). In terms of patient safety, weekly monitoring is important; any deterioration in the patient's condition can be detected promptly and managed appropriately.

To protect privacy and the confidentiality of patient records, Internet-based psychotherapy should be conducted in secure, closed contact management systems (Bennett et al., 2010). Such systems often resemble the procedures used for sensitive online financial transactions, with encryption and double authentication required at login. This can reduce the probability of identity theft by demanding a personal password to log in and also a unique single-use password that is sent automatically to the person's mobile phone. All communication with the patient, including the collection of completed homework and the delivery of feedback, is then held within the closed system and not the patient's or therapist's personal e-mail or texting platform. If e-mail or text messages have to be used, they should be crafted in a way to cause no harm if they were read by an unauthorized person. Finally, the security systems should be continuously updated with frequent upgrades to meet the latest security requirements.

After securely logging in, patients or study subjects can access the actual treatment content. Many Internet treatments are adaptations of self-help books, even if the Internet format allows flexibility that is not possible in books (Andersson et al., 2009a). For example, a self-help text can be presented online in a condensed, easy-to-read version that is expandable if the client wants to read more. Like evidence-based "manualized" psychotherapies, the treatment program content is organized into "lessons" or "modules." Thus, programs often start with psycho-education, followed by specific interventions based on the diagnosis and symptom-atology (e.g., behavioral activation for depression, exposure for anxiety disorders, stress management, mindfulness, problem solving). The general structure is to present information about the treatment technique for the week (e.g., interoceptive exposure exercises in the treatment of panic disorder), then discuss how the technique might apply in real life (how practice can lead to decreased anxiety), and finally assign homework (to be turned in later and commented on by the guiding therapist). More content, such as case examples, information on hurdles to expect, quizzes on the content, and film or audio files may also be included. Programs vary in their level of interactivity, and features, such as the ability to build one's own personalized model for social anxiety, are included in some. The duration of treatment programs is usually short—8 to 15 weeks. A deadline for completion and a post-treatment follow-up interview are set before the program begins (Andersson et al., 2013b), which seems to encourage adherence and prevent dropout (Nordin et al., 2010). The final module typically includes advice on relapse prevention. "Booster" modules are sometimes included as well.

The self-help materials mostly consist of text and should be engaging and easy to read by the average user, and they should convey empathy (Richardson et al., 2010). This can be achieved via a clear style that interacts with the reader, the use of case examples, and the reliance on the therapist's clinical experience as gleaned from traditional therapy situations. For example, a representative segment from a depression text might read: "Many persons who suffer from depression become passive and withdrawn. But there are also exceptions where instead, the person may become irritable and stressed. Indeed, we know that some of you who are reading this may recognize this emotion from the experience of being stressed at work. The stress that sometimes accompanies depression may feel like a magnified version of that emotion."

Like "manualized" psychotherapies, Internet treatments are informed by psychological theories, even if the content of Internet treatments is more controlled (i.e., the text does not change from patient to patient, whereas a therapist may be more likely to diverge from a treatment manual) (Waller, 2009). Most Internet treatments are based on CBT, with some being more behaviorally oriented, some more based on a cognitive approach, and some offering a mix. In addition to the predominant CBT orientation, a few Internet treatment programs are based on acceptance and commitment therapy (Buhrman et al., 2013), interpersonal psychotherapy (Dagöö et al., 2014), mindfulness (Boettcher et al., 2014a), and psychodynamic psychotherapy (Andersson et al., 2012c; Johansson et al., 2012a). More recently, Internet treatments have been developed based on information processing paradigms such as attention training (Boettcher et al., 2013a), but these are different in that they rely more on pictures and reaction times, rather than text.

Internet psychotherapy programs have been developed and tested in several psychiatric disorders (Hedman et al., 2012b) and in some physical conditions as well, including tinnitus (Andersson et al., 2002), diabetes (van Bastelaar et al., 2011), chronic pain (Buhrman et al., 2004), and irritable bowel syndrome (Ljótsson et al., 2011). In the field of mental health, several programs that target specific disorders are available and will be discussed in the next sections. Transdiagnostic approaches, where treatment ingredients that are shared between treatment protocols are used for different disorders, have also been developed. For example, a patient with panic disorder and another with major depressive disorder may share the symptoms of "stress" and insomnia, both of which can be treated with ICBT (Carlbring et al., 2010; Johansson et al., 2012b). Another approach to transdiagnostic ICBT focuses on common features of CBT (e.g., cognitive restructuring that may apply across several symptoms and diagnoses), and there is the option of accessing additional treatment material (Titov et al., 2011). Tailored treatment builds on the idea that it is possible to tailor treatment content according to the specific symptoms and regardless of the exact diagnosis; in this case, each patient receives different treatment.

THE ROLE OF THE THERAPIST

The roles of the therapist and his or her level of experience are undeniably important in face-to-face psychotherapy (Fairburn and Cooper, 2011) but probably less crucial in Internet-based psychotherapy, where most of the treatment lies in the program (mostly text, but also any accompanying features such as video and audio files). In Internet-based psychotherapy with minimal guidance, the role of the therapist is mainly to provide support and encouragement (Sanchez-Ortiz et al., 2011b). Perhaps surprisingly to some, who the therapist is appears to have a very small or nonexistent effect when studied (Almlöv et al., 2009, 2011). In other words, the variance explained by the therapist factor is very small, and much smaller than the usual 5% found in studies of face-to-face psychotherapy (Wampold and Brown, 2005). But that is not to say that what the guiding/supportive therapist writes in the feedback given to patients is irrelevant. In a study of ICBT involving 44 subjects with generalized anxiety disorder (GAD), 490 e-mails from three therapists were analyzed, and a lenient attitude toward homework assignments was found to be associated with a worse treatment outcome (Paxling et al., 2013). Thus, the role of the therapist cannot be completely dismissed, and a poor patient-therapist match may have negative consequences. Still, a series of studies by Titov and others have shown that the guidance provided can be mainly "technical" and practical and that specific therapy skills may not be necessary (Titov et al., 2009a, 2010a; Robinson et al., 2010). This opens up the possibility of scaling up Internet interventions; lay people could potentially be recruited to offer support and guidance, provided that adequate supervision and back-up are available from skilled clinicians (Andersson and Titov, 2014).

However, many psychotherapy researchers argue that the therapeutic alliance between therapist and patient is a determining factor for therapy success (e.g., Wampold, 2001). Therapeutic alliance has been assessed in Internet intervention studies; although high ratings of alliance are generally provided by patients, they do not tend to be associated with outcome (Sucala et al., 2012), even if exceptions do exist (Wagner et al., 2012a; Bergman Nordgren et al., 2013). In the largest study, 49 depressed subjects, 35 with GAD, and 90 with social anxiety disorder completed the Working Alliance Inventory early in the treatment. The results did not show any significant associations between patient-therapist alliance and subsequent outcome (Andersson et al., 2012d).

TREATMENT OUTCOMES IN RANDOMIZED CONTROLLED TRIALS
Major Depression and Depressive Symptoms

There is a rather large literature (Johansson and Andersson, 2012) on the use of ICBT in 6- to 15-week programs to treat depression. Several meta-analyses have focused on many types of computerized or online interventions and have not isolated Internet studies (Andersson and Cuijpers, 2009; Richards and Richardson, 2012). However, a review of Internet-delivered treatments only in which there was contact with a clinician and including a total of 25 controlled trials with 5509 participants found a between-group effect size of Cohen's d of 0.76 (Johansson and Andersson, 2012). The studies covered by the review constituted a range of CBT interventions (e.g., problem-solving therapy) within the broad category of Internet-delivered therapy with minimal therapist guidance. For comparison purposes, the between-group effect size in the nine studies where there was no therapist contact was much smaller (Cohen's $d = 0.21$) and clearly inferior to what is usually found in regular face-to-face treatment studies (Cuijpers et al., 2011a). However, this does not necessarily mean that self-guided treatments are without value (Cuijpers et al., 2011b), because they can be provided at very low cost once the treatment platform is in place (Gerhards et al., 2010). Indeed, small and occasionally moderate effects on depressive symptoms have been reported from self-guided programs (Andersson and Titov, 2014). These trials have often been large, exceeding 200 participants (Johansson and Andersson, 2012).

Although most studies have involved middle-aged adults with mild to moderate depression, one controlled study of guided ICBT was conducted in a sample of 84 subjects with partially remitted depression. Results showed that relapse could be prevented compared with the no-treatment control group (Holländare et al., 2011). Furthermore, the benefit was maintained at a 2-year follow-up where 14% of the ICBT group had relapsed compared to 61% in the control group (Holländare et al., 2013).

Internet CBT research trials have been conducted in adolescents with depression as well (Calear et al., 2009), but these are mostly in a self-guided format, without clinician involvement. A pilot trial of ICBT in depressed older adults has also been conducted (Dear et al., 2013), as have trials in non-Western countries such as China (Choi et al., 2012). To the best of this author's knowledge, there are no controlled ICBT trials in chronic depression or dysthymia and only a few preliminary studies in bipolar disorder (Smith et al., 2011).

As mentioned, most studies in the field of Internet interventions have been based on CBT (Andersson, 2009). However, in one controlled trial in 92 subjects with major depressive disorder, a very large effect was seen when psychodynamic Internet treatment (a guided self-help treatment based on psychodynamic principles) was compared against the weekly Internet supportive contact control (between-group effect size of Cohen's $d = 1.11$) (Johansson et al., 2012a). Moreover, treatment effects were maintained at a 10-month follow-up.

Anxiety Disorders

Controlled trials of guided ICBT have been conducted in several anxiety disorders, and the results generally tend to replicate what has been found in face-to-face treatments (Andersson, 2014b). The earliest controlled trials focused on panic disorder (Carlbring et al., 2001), and at least 10 trials on panic disorder or panic symptoms have been conducted since (Hedman et al., 2012b) in countries as diverse as Sweden (Carlbring et al., 2001), Australia (Klein and Richards, 2001; Wims et al., 2010), the United Kingdom (Schneider et al., 2005), Norway (Nordgreen et al., 2010), and Switzerland (Berger et al., 2014). Trial samples ranged from 20 to 104 patients, and treatment program duration ranged from 6 to 15 weeks. The largest controlled trial to date in panic disorder included 104 patients (Bergström et al., 2010) who were randomized to either therapist-guided ICBT or offline group CBT. Large within-group effects were observed for both treatment formats ($d = 1.73$ and 1.63 for ICBT and group treatment, respectively). The difference between the two formats was minimal. In addition, ICBT was more cost-effective than group CBT with respect to therapist time.

Social anxiety disorder is probably the anxiety disorder that has received the most research attention (Andersson et al., 2014a), with nearly 20 controlled trials testing ICBT in its treatment. In a meta-analysis of eight trials enrolling a total of 707 subjects, the average between-group effect size was $d = 0.86$ (Tulbure, 2011). Larger studies have been conducted since the publication of this meta-analysis. One of the largest enrolled 201 participants and tested knowledge acquisition about social anxiety and its treatment. The trial showed that confidence in knowledge about social anxiety and its treatment increased following the intervention (Andersson et al., 2012b). Improvement in knowledge, however, only correlated with improvement on one measure of social anxiety ($r = .26, p = .01$).

Posttraumatic stress disorder (PTSD) has been studied in several controlled ICBT trials (Andersson, 2010). Although no systematic review or meta-analysis of guided Internet treatment alone has been published (Amstadter et al., 2009), a meta-analysis with a broader focus that included guided ICBT studies and other computerized treatments found large effects ($d = 1.01$) when comparing against no treatment (Sloan et al., 2011). Also, Hedman et al. (2012b) identified six controlled PTSD trials in their review of a total of 193 subjects and found within-group effect sizes against no treatment ranging from 0.89 to 1.69. Finally, in an interesting German pilot study, subjects with PTSD residing in Iraq were treated remotely with guided ICBT (Wagner et al., 2012b). Results showed large within-group effects (for example, $d = 1.23$ for avoidance symptoms and $d = 1.44$ for intrusions).

There are fewer controlled trials and guided ICBT programs devoted to GAD (Hedman et al., 2012b), but four published controlled trials have shown the same promising outcomes as in other therapist-guided ICBT studies (Titov et al., 2009b; Robinson et al., 2010; Paxling et al., 2011; Andersson et al., 2012c), with moderate to large effect sizes. In addition, a series of trials on transdiagnostic ICBT (Titov et al., 2010b) and tailored ICBT (Carlbring et al., 2010) included subjects with GAD.

Other anxiety disorders have received less research attention, but two separate groups have tested guided ICBT in obsessive-compulsive disorder (OCD) in a Swedish controlled trial involving 101 subjects (Andersson et al., 2012a) and in an Australian controlled trial with 56 subjects (Wootton et al., 2013). Moderate to large effects were reported in both studies. Another controlled trial in 81 subjects with hypochondriasis showed large treatment effects (Cohen's $d = 1.52$ to 1.62) (Hedman et al., 2011b). The intervention, which lasted 12 weeks, consisted of 12 text-based treatment modules. The therapist involvement was provided as in other trials (e.g., weekly support and feedback totaling 10 minutes per client per week). Surprisingly few trials have been conducted in individuals with specific phobias, with only two small trials comparing ICBT against state-of-the-art one-session exposure therapy (Andersson et al., 2009b, 2013c). The results of both trials showed that the one-session treatment was slightly superior.

Other Psychiatric Conditions

In addition to anxiety disorders and mild to moderate depression, guided ICBT has been preliminarily explored in other conditions, including eating disorders (Sanchez-Ortiz et al., 2011a), insomnia (Ström et al., 2000), pathological gambling (Carlbring and Smit, 2008), and substance use disorders (Riper et al., 2011; Tait et al., 2013). Results of these studies have been promising, with moderate to large effects. It is striking, however, that guided ICBT has not yet been developed and tested for other relatively common and/or severe conditions, such as bipolar disorder, schizophrenia, chronic or severe depression, and personality disorders.

AS EFFECTIVE AS TRADITIONAL PSYCHOTHERAPY?

Few direct comparisons with face-to-face traditional therapy have been conducted. One recent meta-analysis (total N = 1053) assessed 13 controlled trials of guided ICBT versus face-to-face treatment in which participants were randomized to receive either treatment format (Andersson et al., 2014b). Three studies were conducted in individuals with social anxiety disorder (Botella et al., 2010; Andrews et al., 2011; Hedman et al., 2011c), three in those with panic disorder (Carlbring et al., 2005; Kiropoulos et al., 2008; Bergström et al., 2010), two in those with depressive symptoms (Spek et al., 2007; Wagner et al., 2014), two in individuals with body dissatisfaction symptoms associated with eating disorders (Gollings and Paxton, 2006; Paxton et al., 2007), one in those suffering from tinnitus (Kaldo et al., 2008), one in men with sexual dysfunction (Schover et al., 2012), and one in individuals with spider phobia (Andersson et al., 2009b). Traditional face-to-face CBT was administered either in the individual (six studies) or group (seven studies) format. The pooled effect size at post-treatment suggested that ICBT and face-to-face treatment produced similar overall effects (Hedges $g = -0.01$; 95% confidence interval -0.13 to 0.12). These findings are in line with those of a previous meta-analysis comparing guided self-help (including ICBT studies) and face-to-face psychotherapy (Cuijpers et al., 2010), which included 21 studies with a total of 810 participants.

Although these data may surprise clinicians trained in traditional psychotherapy, they should not be taken as indication that ICBT can or should replace regular psychotherapy. They do, however, suggest that outcomes can be similar and that bringing technology to the aid of traditional therapy can provide benefit to many patients and should not be met with immediate dismissiveness or doubt. Larger trials are still needed but overall, the evidence to date clearly implies that guided ICBT can be as effective as face-to-face therapy in social anxiety disorder, panic disorder, and some forms of depression. There is a need for more studies in other areas, including severe and chronic depression, bipolar affective disorder, PTSD, psychotic illnesses, and personality disorders, and research should be conducted in age groups other than adults.

TREATMENT OUTCOMES IN EFFECTIVENESS TRIALS

Internet-based interventions are becoming more popular, especially in countries such as Sweden and Australia. This raises the need to evaluate how well they work in real-world practice settings. These evaluations are often referred to as "effectiveness" studies (in contrast with "efficacy" trials, conducted in a select group of study subjects recruited based on stringent criteria). Their goal is to assess the external validity of the research findings (Lutz, 2003). One review of guided ICBT effectiveness studies has been published (Andersson and Hedman, 2013). It included four controlled trials and eight open studies conducted in a total of 3888 patients with panic disorder, social anxiety disorder, GAD, PTSD, depression, tinnitus, and irritable bowel syndrome. The review suggests that it is feasible to transfer ICBT to clinical practice with sustained benefits and moderate to large effect sizes. More recently, a large noncontrolled effectiveness study conducted in Sweden included 1203 patients with major depressive disorder (Hedman et al., 2014). Subjects had received guided ICBT and results showed large pretreatment to post-treatment within-group effects ($d = 1.27$).

NEGATIVE EFFECTS OF TREATMENT

There have been few reports of the possible negative effects of ICBT, although concerns about confidentiality, data security, and the risk of deterioration have been voiced (Dever Fitzgerald et al., 2010). In general, it is thought that side effects are relatively rare but can occur (Boettcher et al., 2014b). For example, in a study of individuals with social anxiety disorder, 19 out of 133 participants described unwanted negative events that they related to treatment (Boettcher et al., 2014b). The most common was the emergence of new symptoms, followed by a worsening of baseline social anxiety symptoms. Although it has been argued that Internet-derived treatment may hurt patients by preventing them from receiving "better" treatment (such as face-to-face CBT), there is little support for this claim. In general, it is strongly recommended that future trials of Internet-derived and traditional psychotherapy pay more attention to assessing and reporting side effects (Dimidjian and Hollon, 2010).

WHAT WORKS FOR WHOM?

As with traditional psychotherapy research, the literature on predictors, moderators, and mediators of outcome is scattered, with few consistent findings reported. In a secondary report from the first Swedish depression trial (Andersson et al., 2005), data from 71 subjects who completed a 6-month follow-up were analyzed (Andersson et al., 2004). A small, but statistically significant, negative correlation was found between the number of previous depression episodes and outcome, indicating that individuals with fewer previous depression episodes may benefit more. Also, a Dutch depression study (Spek et al., 2008) reported that higher baseline Beck Depression Inventory scores, female gender, and lower neuroticism scores predicted better outcome, although there is an overall dearth of data for severe depression. In contrast to what might be expected, there is little evidence that severity of depression (i.e., mild to moderate) makes a difference in depression trials (Bower et al., 2013).

Several predictor studies exist for anxiety disorders, including panic disorder (Andersson et al., 2008b; El Alaoui et al., 2013), PTSD (Knaevelsrud and Maercker, 2006), health-related anxiety (Hedman et al., 2013b), and social anxiety disorder (Nordgreen et al., 2012). The studies are not conclusive, but baseline anxiety symptom severity tends to predict positive outcomes, whereas comorbid depression severity tends to predict negative outcomes.

Not surprisingly, treatment adherence appears to be associated with better results in several studies (e.g., Hilvert-Bruce et al., 2012). To the extent that they have been studied, genetic factors have shown no consistent association with outcome (Hedman et al., 2012a; Andersson et al., 2013a), and neither have patient expectations and patient-rated credibility of the treatment (Boettcher et al., 2013b).

DISCUSSION AND FUTURE DIRECTIONS

In a relatively short period of time, Internet-delivered psychotherapy has accumulated a substantial body of evidence that supports its wider use. This author predicts that novel psychotherapies will be developed with the Internet in mind and not simply adapted to the Internet from established face-to-face, office-based psychotherapies. Also, the cost-effectiveness of guided ICBT will become more apparent (Andersson et al., 2011; Hedman et al., 2011a, 2013a). In addition, the rapid pace of technology evolution and the ubiquity of smartphones may reinvent yet again the delivery of psychotherapy (Donker et al., 2013). To that end, early tests of smartphone-delivered therapy have been promising (Luxton et al., 2011; Ly et al., 2012, 2014; Watts et al., 2013) (see Chapter 13).

Furthermore, one would expect online therapy with real-time, full therapist involvement (with or without camera) to receive more attention in the future. Although limited in number and scope, published trials have been promising. In one multicenter study conducted in the United Kingdom in 297 subjects with major depressive disorder, 38% of subjects assigned to real-time online CBT (without camera) responded at 4 months versus 24% in the wait list group ($p = 0.011$), with benefits maintained at the 8-month assessment point (42% versus 26%; $p = 0.023$) (Kessler et al., 2009). Also, in a randomized trial in 31 youths with OCD, real-time online CBT with full therapist involvement delivered via webcam was compared to a wait list control. Webcam-delivered CBT was superior to the wait list control on all primary outcome measures with large effect sizes (Cohen's $d \geq 1.36$), whereby 81% in the active arm responded versus 13% in the wait list arm, and 56% versus 13% met remission criteria. Gains were generally maintained at 3-month follow-up for those randomized to webcam-delivered CBT (Storch et al., 2011).

Indeed, all delivery methods may have something to offer, and blended treatment formats are likely to become part of the future of care delivery. Some of this is already happening. Traditional therapists increasingly allow a certain degree of online communication with their patients and some are gradually bringing Internet treatment to the office by having parts of the treatment delivered via an online platform (Månsson et al., 2013).

Finally, the attitudes surrounding the use of new technologies in psychotherapy will continue to change as people become more familiar with other health care solutions being provided online and as technology becomes even more a part of normal daily life. Despite some differences based on country (Mohr et al., 2010) and on the health care funding entity, it appears that patients are probably more positive about online therapy than therapists (Stallard et al., 2010; Gun et al., 2011; Spence et al., 2011; Wootton et al., 2011). This author expects that this will change as research such as the one presented in this chapter is more broadly disseminated, and as better designed, larger, and more representative studies are conducted.

DISCLOSURE STATEMENT

The preparation of this chapter was funded in part by the Swedish Research Council, FORTE, and Linköping University. The author discloses no relationships with commercial entities and professional activities that may bias his views.

REFERENCES

Almlöv J, Carlbring P, Berger T, et al (2009). Therapist factors in Internet-delivered CBT for major depressive disorder. Cognitive Behaviour Therapy 38: 247–254.

Almlöv J, Carlbring P, Källqvist K, et al (2011). Therapist effects in guided Internet-delivered CBT for anxiety disorders. Behavioural and Cognitive Psychotherapy 39: 311–322.

Amstadter AB, Broman-Fulks J, Zinzow H, et al (2009). Internet-based interventions for traumatic stress-related mental health problems: a review and suggestion for future research. Clinical Psychology Review 29: 410–420.

Andersson E, Enander J, Andrén P, et al (2012a). Internet-based cognitive behaviour therapy for obsessive-compulsive disorder: a randomised controlled trial. Psychological Medicine 42: 2193–2203.

Andersson E, Ljótsson B, Smit F, et al (2011). Cost-effectiveness of Internet-based cognitive behavior therapy for irritable bowel syndrome: results from a randomized controlled trial. BMC Public Health 11: 215.

Andersson E, Rück C, Lavebratt C, et al (2013a). Genetic polymorphisms in monoamine systems and outcome of cognitive behavior therapy for social anxiety disorder. PLoS One 8: e79015.

Andersson G (2009). Using the Internet to provide cognitive behaviour therapy. Behaviour Research and Therapy 47: 175–180.

Andersson G (2010). Guided Internet-delivered cognitive behavior therapy for posttraumatic stress disorder and other comorbid anxiety disorders. In Brunet A, Ashbaugh AR, Herbert CF, Editors. Internet Use in the Aftermath of Trauma. IOS Press, Amsterdam, the Netherlands, pp. 243–254.

Andersson G (2014a). The Internet and CBT: A Clinical Guide. CRC Press, Boca Raton, FL.

Andersson G (2014b). Guided Internet treatment of anxiety disorders in adults. In Emmelkamp PMG, Ehring T, Editors. The Wiley Handbook of Anxiety Disorders. Wiley-Blackwell, New York, NY, pp. 1279–1296.

Andersson G, Bergström J, Buhrman M, et al (2008a). Development of a new approach to guided self-help via the Internet. The Swedish experience. Journal of Technology in Human Services 26: 161–181.

Andersson G, Bergström J, Holländare F, et al (2004). Delivering CBT for mild to moderate depression via the Internet. Predicting outcome at 6-months follow-up. Verhaltenstherapie 14: 185–189.

Andersson G, Bergström J, Holländare F, et al (2005). Internet-based self-help for depression: a randomised controlled trial. British Journal of Psychiatry 187: 456–461.

Andersson G, Carlbring P, Berger T, et al (2009a). What makes Internet therapy work? Cognitive Behaviour Therapy 38: 55–60.

Andersson G, Carlbring P, Furmark T (2014a). Internet-delivered treatments for social anxiety disorder In Weeks J, Editor. Handbook of Social Anxiety Disorder. Wiley-Blackwell, New York, NY, pp. 569–587.

Andersson G, Carlbring P, Furmark T, et al (2012b). Therapist experience and knowledge acquisition in Internet-delivered CBT for social anxiety disorder: a randomized controlled trial. PLoS One 7: e37411.

Andersson G, Carlbring P, Grimlund A (2008b). Predicting treatment outcome in Internet versus face to face treatment of panic disorder. Computers and Human Behavior 24: 1790–1801.

Andersson G, Carlbring P, Holmström A, et al (2006). Internet-based self-help with therapist feedback and in-vivo group exposure for social phobia: a randomized controlled trial. Journal of Consulting and Clinical Psychology 74: 677–686.

Andersson G, Carlbring P, Ljótsson B, et al (2013b). Guided Internet-based CBT for common mental disorders. Journal of Contemporary Psychotherapy 43: 223–233.

Andersson G, Cuijpers P (2009). Internet-based and other computerized psychological treatments for adult depression: a meta-analysis. Cognitive Behaviour Therapy 38: 196–205.

Andersson G, Cuijpers P, Carlbring P, Riper H, Hedman E (2014b). Internet-based vs. face-to-face cognitive behaviour therapy for psychiatric and somatic disorders: a systematic review and meta-analysis. World Psychiatry 13: 288–295.

Andersson G, Hedman E (2013). Effectiveness of guided Internet-delivered cognitive behaviour therapy in regular clinical settings. Verhaltenstherapie 23: 140–148.

Andersson G, Paxling B, Roch-Norlund P, et al (2012c). Internet-based psychodynamic vs. cognitive behavioural guided self-help for generalized anxiety disorder: a randomised controlled trial. Psychotherapy and Psychosomatics 81: 344–355.

Andersson G, Paxling B, Wiwe M, et al (2012d). Therapeutic alliance in guided Internet-delivered cognitive behavioral treatment of depression, generalized anxiety disorder and social anxiety disorder. Behaviour Research and Therapy 50: 544–550.

Andersson G, Strömgren T, Ström L, et al (2002). Randomised controlled trial of Internet based cognitive behavior therapy for distress associated with tinnitus. Psychosomatic Medicine 64: 810–816.

Andersson G, Titov N (2014). Advantages and limitations of Internet-based interventions for common mental disorders. World Psychiatry 13: 4–11.

Andersson G, Waara J, Jonsson U, et al (2009b). Internet-based self-help vs. one-session exposure in the treatment of spider phobia: a randomized controlled trial. Cognitive Behaviour Therapy 38: 114–120.

Andersson G, Waara J, Jonsson U, et al (2013c). Internet-based vs. one-session exposure treatment of snake phobia: a randomized controlled trial. Cognitive Behaviour Therapy 42: 284–291.

Andrews G, Davies M, Titov N (2011). Effectiveness randomized controlled trial of face to face versus Internet cognitive behaviour therapy for social phobia. Australian and New Zealand Journal of Psychiatry 45: 337–340.

Bennett K, Bennett AJ, Griffiths KM (2010). Security considerations for e-mental health interventions. Journal of Internet Medical Research 12: e61.

Berger T, Boettcher J, Caspar F (2014). Internet-based guided self-help for several anxiety disorders: a randomized controlled trial comparing a tailored with a standardized disorder-specific approach. Psychotherapy 51: 207–219.

Berger T, Hämmerli K, Gubser N, et al (2011). Internet-based treatment of depression: a randomized controlled trial comparing guided with unguided self-help. Cognitive Behaviour Therapy 40: 251–266.

Bergman Nordgren L, Carlbring P, Linna E, et al (2013). Role of the working alliance on treatment outcome in tailored Internet-based cognitive behavioural therapy for anxiety disorders: randomized controlled pilot trial. Journal of Internet Medical Research Protocols 2: e4.

Bergström J, Andersson G, Ljótsson B, et al (2010). Internet- versus group-administered cognitive behaviour therapy for panic disorder in a psychiatric setting: a randomised trial. BMC Psychiatry 10: 54.

Boettcher J, Åström V, Påhlsson D, et al (2014a). Internet-based mindfulness treatment for anxiety disorders: a randomised controlled trial. Behavior Therapy 45: 241–253.

Boettcher J, Leek L, Matson L, et al (2013a). Internet-based attention modification for social anxiety: a randomised controlled comparison of training towards negative and training towards positive cues. PLoS One 8: e71760.

Boettcher J, Renneberg B, Berger T (2013b). Patient expectations in Internet-based self-help for social anxiety. Cognitive Behaviour Therapy 42: 203–214.

Boettcher J, Rozental A, Andersson G, et al (2014b). Side effects in Internet-based interventions for social anxiety disorder. Internet Interventions 1: 3–11.

Botella C, Gallego MJ, Garcia-Palacios A, et al (2010). An Internet-based self-help treatment for fear of public speaking: a controlled trial. Cyberpsychology, Behavior, and Social Networking 13: 407–421.

Bower P, Kontopantelis E, Sutton AP, et al (2013). Influence of initial severity of depression on effectiveness of low intensity interventions: meta-analysis of individual patient data. British Medical Journal 346: f540.

Buchanan T (2003). Internet-based questionnaire assessment: appropriate use in clinical contexts. Cognitive Behaviour Therapy 32: 100–109.

Buhrman M, Fältenhag S, Ström L, et al (2004). Controlled trial of Internet-based treatment with telephone support for chronic back pain. Pain 111: 368–377.

Buhrman M, Skoglund A, Husell J, et al (2013). Guided Internet-delivered acceptance and commitment therapy for chronic pain patients: a randomized controlled trial. Behaviour Research and Therapy 51: 307–315.

Cacciola JS, Alterman AI, Rutherford MJ, et al (1999). Comparability of telephone and in-person structured clinical interview for DSM-III-R (SCID) diagnoses. Assessment 6: 235–242.

Calear AL, Christensen H, Mackinnon A, et al (2009). The YouthMood Project: a cluster randomized controlled trial of an online cognitive behavioral program with adolescents. Journal of Consulting and Clinical Psychology 77: 1021–1032.

Carlbring P, Brunt S, Bohman S, et al (2007). Internet vs. paper and pencil administration of questionnaires commonly used in panic/agoraphobia research. Computers and Human Behavior 23: 1421–1434.

Carlbring P, Forslin P, Ljungstrand P, et al (2002). Is the Internet-administered CIDI-SF equivalent to a human SCID-interview? Cognitive Behaviour Therapy 31: 183–189.

Carlbring P, Maurin L, Törngren C, et al (2010). Individually tailored Internet-based treatment for anxiety disorders: a randomized controlled trial. Behaviour Research and Therapy 49: 18–24.

Carlbring P, Nilsson-Ihrfelt E, Waara J, et al (2005). Treatment of panic disorder: live therapy vs. self-help via Internet. Behaviour Research and Therapy 43: 1321–1333.

Carlbring P, Smit F (2008). Randomized trial of Internet-delivered self-help with telephone support for pathological gamblers. Journal of Consulting and Clinical Psychology 76: 1090–1094.

Carlbring P, Westling BE, Ljungstrand P, et al (2001). Treatment of panic disorder via the Internet—a randomized trial of a self-help program. Behavior Therapy 32: 751–764.

Choi I, Zou J, Titov N, et al (2012). Culturally attuned Internet treatment for depression amongst Chinese Australians: a randomised controlled trial. Journal of Affective Disorders 136: 459–468.

Christensen H, Griffiths KM, Mackinnon AJ, et al (2006). Online randomized trial of brief and full cognitive behaviour therapy for depression. Psychological Medicine 36: 1737–1746.

Cuijpers P, Andersson G, Donker T, et al (2011a). Psychological treatments of depression: results of a series of meta-analyses. Nordic Journal of Psychiatry 65: 354–364.

Cuijpers P, Donker T, Johansson R, et al (2011b). Self-guided psychological treatment for depressive symptoms: a meta-analysis. PLoS One 6: e21274.

Cuijpers P, Donker T, van Straten A, et al (2010). Is guided self-help as effective as face-to-face psychotherapy for depression and anxiety disorders? A meta-analysis of comparative outcome studies. Psychological Medicine 40: 1943–1957.

Dagöö J, Persson Asplund R, Bsenko AH, et al (2014). Cognitive behavior therapy versus interpersonal psychotherapy for social anxiety disorder delivered via smartphone and computer: a randomized controlled trial. Journal of Anxiety Disorders 28: 410–417.

Dear BF, Zou J, Titov N, et al (2013). Internet-delivered cognitive behavioural therapy for depression: a feasibility open trial for older adults. Australian and New Zealand Journal of Psychiatry 47: 169–176.

Dever Fitzgerald T, Hunter PV, Hadjistavropoulos T, et al (2010). Ethical and legal considerations for Internet-based psychotherapy. Cognitive Behaviour Therapy 39: 173–187.

Dimidjian S, Hollon SD (2010). How would we know if psychotherapy were harmful? American Psychologist 65: 21–33.

Donker T, Griffiths KM, Cuijpers P, et al (2009). Psychoeducation for depression, anxiety and psychological distress: a meta-analysis. BMC Medicine 7: 79.

Donker T, Petrie K, Proudfoot J, et al (2013). Smartphones for smarter delivery of mental health programs: a systematic review. Journal of Internet Medical Research 15: e247.

El Alaoui S, Hedman E, Ljótsson B, et al (2013). Predictors and moderators of Internet- and group-based cognitive behaviour therapy for panic disorder. PLoS One 8: e79024.

Emmelkamp PM (2005). Technological innovations in clinical assessment and psychotherapy. Psychotherapy and Psychosomatics 74: 336–343.

Fairburn CG, Cooper Z (2011). Therapist competence, therapy quality, and therapist training. Behaviour Research and Therapy 49: 373–378.

Gerhards SA, de Graaf LE, Jacobs LE, et al (2010). Economic evaluation of online computerised cognitive-behavioural therapy without support for depression in primary care: randomised trial. British Journal of Psychiatry 196: 310–318.

Gollings EK, Paxton SJ (2006). Comparison of Internet and face-to-face delivery of a group body image and disordered eating intervention for women: a pilot study. Eating Disorders 14: 1–15.

Gun SY, Titov N, Andrews G (2011). Acceptability of Internet treatment of anxiety and depression. Australasian Psychiatry 19: 259–264.

Hedman E, Andersson E, Lindefors N, et al (2013a). Cost-effectiveness and long-term effectiveness of Internet-based cognitive behaviour therapy for severe health anxiety. Psychological Medicine 43: 363–374.

Hedman E, Andersson E, Ljótsson B, et al (2011a). Cost-effectiveness of Internet-based cognitive behavior therapy vs. cognitive behavioral group therapy for social anxiety disorder: results from a randomized controlled trial. Behaviour Research and Therapy 49: 729–736.

Hedman E, Andersson E, Ljótsson B, et al (2012a). Clinical and genetic outcome determinants of Internet- and group-based cognitive behavior therapy for social anxiety disorder. Acta Psychiatrica Scandinavica 126: 126–136.

Hedman E, Andersson G, Ljótsson B, et al (2011b). Internet-based cognitive-behavioural therapy for severe health anxiety: randomised controlled trial. British Journal of Psychiatry 198: 230–236.

Hedman E, Andersson G, Ljótsson B, et al (2011c). Internet-based cognitive behavior therapy vs. cognitive behavioral group therapy for social anxiety disorder: a randomized controlled non-inferiority trial. PLoS One 6: e18001.

Hedman E, Lindefors N, Andersson G, et al (2013b). Predictors of outcome in Internet-based cognitive behavior therapy for severe health anxiety. Behaviour Research and Therapy 51: 711–717.

Hedman E, Ljótsson B, Kaldo V, et al (2014). Effectiveness of Internet-based cognitive behaviour therapy for depression in routine psychiatric care. Journal of Affective Disorders 155: 49–58.

Hedman E, Ljótsson B, Lindefors N (2012b). Cognitive behavior therapy via the Internet: a systematic review of applications, clinical efficacy and cost-effectiveness. Expert Review of Pharmacoeconomics and Outcomes Research 12: 745–764.

Hedman E, Ljótsson B, Rück C, et al (2010). Internet administration of self-report measures commonly used in research on social anxiety disorder: a psychometric evaluation. Computers and Human Behavior 26: 736–740.

Hilvert-Bruce Z, Rossouw PJ, Wong N, et al (2012). Adherence as a determinant of effectiveness of Internet cognitive behavioural therapy for anxiety and depressive disorders. Behaviour Research and Therapy 50: 463–468.

Holländare F, Andersson G, Engström I (2010). A comparison of psychometric properties between Internet and paper versions of two depression instruments (BDI-II and MADRS-S) administered to clinic patients. Journal of Internet Medical Research 12: e49.

Holländare F, Johnsson S, Randestad M, et al (2011). Randomized trial of Internet-based relapse prevention for partially remitted depression. Acta Psychiatrica Scandinavica 124: 285–294.

Holländare F, Johnsson S, Randestad M, et al (2013). Two-year outcome for Internet-based relapse prevention for partially remitted depression. Behaviour Research and Therapy 51: 719–722.

Johansson R, Andersson G (2012). Internet-based psychological treatments for depression. Expert Review of Neurotherapeutics 12: 861–870.

Johansson R, Ekbladh S, Hebert A, et al (2012a). Psychodynamic guided self-help for adult depression through the Internet: a randomised controlled trial. PLoS One 7: e38021.

Johansson R, Sjöberg E, Sjögren M, et al (2012b). Tailored vs. standardized Internet-based cognitive behavior therapy for depression and comorbid symptoms: a randomized controlled trial. PLoS One 7: e36905.

Kaldo V, Levin S, Widarsson J, et al (2008). Internet versus group cognitive-behavioral treatment of distress associated with tinnitus. A randomised controlled trial. Behavior Therapy 39: 348–359.

Kessler D, Lewis G, Kaur S, et al (2009). Therapist-delivered Internet psychotherapy for depression in primary care: a randomised controlled trial. Lancet 374: 628–634.

Kiropoulos LA, Klein B, Austin DW, et al (2008). Is Internet-based CBT for panic disorder and agoraphobia as effective as face-to-face CBT? Journal of Anxiety Disorders 22: 1273–1284.

Klein B, Richards JC (2001). A brief Internet-based treatment for panic disorder. Behavioural and Cognitive Psychotherapy 29: 113–117.

Knaevelsrud C, Maercker A (2006). Does the quality of the working alliance predict treatment outcome in online psychotherapy for traumatized patients? Journal of Internet Medical Research 8: e31.

Ljótsson B, Hedman E, Andersson E, et al (2011). Internet-delivered exposure based treatment vs. stress management for irritable bowel syndrome: a randomized trial. American Journal of Gastroenterology 106: 1481–1491.

Ljótsson B, Hesser H, Andersson E, et al (2013). Mechanisms of change in exposure-based Internet-treatment for irritable bowel syndrome Journal of Consulting and Clinical Psychology 81: 1113–1126.

Lutz W (2003). Efficacy, effectiveness, and expected treatment response in psychotherapy. Journal of Clinical Psychology 59: 745–750.

Luxton DD, McCann RA, Bush NE, et al (2011). mHealth for mental health: integrating smartphone technology in behavioral healthcare. Professional Psychology: Research and Practice 42: 505–512.

Ly KH, Dahl J, Carlbring P, et al (2012). Development and initial evaluation of a smartphone application based on acceptance and commitment therapy. SpringerPlus 1: 11.

Ly KH, Trüschel A, Jarl L, et al (2014). Behavioral activation vs. mindfulness-based guided self-help treatment administered through a smartphone application: a randomized controlled trial. British Medical Journal Open 4: e003440.

Månsson KNT, Ruiz E, Gervind E, et al (2013). Development and initial evaluation of an Internet-based support system for face to face cognitive behavior therapy: a proof of concept study. Journal of Internet Medical Research 15: e280.

Marks IM, Shaw S, Parkin R (1998). Computer-assisted treatments of mental health problems. Clinical Psychology: Science and Practice 5: 51–170.

Melville KM, Casey LM, Kavanagh DJ (2010). Dropout from Internet-based treatment for psychological disorders. British Journal of Clinical Psychology 49: 455–471.

Mohr DC, Siddique J, Ho J, et al (2010). Interest in behavioral and psychological treatments delivered face-to-face, by telephone, and by Internet. Annals of Behavioral Medicine 40: 89–98.

Nordgreen T, Havik OE, Öst L-G, et al (2012). Outcome predictors in guided and unguided self-help for social anxiety disorder. Behaviour Research and Therapy 50:13–21.

Nordgreen T, Standal B, Mannes H, et al (2010). Guided self-help via Internet for panic disorder: dissemination across countries. Computers and Human Behavior 26: 592–596.

Nordin S, Carlbring P, Cuijpers P, et al (2010). Expanding the limits of bibliotherapy for panic disorder. Randomized trial of self-help without support but with a clear deadline. Behavior Therapy 41: 267–276.

Palmqvist B, Carlbring P, Andersson G (2007). Internet-delivered treatments with or without therapist input: does the therapist factor have implications for efficacy and cost? Expert Review of Pharmacoeconomics & Outcomes Research 7: 291–297.

Paxling B, Almlöv J, Dahlin M, et al (2011). Guided Internet-delivered cognitive behavior therapy for generalized anxiety disorder: a randomized controlled trial. Cognitive Behaviour Therapy 40: 159–173.

Paxling B, Lundgren S, Norman A, et al (2013). Therapist behaviours in Internet-delivered cognitive behaviour therapy: analyses of e-mail correspondence in the treatment of generalized anxiety disorder. Behavioural and Cognitive Psychotherapy 41: 280–289.

Paxton SJ, McLean SA, Gollings EK, et al (2007). Comparison of face-to-face and Internet interventions for body image and eating problems in adult women: an RCT. International Journal of Eating Disorders 40: 692–704.

Richards D, Richardson T (2012). Computer-based psychological treatments for depression: a systematic review and meta-analysis. Clinical Psychology Review 32: 329–342.

Richards D, Vigano N (2013). Online counseling: a narrative and critical review of the literature. Journal of Clinical Psychology 69: 994–1011.

Richardson R, Richards DA, Barkham M (2010). Self-help books for people with depression: the role of the therapeutic relationship. Behavioural and Cognitive Psychotherapy 38:67–81.

Riper H, Spek V, Boon B, et al (2011). Effectiveness of E-self-help interventions for curbing adult problem drinking: a meta-analysis. Journal of Internet Medical Research 13: e42.

Robinson E, Titov N, Andrews G, et al (2010). Internet treatment for generalized anxiety disorder: a randomized controlled trial comparing clinician vs. technician assistance. PLoS One 5: e10942.

Sanchez-Ortiz VC, Munro C, Stahl D, et al (2011a). A randomized controlled trial of Internet-based cognitive-behavioural therapy for bulimia nervosa or related disorders in a student population. Psychological Medicine 41: 407–417.

Sanchez-Ortiz VC, Munro C, Startup H, et al (2011b). The role of email guidance in Internet-based cognitive-behavioural self-care treatment for bulimia nervosa. European Eating Disorders Review 19: 342–348.

Schneider AJ, Mataix-Cols D, Marks IM, et al (2005). Internet-guided self-help with or without exposure therapy for phobic and panic disorders. Psychotherapy and Psychosomatics 74: 154–164.

Schover LR, Canada AL, Yuan Y, et al (2012). A randomized trial of Internet-based versus traditional sexual counseling for couples after localized prostate cancer treatment. Cancer 118: 500–509.

Sheehan DV, Lecrubier Y, Sheehan KH, et al (1998). The Mini-International Neuropsychiatric Interview (M.I.N.I.): the development and validation of a structured diagnostic psychiatric interview for DSM-IV and ICD-10. Journal of Clinical Psychiatry 59(Suppl 20): 22–33.

Sloan DM, Gallagher MW, Feinstein BA, et al (2011). Efficacy of telehealth treatments for posttraumatic stress-related symptoms: a meta-analysis. Cognitive Behaviour Therapy 40: 111–125.

Smith DJ, Griffiths E, Poole R, et al (2011). Beating Bipolar: exploratory trial of a novel Internet-based psychoeducational treatment for bipolar disorder. Bipolar Disorders 13: 571–577.

Spek V, Nyklicek I, Cuijpers P, et al (2008). Predictors of outcome of group and Internet-based cognitive behavior therapy. Journal of Affective Disorders 105: 137–145.

Spek V, Nyklicek I, Smits N, et al (2007). Internet-based cognitive behavioural therapy for subthreshold depression in people over 50 years old: a randomized controlled clinical trial. Psychological Medicine 37: 1797–1806.

Spence J, Titov N, Solley K, et al (2011). Characteristics and treatment preferences of people with symptoms of posttraumatic stress disorder: an Internet survey. PLos One 6: e21864.

Stallard P, Richardson T, Velleman S (2010). Clinicians' attitudes towards the use of computerized cognitive behaviour therapy (cCBT) with children and adolescents. Behavioural and Cognitive Psychotherapy 38: 545–560.

Storch EA, Caporino NE, Morgan JR, et al (2011). Preliminary investigation of web-camera delivered cognitive-behavioral therapy for youth with obsessive-compulsive disorder. Psychiatry Research 189: 407–412.

Ström L, Pettersson R, Andersson G (2000). A controlled trial of self-help treatment of recurrent headache conducted via the Internet. Journal of Consulting and Clinical Psychology 68: 722–727.

Sucala M, Schnur JB, Constantino MJ, et al (2012). The therapeutic relationship in e-therapy for mental health: a systematic review. Journal of Internet Medical Research 14: e110.

Tait RJ, Spijkerman R, Riper H (2013). Internet and computer based interventions for cannabis use: a meta-analysis. Drug and Alcohol Dependence 133: 295–304.

Titov N, Andrews G, Choi I, et al (2008). Shyness 3: randomized controlled trial of guided versus unguided Internet-based CBT for social phobia. Australian and New Zealand Journal of Psychiatry 42: 1030–1040.

Titov N, Andrews G, Davies M, et al (2010a). Internet treatment for depression: a randomized controlled trial comparing clinician vs. technician assistance. PLoS One 5: e10939.

Titov N, Andrews G, Johnston L, et al (2010b). Transdiagnostic Internet treatment for anxiety disorders: a randomized controlled trial. Behaviour Research and Therapy 48: 890–899.

Titov N, Andrews G, Schwencke G, et al (2009a). An RCT comparing the effects of two types of support on severity of symptoms for people completing Internet-based cognitive behaviour therapy for social phobia. Australian and New Zealand Journal of Psychiatry 43: 920–926.

Titov N, Dear BF, Schwencke G, et al (2011). Transdiagnostic Internet treatment for anxiety and depression: a randomised controlled trial. Behaviour Research and Therapy 49: 441–452.

Titov N, Gibson M, Andrews G, et al (2009b). Internet treatment for social phobia reduces comorbidity. Australian and New Zealand Journal of Psychiatry 43: 754–759.

Tulbure BT (2011). The efficacy of Internet-supported intervention for social anxiety disorder: a brief meta-analytic review. Procedia—Social and Behavioral Sciences 30: 552–557.

van Bastelaar KM, Pouwer F, Cuijpers P, et al (2011). Web-based depression treatment for type 1 and type 2 diabetic patients: a randomized, controlled trial. Diabetes Care 34: 320–325.

Wagner B, Brand J, Schulz W, et al (2012a). Online working alliance predicts treatment outcome for posttraumatic stress symptoms in Arab war-traumatized patients. Depression and Anxiety 29: 646–651.

Wagner B, Horn AB, Maercker A (2014). Internet-based versus face-to-face cognitive-behavioral intervention for depression: a randomized controlled non-inferiority trial. Journal of Affective Disorders 152-154: 113–121.

Wagner B, Schulz W, Knaevelsrud C (2012b). Efficacy of an Internet-based intervention for posttraumatic stress disorder in Iraq: a pilot study. Psychiatry Research 195: 85–88.

Waller G (2009). Evidence-based treatment and therapist drift. Behaviour Research and Therapy 47: 119–127.

Wampold BE (2001). The Great Psychotherapy Debate. Models, Methods, and Findings. Lawrence Erlbaum, Mahwah, NJ.

Wampold BE, Brown GS (2005). Estimating the variability outcome attributable to therapists: a naturalistic study of outcomes in managed care. Journal of Consulting and Clinical Psychology 73: 914–923.

Warmerdam L, Riper H, Klein M, et al (2012). Innovative ICT solutions to improve treatment outcomes for depression: the ICT4Depression project. Studies in Health Technology and Informatics 181: 339–343.

Watkins PL (2008). Self-help therapies: past and present. In Watkins PL, Clum GA, Editors. Handbook of Self-help Therapies. Routledge, New York, NY, pp. 1–24.

Watts S, Mackenzie A, Thomas C, et al (2013). CBT for depression: a pilot RCT comparing mobile phone vs. computer. BMC Psychiatry 13: 49.

Wims E, Titov N, Andrews G, et al (2010). Clinician-assisted Internet-based treatment is effective for panic: a randomized controlled trial. Australian and New Zealand Journal of Psychiatry 44: 599–607.

Wootton BM, Dear BF, Johnston L, et al (2013). Remote treatment of obsessive-compulsive disorder: a randomized controlled trial. Journal of Obsessive-Compulsive and Related Disorders 2: 375–384.

Wootton BM, Titov N, Dear BF, et al (2011). The acceptability of Internet-based treatment and characteristics of an adult sample with obsessive compulsive disorder: an Internet survey. PLoS One 6: e20548.

11 Software-Based Psychotherapy

The Example of Computerized Cognitive-Behavioral Therapy

Lina Gega and Simon Gilbody

INTRODUCTION

Software-based psychotherapy is a standardized, automated, self-directed, psychological intervention, which uses electronic information and digital communication technology to help a patient work through a comprehensive therapy program independently of a therapist. Software-based psychotherapy programs collect; store and retrieve clinical information; deliver standardized therapy instructions via text, voice files, or video clips; and guide patients in the application of therapeutic techniques to achieve personalized goals. It is important to note that although software-based psychotherapy can be delivered independently of a therapist, software and therapists are not mutually exclusive, and some professional support or guidance can still be offered as an optional adjunct to the software program.

Cognitive-behavioral therapy (CBT) lends itself well to software-based delivery because of its brief and structured approach. According to the CBT model, treatment of a mental health problem entails targeting certain beliefs and behaviors that maintain the distressing feelings or disabling symptoms associated with this problem (e.g., Butler et al., 2006; Roth and Fonagy, 2008). CBT places emphasis on activities completed by patients outside therapy sessions; this is commonly referred to as "homework" (e.g., Kazantzis and L'Abate, 2007) and fits well with the self-directed nature of software-based psychotherapy.

Software-based CBT, or, as commonly called, computerized CBT (cCBT), has three defining elements shown in Figure 11.1: self-help, computerization, and bona fide CBT.

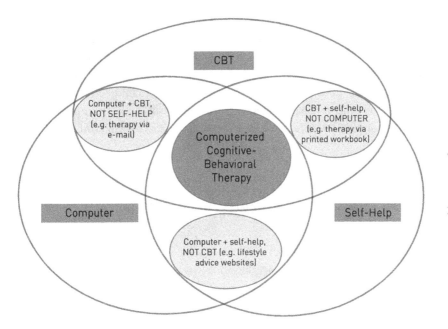

FIGURE 11.1

Elements of computerized cognitive-behavioral therapy (CBT) and relationships with related forms of psychotherapy and self-help.

(1) Self-help. This component relates to the delivery of cCBT independently of a therapist and is not to be mistaken with nonprofessional, peer-organized online support groups (Griffiths et al., 2009). In the context of self-help, patients are autonomous and can complete cCBT without therapist input; however, adjunct support and guidance can be offered by trained therapists, by professionals without formal therapy training (e.g., nurses), or by lay volunteers. Adjunct support can be offered by phone, e-mail/online chat, text messaging, postal mail, or face-to-face.

(2) Computerization. This aspect of cCBT denotes both the software that delivers the cCBT program and the digital media and hardware that allow for its content to be accessed. Examples of media that deliver cCBT are the Internet, portable devices (e.g., CD-ROMs), or telephones (e.g., interactive voice response systems and smartphone apps).

(3) Bona fide CBT. This suggests that the intervention builds on a CBT model, which includes an assessment, personalized goals, CBT techniques, homework, and a relapse prevention blueprint. Bona fide CBT techniques adhere to evidence-based or common practice guidelines for the specific problem that the cCBT program aims to treat (e.g., exposure therapy for phobic disorders, behavioral activation and cognitive restructuring for depression, and applied relaxation/progressive muscle relaxation training for generalized anxiety) (Hawton et al., 1989; Wright et al., 2010).

Programs of cCBT have been developed for anxiety disorders, including phobias and panic disorder (Marks et al., 2004), obsessive-compulsive disorder (Greist et al., 2002), depression (Proudfoot et al., 2004), and general anxiety/stress (Kenardy et al., 2003). Such programs also exist for physical health problems (Cuijpers et al., 2008; van Beugen et al., 2014) and for children and adolescents (e.g., Headstrong, for management of recurrent headache in children [Connelly et al., 2006] and BRAVE, a web-based CBT program for childhood anxiety [Spence et al., 2006]).

COMPUTERIZED COGNITIVE-BEHAVIORAL THERAPY IN THE CONTEXT OF COMPUTER-ASSISTED INTERVENTIONS

A review by Barak et al. (2009) offers a useful guide to terms used to describe different computer-assisted interventions that may share features with cCBT but are not synonymous with it. Examples include "computer therapy" (Andrews et al., 2010), "Internet interventions" (Griffiths et al., 2010), "computer-aided psychotherapy" (Cuijpers et al., 2009), "telemedicine" (Garcia-Lizana and Munoz-Mayorga, 2010), "e-therapy" (Postel et al., 2008), "media-delivered CBT" (Mayo-Wilson and Montgomery, 2013), "web-based interventions" (Wantland et al., 2004), or simply "technologies" (Farrer et al., 2013; Mohr et al., 2013).

Not all computer-assisted CBT is considered cCBT. Figure 11.2 illustrates how different computer-assisted CBT programs can be placed in a continuum of varying levels of standardization, self-help, and therapist involvement. At one end of the continuum, stand-alone cCBT entails standardized, software-based self-help that is independent of a therapist (e.g., Powell et al., 2012). At the other end of the continuum, online CBT depends on a therapist using synchronous "free-style" communication via e-mail/chat room and has no software or standardization (e.g., Kessler et al., 2009). In the middle of the continuum, hybrids of software-based self-help and therapist contact are referred to as supported or guided cCBT (e.g., Berger et al., 2011). Two further examples of hybrids, yet not strictly speaking cCBT, are Interapy (Ruwaard et al., 2011) and Calm Tools for Living (Craske et al., 2011). Both have a standardized, software-based therapeutic content but depend

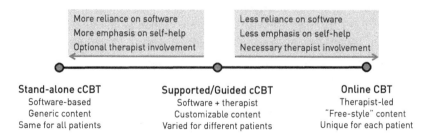

FIGURE 11.2

Computer-assisted cognitive-behavioral therapy (CBT) continuum.

cCBT, computerized cognitive-behavioral therapy.

on a therapist to administer the program or guide the patient through it; therefore, they are not cCBT, according to its strict definition.

Some cCBT programs have been used for clinical training and professional education. These programs have either been designed exclusively for professional education (Bennett-Levy et al., 2012) or adapted from their original therapeutic version to a condensed professional educational version (Gega et al., 2007).

Another example of computer-assisted CBT self-help that is not necessarily cCBT pertains to the use of electronic books or online therapy manuals (Carlbring et al., 2006). Those could be considered electronic bibliotherapy, but its distinction with cCBT is not always clear. Such bibliotherapy does not require sophisticated software if the computer is merely used to read through information or download a document. On the other hand, electronic bibliotherapy can be similar to cCBT when it includes interactive web pages and requires some degree of information processing (e.g., administration of questionnaires and interpretation of scores).

Also, cCBT is different from informative or educational websites that do not deliver a therapy program. Examples of the latter are BluePages (http://www.bluepages.anu.edu.au) and MoodGYM (http://moodgym.anu.edu.au; Christensen et al., 2004).

Some computerized programs deliver psychological interventions that are not based on CBT. These include problem-solving training (Warmerdam et al., 2010), interpersonal therapy (Donker et al., 2013), and psychodynamic therapy (Johansson et al., 2012). Other programs may partially use CBT principles to change lifestyle behaviors (Kohl et al., 2013), help weight control (Neve et al., 2010), and reduce smoking (Walters et al., 2006), drug use (Wood et al., 2014) or alcohol use (White et al., 2010).

CLINICAL EVIDENCE
Overview of Outcomes of Computerized Cognitive-Behavioral Therapy

A monograph by Marks et al. (2007) reviewed 97 computer-assisted psychotherapy programs in 175 studies for more than 30 types of mental health and psychosomatic problems. Since then, the number of computer-assisted psychological interventions, including cCBT, has increased exponentially. As shown in Figure 11.2, computer-assisted CBT can be divided into three broad categories: stand-alone cCBT (standardized self-help with no therapist contact), supported/guided cCBT (standardized self-help with optional therapist contact), and online CBT (therapist-administered intervention with some or no standardized self-help elements).

The first question asked by patients, clinicians, and health care organizations in relation to cCBT is: "does it work?" The caveat of using published evidence to answer this question is that most reviews, meta-reviews, or meta-analyses (1) do not differentiate between stand-alone and supported or guided cCBT and (2) include cCBT along with online CBT. This chapter discusses reviews that pool together cCBT and online CBT if the cCBT studies make up the majority of the review. Reviews that combine studies of cCBT with studies of CBT-based self-help that is not computerized (e.g., delivered with a manual or by phone as in Cuijpers et al., 2010 or Mayo-Wilson and Montgomery, 2013) and reviews of studies of computerized non–CBT-based self-help (e.g., computerized interpersonal therapy in Donker et al., 2013) are excluded.

A metareview of computer-assisted interventions for depression (Foroushani et al., 2011) drew on 10 reviews, the majority of which were about cCBT, and concluded that cCBT could reduce symptoms more than usual care or being in a wait list control and to a similar extent as therapist-delivered face-to-face CBT. A subsequent review of 14 cCBT-specific trials by So et al. (2013) concluded that, although cCBT for depression was effective in reducing depressive symptoms on a short-term basis, it failed to demonstrate long-term effects and any benefit for the functional recovery of patients. These contradictory findings may be accounted for by the fact that the meta-review by Foroushani et al. (2011) was more inclusive, whereas the review by So et al. (2013) excluded many studies on the basis of poor methodological quality, extended therapist contact, or lack of outcome measures for functioning.

Another systematic review examined psychosocial/functioning outcomes with web-based interventions for chronic physical and psychiatric conditions and included both cCBT and online CBT (Paul et al., 2013). This review found that 20 out of the 36 studies demonstrated a significant effect in favor of web-based intervention, most of which were cCBT for depression. A review of 22 studies of computer therapy by Andrews et al. (2010) concluded: "computerised CBT for major depression, social phobia, panic disorder or generalized anxiety disorder showed superiority in outcome over control groups. The effect sizes are substantial, and the results indicate both short term and long term benefits" (p. 4). The majority of the included studies used cCBT, and only five studies pertained to clinician-administered CBT (via e-mail consultations or with computerized self-help tasks supplementing face-to-face CBT).

Barak et al. (2008) found no difference between face-to-face and Internet interventions based on 14 studies across different conditions. Another systematic review (Hedman et al., 2012) identified 12 randomized controlled trials (RCTs) that compared Internet-based CBT with conventional face-to-face CBT and found no difference in their effects. Both reviews included studies of cCBT and online CBT, but the majority of the studies used cCBT with or without adjunct support.

In children and adolescents, a systematic review of 10 studies, including RCTs, single pre-post group comparisons and case series, found cCBT for depression and anxiety to be an effective intervention (Richardson et al., 2010). Three other reviews (Calear and Christensen, 2009, 2010; Neil and Christensen, 2009) supported the effectiveness of Internet-based prevention, early intervention, and treatment for anxiety and depression in children and adolescents, especially for pupils with elevated depression symptoms at baseline and for cCBT that was school-based and was facilitated by a mental health professional. These four reviews all included studies of cCBT and online CBT, but the majority were studies of cCBT self-help with some adjunct professional support.

A clinical guidance by the National Institute for Health and Care Excellence in the United Kingdom (National Institute for Health and Care Excellence, 2009) recommends cCBT for persistent subthreshold depression and mild to moderate depression as long as it is "supported by a trained practitioner who reviews progress and outcome" (p. 14). Other clinical guidance for phobias (National Institute for Health and Care Excellence, 2013b) recommends to "not routinely offer computerized CBT to treat specific phobias in adults" (p. 32). This recommendation was made on the basis of having relatively few cCBT studies dedicated exclusively to specific phobias and despite having ample evidence for large effects of supported cCBT across a pooled population with anxiety disorders (Cuijpers et al., 2009; Reger and Gahm, 2009).

Also, cCBT has been used as a priming intervention for patients waiting to see a therapist. A naturalistic study by Learmonth and Rai (2008) found significant therapeutic gains from using computerized self-help as a first step in treating severe, chronic depression. Another observational study (Kenter et al., 2013) reported that computerized self-help, albeit not CBT but problem-solving training, was used by just over half of the patients to whom it was offered, and it expedited their recovery with subsequent face-to-face therapy. Finally, cCBT has been used as a continuation of conventional therapy to prevent relapse in patients with partially remitted depression (Holländare et al., 2013); at the 2-year follow-up, the relapse rate for cCBT users was 14% versus 61% in the control group.

Stand-alone cCBT without any therapist involvement may be a promising tool for health promotion across nonclinical and nonrisk populations and for primary prevention in at-risk populations. A study by Powell et al. (2012) showed that stand-alone cCBT produced a positive shift in the population distribution of mental well-being. Another study (Lintvedt et al., 2013) demonstrated that stand-alone cCBT helped people recognize the warning signs of a problem, improved mental health literacy, and encouraged help seeking in individuals with subclinical symptoms that would have deteriorated if left untreated.

Factors Influencing Outcomes of Computerized Cognitive-Behavioral Therapy

Factors that moderate or predict outcomes of cCBT are important sources of variance in clinical studies. Examples of variables explored in the cCBT literature as potential effect moderators or predictors of outcome include the type and severity of the problem, the type and amount of adjunct therapist support, patient compliance with therapeutic elements of cCBT, and the features of the cCBT program itself.

There is very little evidence about the potential superiority of particular cCBT programs over others. One large-scale multisite study in the United Kingdom, the "Randomised Evaluation of the Effectiveness and Acceptability of Computerised Therapy" (REEACT) (Gilbody, personal communication), was recently completed and is the first independent comparison of a free cCBT program against a commercially available one. Patients who were randomized to either cCBT program continued to receive usual care and were offered technical support, but no thera-peutic assistance, as an adjunct to cCBT. The study found no differences between the two cCBT programs for depression symptoms at 4 months follow-up from randomization.

Effect sizes for cCBT for anxiety disorders were found to be higher than those for cCBT for depression (Spek et al., 2007). Baseline severity of depression and anx-iety can also influence clinical outcomes with cCBT; greater effects have been asso-ciated with higher baseline severity (Bower et al., 2013; Christensen et al., 2006). This is slightly paradoxical given that most cCBT programs have been developed for depression rather than anxiety and that they are generally recommended for mild to moderate rather than severe problems.

Adjunct support is an important source of heterogeneity of findings across cCBT studies (see Chapter 10 for further discussion of minimally supported online therapy). Unsupported cCBT seems to have a small effect on depression (Cuijpers et al., 2011), as opposed to supported cCBT whose effect seems comparable to that of face-to-face therapy (Cuijpers et al., 2010). A meta-analysis covering depres-sion and anxiety disorders found that Internet-delivered CBT was four times more effective with online therapist support than without any therapist contact (Spek et al., 2007).

Two further meta-analyses (Palmqvist et al., 2007; Cuijpers et al., 2009) indi-cated that the longer the therapist input, the better the clinical outcomes with cCBT. Another review found that supported computerized interventions for depression yielded better outcomes than unsupported ones (Reger and Gahm, 2009). Two RCTs of social phobia found that (1) cCBT with personalized thera-pist guidance by e-mail (and occasionally by phone) was superior to unguided cCBT (Titov et al., 2008) and (2) an Internet-accessed CBT self-help manual had better outcomes when supplemented by an online discussion group (Furmark et al., 2009).

The relationship between greater therapist input and improved outcomes with cCBT has not always been strong. A three-arm RCT of stand-alone cCBT (N = 25), guided cCBT (N = 25) and wait list controls (N = 26) found a trend (not reaching statistical significance) for better outcomes in depression with guided cCBT (sup-plementation of cCBT with generic weekly e-mails that only offered encourage-ment) compared to stand-alone cCBT (Berger et al., 2011). In another study, online CBT (entirely therapist-delivered intervention) was only marginally superior to supported cCBT (self-help with brief therapist support) on reduction of depression symptoms at 6 months from randomization, with moderate to large effect sizes reported for both interventions (Vernmark et al., 2011).

Some studies found that additional monitoring or therapist contact did not influence outcomes. Having three face-to-face support sessions with a therapist as an adjunct to cCBT for bulimia nervosa did not enhance outcomes compared to cCBT with "minimal" administrative guidance (Murray et al., 2007). Also, weekly telephone tracking for cCBT for depression did not have an advantage over stand-alone cCBT (Farrer et al., 2011). Finally, more frequent therapist contact via e-mail (three times versus once per week) did not improve outcomes with cCBT for panic (Klein et al., 2009).

How can these findings about the influence of adjunct human support on cCBT outcomes be interpreted? There is robust evidence to suggest that effect sizes drop with a larger self-help element of cCBT and rise with more professional input; however, studies that did not find an association between available or increased therapist support, and better outcomes suggest that the type of offered support might be important. First, it appears that support should have a personal therapeutic element to it, rather than just consist of generic tracking or monitoring. Second, support should be connected to the cCBT program and not constitute independent therapy sessions. Finally, there seems to be a relatively low level of support that is able to influence outcomes, whereas support beyond a certain level does not seem to lead to proportionally better outcomes.

Better outcomes have also been associated with better adherence to the cCBT program (Donkin et al., 2011; Hilvert-Bruce et al., 2012). However, a cause-and-effect relationship between adherence and outcome is not always clear. Patients may do well because they adhere to cCBT, but, equally, patients may be more likely to adhere to cCBT if they find it beneficial.

ADOPTION AND ATTRITION

A comprehensive review reported that a median of 56% of cCBT users (range, 12%–100%) completed the intervention and a median of 83% of participants who started the intervention (range, 26%–100%) completed outcome measures at follow-up, whether or not they completed the intervention (Waller and Gilbody, 2009). Another review of adherence to Internet interventions, which included both cCBT and online CBT, reported a 1% to 50% range of attrition in RCTs (Christensen et al., 2009). A third review reported a weighted average of 31% (range, 2%–83%) of dropout from Internet-based therapy, which included stand-alone cCBT, supported cCBT, and online CBT (Melville et al., 2010). Finally, a review of cCBT for children and adolescents reported a range of 33% to 70% completion rates across different programs (Richardson et al., 2010).

Qualitative data give some insight into the reasons for nonadoption and dropout from cCBT studies (Murray et al., 2003; Kaltenhaler et al., 2008; Christensen et al., 2009; Waller and Gilbody, 2009; Postel et al., 2010; Richardson et al., 2010). In brief, patients who do not adopt cCBT doubt that the program could be as helpful as talking to a person or are anxious about using a computer. Patients who discontinue cCBT attribute it to:

(1) The intervention itself (technical difficulties, not liking the program, lack of human contact, lack of benefit, or finding it too difficult)
(2) The patient's own psychological and physical state (feeling better, lack of motivation, physical problems, or an exacerbation of mental health problems)
(3) External factors (moving away, not having enough time)

Factors Influencing Adoption of and Attrition from Computerized Cognitive-Behavioral Therapy

The variance of follow-up (range, 26%–100%) and completion (range, 12%–100%) rates in cCBT is striking. To explain this variance, studies explored factors associated with cCBT adoption, completion, and dropout. These factors can be broadly grouped into three categories: person-related, intervention-related and methodological factors.

Person-Related Factors

Better adherence is associated with younger age, living in a rural location, and having less knowledge of psychological treatments (Christensen et al., 2009; Neil et al., 2009; Calear et al., 2013). Individuals with higher self-esteem and more independent personalities are more likely to adopt and adhere to cCBT (Vangberg et al., 2012; Calear et al., 2013). Higher baseline depression severity is linked with better adoption and program usage (Neil et al., 2009; Vangberg et al., 2012; Calear et al., 2013), whereas lower baseline depression severity is associated with program completion (Christensen et al., 2009). Better adherence has also been associated with positive expectations at baseline about potential usefulness of cCBT (Murray et al., 2007; Kaltenhaler et al., 2008) and with patient preference for CBT rather than psychodynamic therapy when given the choice between the two (Johansson et al., 2013).

Intervention-Related Factors

Adapting the cCBT program itself, such as adding motivational enhancement strategies (Titov et al., 2010) and using persuasive design features (Chatterjee and Price, 2009; van Gemert-Pijnen et al., 2011; Kelders et al., 2012) can have a positive impact on adherence. Implementing cCBT in monitored settings, such as schools, rather than open-access websites in the community (Neil et al., 2009), and offering adjunct support via phone, e-mail, or face-to-face contact (Palmqvist et al., 2007; Cuijpers et al., 2009; Gerhards et al., 2011) are also associated with higher adherence and completion rates.

Methodological Factors

These relate to the design of a particular cCBT study, the way participants are followed up, and the way adherence is defined in the context of the study. Attrition is found to be much lower in restricted-access cCBT programs and RCTs than in open access websites and observational studies (Christensen et al., 2009; Waller and Gilbody, 2009; Kelders et al., 2012). Also, strategies to enhance follow-up rates, such as financial incentives (An et al., 2008), may result in better adherence.

Comparison to Other Interventions

Does cCBT suffer from higher attrition than other interventions, and what do the rates of different types of attrition tell us about cCBT? Overall, based on review by Waller and Gilbody (2009), a median of 83% of patients complete outcome measures at follow-up irrespective of whether they adhere to the treatment protocol. This fits with the 20% rule of acceptable "loss to follow-up" for a study to maintain its internal validity (Schulz and Grimes, 2002), suggesting that cCBT studies have credible results. According to the same review (Waller and Gilbody, 2009), cCBT interventions have a median of 56% intervention adherence rate (patients adhere to the treatment protocol by using the intervention as it is intended to be used whether or not they complete outcome measures at follow-up), which is similar to or better than that reported for psychological therapies in routine practice (Gyani et al., 2013).

Given the consistent message that RCTs have better adherence and completion rates than observational studies, strategies commonly used in RCTs may have some value in minimizing overall attrition; examples include screening participants for suitability, careful monitoring, and frequent contact with a researcher (Brueton et al., 2014). That said, using strategies to enhance follow-up rates reflects the success of the retention efforts rather than the engagement qualities of the cCBT program itself. The program needs to use an approach combining persuasive technology and self-help with human contact and therapeutic guidance. Four main strategies to improve adherence with cCBT, and ultimately clinical outcomes, arise from the literature: (1) explaining the value, limitations, and requirements of cCBT to patients at the outset; (2) providing scheduled adjunct help with the application of therapeutic techniques and offering emotional support as needed; (3) tailoring the cCBT program to suit the patient's needs and preferences; and (4) keeping the program brief but inclusive of all the necessary therapeutic ingredients (such as homework and behavioral tasks).

ECONOMIC EVIDENCE
Overview of Economic Evaluations of Computerized Cognitive-Behavioral Therapy

Computerized CBT is often promoted as a "low-cost" intervention on the basis that it saves clinician time compared to conventional face-to-face therapy (Marks et al., 2004). Formal economic evaluations are the best sources of evidence as to whether cCBT is "good value for money"; they involve cost-effectiveness analyses, which compare the costs and effects of cCBT to those of alternative options, such as nontreatment (e.g., wait list or placebo), usual care (e.g., monitoring from a family physician), noncomputerized self-help (e.g., bibliotherapy), and clinician-delivered therapy (e.g., face-to-face or online CBT).

"Costs" in economic evaluations are expressed as the monetary value of resources used in connection with both the problem and the studied intervention (e.g., software and hardware set-up, clinician time, income support, health care costs). "Effects" in economic evaluations are usually expressed in quality-adjusted life years gained (QALYs), rather than in condition-specific measurement units (e.g., improvement in depression scores), to allow for economic comparisons across different conditions and different outcome measures (National Institute for Health and Care Excellence, 2013a).

The first systematic review of economic evaluations specific to cCBT was completed by the National Institute for Health and Care Excellence (NICE) in the United Kingdom (Kaltenthaler et al., 2006); it concluded that cCBT was more cost-effective than face-to-face therapy for depression using economic modeling on the basis of only one cost-effectiveness study available at the time (McCrone et al., 2004). The only other review of economic evaluations of cCBT to date (Hedman et al., 2012) has major limitations, because it does not use any quality assessment and does not include all available studies in the field.

Since the first economic evaluation of cCBT (McCrone et al., 2004), at least a dozen more have appeared. Figure 11.3 is a visual representation of these economic evaluations (Black, 1990). The four quadrants of the figure represent all four possible combinations of relative costs and effects between cCBT and its comparators. The economic evaluations are plotted in a particular quadrant depending on whether they found cCBT to be more effective and less costly (southeast quadrant), more effective and more costly (northeast quadrant), less effective and less costly (southwest quadrant), or less effective and more costly (northwest quadrant).

Seven economic evaluations occupy the southeast quadrant of Figure 11.3 (Bergström et al., 2010; Gerhards et al., 2010; Andersson et al., 2011; Hedman et al., 2011, 2013; Ljótsson et al., 2011; van Spijker et al., 2012). These found cCBT for

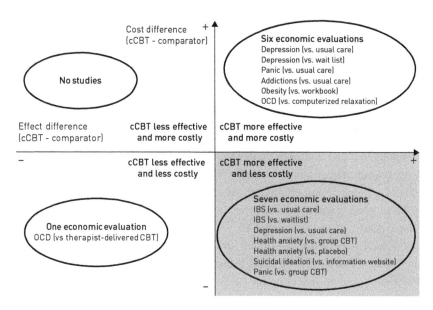

FIGURE 11.3

Computerized cognitive-behavioral therapy (cCBT): relative costs and effects against comparators. OCD, obsessive-compulsive disorder; IBS, irritable bowel syndrome.

irritable bowel syndrome, depression, health anxiety, suicidal ideation, and panic to be more effective and less costly than its comparators, which included usual care, group CBT, wait list, and psychological placebo (a peer-support online forum and an information website with no therapeutic advice). The lower cost of cCBT in these studies was the result of less health care utilization and less absence from work by users.

Six studies occupy the northeast quadrant of Figure 11.3 (Wylie-Rosett et al., 2001; McCrone et al., 2004, 2007; Mihalopoulos et al., 2005; Olmstead et al., 2010; Warmerdam et al., 2010). These found cCBT for depression, panic, addictions, obesity, and obsessive-compulsive disorder (OCD) to be more effective but also more costly compared to usual care, wait list, workbook, and psychological placebo (computerized relaxation for OCD).

Finally, a cost-effectiveness comparison in one of the above studies (McCrone et al., 2007) found cCBT for OCD to be less costly but also less effective than therapist-delivered CBT and is therefore plotted on the southwest quadrant of Figure 11.3. The northwest quadrant is empty, because there are no published studies that reported cCBT to be less effective and more costly than another management option.

Critical Review and Interpretation of Economic Evaluations of Computerized Cognitive-Behavioral Therapy

How are economic evaluations of cCBT to be interpreted? Based on the seven economic evaluations where cCBT was shown to be more effective and less costly than its comparators, the straightforward conclusion is that cCBT is the most cost-effective option. In practical terms, this means that using cCBT instead of another intervention might give those who pay for health care (patients themselves, insurance companies, or national health services) a "bigger bang for their buck."

A complication with interpreting economic evaluations of cCBT arises when the comparator is usual care (Gerhards et al., 2010; Andersson et al., 2011) that cannot be withdrawn or replaced by cCBT (e.g., when a general practitioner/family physician needs to evaluate the patient, facilitate access to cCBT, and monitor general health). In this case, demonstrating cost-effectiveness of cCBT as a stand-alone intervention against usual care is a moot point; it would make sense that economic evaluations consider cCBT as an adjunct to usual care and not independently, but this may change the cost-effectiveness conclusions. As a case in point, the study by Gerhards et al. (2010) found cCBT alone to be more cost-effective than usual care for depression, but it did not reach the same conclusion when cCBT was evaluated as an adjunct to usual care.

With regard to the six economic evaluations that found cCBT to be more costly and more effective than its comparators, decisions as to whether cCBT is a cost-effective option depend on how much people are willing to pay for an extra unit of improvement in the outcome of interest. There are some price benchmarks as to what is acceptable to pay for an intervention (cost-effectiveness threshold) when the outcome of interest is expressed in QALYs gained; widely accepted cost-effectiveness thresholds are $50,000 (Grosse, 2008) and £20,000 (National Institute for Health and Care Excellence, 2013a) per QALY gained. However, the problem with using a specific cost-effectiveness threshold is that not all cCBT economic evaluations estimate QALYs.

Those who bear the cost of health care (patients, insurance companies, or national health services) still need to make a decision as to how much more they are willing to pay for cCBT when it is both more expensive and more effective than other interventions (trade-off). By the same token, with regard to the study that found cCBT to be less costly but also less effective than therapist-delivered CBT (McCrone et al., 2007), value judgments need to be made as to whether people are willing to compromise outcomes for less cost with cCBT or whether they can afford to pay more for better outcomes with therapist-delivered CBT.

An additional problem with interpreting economic evaluations of cCBT is that they are often conducted from a societal perspective (Gerhards et al., 2010; Andersson et al., 2011). The rationale for this is that the benefits from an intervention accrue to all those affected by the problem, including the patient, the health care service, the patient's employers, and any organizations that offer practical and financial support. A societal perspective calculates costs as if they were shared across a large "societal purse," which, of course, is not true. Savings for employers or welfare agencies are often independent of savings for those who pay for health care, so lumping costs and benefits across different societal stakeholders makes it difficult for patients or insurance companies to decide whether they can afford cCBT.

A further issue to consider is that, even when cCBT is cost-effective, it may not reduce health care costs (Bower et al., 2000). If cCBT leads to higher patient demand, it can paradoxically have a higher overall cost, considering its accessibility to those who would otherwise not seek help.

USER PERSPECTIVES
Patient Perspectives on Computerized Cognitive-Behavioral Therapy

Patients' satisfaction with cCBT is generally high (MacGregor et al., 2009). Still, the majority of patients may prefer face-to-face therapy if given the choice; in a survey of 658 primary care patients, most respondents were interested in face-to-face therapy rather than Internet-delivered interventions, except for those who reported lack of time as a barrier in help seeking and were interested in lifestyle changes rather than psychotherapy (Mohr et al., 2010).

Patients report some aspects of cCBT as being helpful, positive, or productive and other aspects of cCBT as hindering, negative, or counterproductive. Interestingly, "the 'same' aspects of computerised therapy could be portrayed as both positive and negative experiences, rather than there being exclusive barriers or facilitators" (Knowles et al., 2014, p. 8). For example, some patients see audiovisual case studies in a cCBT program as helpful because they depict other people with similar problems. Other patients may find the same case studies irrelevant or artificial, because they do not reflect their own experiences and are not recordings of "real people" but actors (Gega et al., 2013).

On the positive side, patients reported that cCBT helped them develop insight into their problems and increased their knowledge of CBT principles and techniques (Bendelin et al., 2011; Gega et al., 2013; Lillevoll et al., 2013). Users of cCBT also valued the flexibility and privacy of the intervention and felt empowered because they were doing something to help themselves (Knowles et al., 2014)

On the negative side, the standardized content of cCBT was often viewed by patients as too basic or irrelevant, and their experience was described as impersonal and isolating (Hind et al., 2010). Patients reported that cCBT lacked a person's genuineness and warmth, even when it tried to emulate human interactions by voicing statements such as "I am sorry to hear this" or "it must have been difficult"; this made patients laugh or irritated them (Gega et al., 2013). Finally, patients reported that lack of success or progress with the self-help materials made them feel like a failure (Murray et al., 2003).

Professional Perspectives on Computerized Cognitive-Behavioral Therapy

Professional views on computerized interventions can affect the wider implementation of cCBT. In Norway, 45% of psychologists who responded to a survey used electronic therapy (e-therapy; albeit not only cCBT) (Wangberg et al., 2007). The majority had an overall neutral rather than enthusiastic stance on e-therapy, with the exception of those who routinely used text messaging and e-mail. Interestingly, a survey in the United States found that practitioners preferred asynchronous e-mail communication (as in cCBT) rather than synchronous web chat (as in online CBT) (Mora et al., 2008).

A survey of British therapists about cCBT reported that only 2.4% used it; the rest were not averse to it and did not rule out using it in the future (Whitfield and Williams, 2004). Cautiously positive views on using cCBT for the prevention or treatment of mild to moderate problems in children and adolescents were also found by a small survey of British clinicians (Stallard et al., 2010). The majority had reservations about using cCBT for more severe presentations and emphasized the need for adjunct professional support. These two British surveys also found that clinicians assumed cCBT to be less effective than face-to-face CBT and saw it as an adjunct rather than an alternative to standard face-to-face therapy.

The above surveys suggest that habit and lack of knowledge rather than resistance may be the barriers to the wider implementation of cCBT. Encouraging clinicians to communicate with their patients by e-mail or text messaging can be the first step toward adopting computerized self-help interventions. Dispelling myths about inferiority of cCBT against face-to-face therapy and clarifying the circumstances under which cCBT can be as effective as face-to-face therapy can also improve clinician attitudes toward cCBT.

CONCLUSION
Benefits of Computerized Cognitive-Behavioral Therapy

One advantage of cCBT is that it offers flexible, round-the-clock therapy to patients who can access it in their own time and at their desired pace. Computerized CBT also aims to give patients autonomy and responsibility for their progress and can minimize stigma, especially when it can be accessed from home, in the community, in primary care venues or at schools, without involving psychiatric services. In addition, cCBT can overcome the tyranny of travelling for those living in rural or remote areas.

Using cCBT can guide clinicians who are not therapists (e.g., nurses, social workers, general practitioners) or novice therapists without much experience to deliver a CBT program that conveys the expertise of the therapists who developed it. The structured format of cCBT may also help with interclinician consistency in delivery (Andersson, 2010). In addition, cCBT can make more efficient use of human resources because it allows a higher patient throughput per therapist. Finally, cCBT has been successfully used as an educational tool to disseminate CBT knowledge and skills to health professionals who do not deliver formal therapy but can incorporate basic CBT principles and techniques into their generic "practice toolbox."

Compared to paper-based or electronic bibliotherapy, which disseminates CBT via self-help books or self-administered treatment manuals that can be printed or read on-screen, cCBT allows interaction between user and computer, individual tailoring of therapeutic choices and feedback, and automated tracking of outcomes. Compared to phone or face-to-face interventions, a computer can potentially ease self-disclosure of sensitive issues (Greist et al., 1973; Robinson and West, 1992; Ferriter, 1993).

Most importantly, cCBT can be highly effective for patients with depression, anxiety disorders and substance use disorders, and, on some occasions, as effective as face-to-face therapy. Not only can it be used as a stand-alone intervention, but also as a "primer" prior to patients receiving face-to-face CBT and as a maintenance or booster intervention to treat residual symptoms or prevent relapse following conventional therapy.

Also, cCBT is a promising public health intervention for the primary prevention of mental health problems in at-risk populations, for individuals with subclinical symptoms, or for those who are unlikely to seek help from mental health professionals. Finally, cCBT can improve mental health literacy and well-being in the general population.

Limitations of Computerized Cognitive-Behavioral Therapy

The biggest limitation of cCBT is that, by and large, it is not readily or freely available. Some notable exceptions are the free-to-access cCBT programs MoodGYM (Australia; www.moodgym.anu.edu.au), e-Couch (Australia; https://ecouch.anu.edu.au/welcome), Living Life to the Full (Scotland; www.llttf.com), and the

Panic Center (http://www.paniccenter.net/). Logistic difficulties relating to lack of resources and limited infrastructure, along with inadequate security and poor electronic data confidentiality (Bennett et al., 2010; Andrewes et al., 2013), may also obstruct implementation of cCBT.

Ethical and legal considerations sit at the heart of implementation of cCBT. Lack of any professional involvement may encourage disclosure but may also be perceived as an absolution of responsibility that could have legal repercussions for organizations.

Another limitation of cCBT is the variance in clinical outcomes, cost-effectiveness, and adoption and adherence rates across studies. This may make clinicians and organizations cautious about rolling out cCBT widely. Also, cCBT may not be able to cater for the range of complexity and comorbidity seen in clinical practice. Furthermore, some patients view standardized content of cCBT as impersonal or irrelevant, and the use of Internet-based therapy from home and lack of personal contact could feel isolating.

Finally, a barrier to the implementation of cCBT is the negative preconceptions and low expectations of cCBT by some patients and professionals, especially compared to alternative interventions such as face-to-face therapy.

Future Directions

Within a stepped care model, which is currently used in the British National Health Service, patients are offered the least intensive and least costly intervention first, followed by a more intensive and costly one in the case of nonresponse or deterioration (Bower and Gilbody, 2005). In this context, cCBT is not offered on a par with therapist-administered CBT (which is considered a "high intensity" intervention); instead, cCBT is intended as one of many low-intensity options, such as bibliotherapy or group CBT, before patients are offered face-to-face therapy.

The problem with using cCBT within a stepped care model is that patients may perceive it as an inferior option (Murray et al., 2003). The answer to this might be a stratified care model (Trusheim et al., 2007), according to which cCBT would be administered to individuals who are more likely to adopt, adhere to, and improve with the intervention. A stratified model would recommend cCBT on the basis that it is the best option (or one of many equally good options) for a particular individual rather than because it is less intensive or less costly across a population. Screening tools (Gega et al., 2005) could help identify individuals for whom cCBT would be recommended with confidence.

Hybrids that combine software-based self-help with therapist contact could help improve the clinical outcomes of and adherence to stand-alone cCBT by incorporating the "human element." It is crucial that future clinical trials of cCBT focus on understanding, not only for whom, but also under what circumstances and with what adjunct support cCBT yields the best possible outcomes with the least possible cost.

DISCLOSURE STATEMENT

The authors disclose no relationships with commercial entities and professional activities that may bias their views.

REFERENCES

An LC, Klatt C, Perry CL, et al (2008). The RealU online cessation intervention for college smokers: a randomized controlled trial. Preventative Medicine 47: 194–199.

Andersson E, Ljótsson B, Smit F, et al (2011). Cost-effectiveness of internet-based cognitive behavior therapy for irritable bowel syndrome: results from a randomized controlled trial. BMC Public Health 7: 215.

Andersson G (2010). The promise and pitfalls of the internet for cognitive behavioral therapy. BMC Medicine 8: 82.

Andrewes H, Kenicer D, McClay C, Williams C (2013). A national survey of the infrastructure and IT policies required to deliver computerised cognitive behavioural therapy in the English NHS. BMJ Open 3: e002277.

Andrews G, Cuijpers P, Craske MG, McEvoy P, Titov N (2010). Computer therapy for the anxiety and depressive disorders is effective, acceptable and practical health care: a meta-analysis. PLoS ONE 5: e13196.

Barak A, Hen L, Boniel-Nissim M, Shapira N (2008). A comprehensive review and a meta-analysis of the effectiveness of Internet-based psychotherapeutic interventions. Journal of Technology in Human Services 26: 109–160.

Barak A, Klein B, Proudfoot JG (2009). Defining internet-supported therapeutic interventions. Annals of Behavioral Medicine 38: 4–17.

Bendelin N, Hesser H, Dahl J, Carlbring P, Nelson KZ, Andersson G (2011). Experiences of guided Internet-based cognitive-behavioural treatment for depression: a qualitative study. BMC Psychiatry 11: 107.

Bennett K, Bennett AJ, Griffiths KM (2010). Security considerations for e-mental health interventions. Journal of Medical Internet Research 12: e61.

Bennett-Levy J, Hawkins R, Perry H, Cromarty P, Mills J (2012). Online cognitive behavioural therapy training for therapists: outcomes, acceptability, and impact of support. Australian Psychologist 47: 174–182

Berger T, Hämmerli K, Gubser N, Andersson G, Caspar F (2011). Internet-based treatment of depression: a randomized controlled trial comparing guided with unguided self-help. Cognitive Behaviour Therapy 40: 251–266.

Bergström J, Andersson G, Ljótsson B, et al (2010). Internet- versus group-administered cognitive behavior therapy for panic disorder in a psychiatric setting: a randomised trial. BMC Psychiatry 10: 54.

Black WC (1990). The CE plane: a graphic representation of cost-effectiveness. Medical Decision Making 10: 212–214.

Bower P, Byford S, Sibbald B, et al (2000). Randomised controlled trial of non-directive counselling, cognitive-behavioural therapy, and usual general practitioner care for patients with depression. II: Cost-effectiveness. British Medical Journal 321: 1389–1392.

Bower P, Gilbody S (2005). Stepped care in psychological therapies: access, effectiveness and efficiency. Narrative literature review. British Journal of Psychiatry 186: 11–17.

Bower P, Kontopantelis E, Sutton A, et al (2013). Influence of initial severity of depression on effectiveness of low intensity interventions: meta-analysis of individual patient data. BMJ 346: f540.

Brueton VC, Tierney JF, Stenning S, et al (2014) Strategies to improve retention in randomised trials: a Cochrane systematic review and meta-analysis. BMJ Open 4: e003821.

Butler AC, Chapman JE, Forman EM, Beck AT (2006). The empirical status of cognitive-behavioral therapy: a review of meta-analyses. Clinical Psychology Review 26: 17–31.

Calear AL, Christensen H (2009). Systematic review of school-based prevention and early intervention programs for depression. Journal of Adolescence 33: 429–438.

Calear AL, Christensen H (2010). Review of internet-based prevention and treatment programs for anxiety and depression in children and adolescents. Medical Journal of Australia 192: S12–S14.

Calear AL, Christensen H, Mackinnon A, Griffiths KM (2013). Adherence to the MoodGYM program: outcomes and predictors for an adolescent school-based population. Journal of Affective Disorders 147: 338–344.

Carlbring P, Bohman S, Brunt S, et al (2006). Remote treatment of panic disorder: a randomized trial of internet-based CBT supplemented with telephone calls. American Journal of Psychiatry 163: 2119–2125.

Chatterjee S, Price A (2009). Healthy living with persuasive technologies: framework, issues, and challenges. Journal of the American Medical Informatics Association 16: 171–178.

Christensen H, Griffiths KM, Farrer L (2009). Adherence in Internet interventions for anxiety and depression: systematic review. Journal of Medical Internet Research 11: e13.

Christensen H, Griffiths KM, Jorm AF (2004). Delivering interventions for depression by using the internet: randomised controlled trial. British Medical Journal 328: 265.

Christensen H, Griffiths KM, Mackinnon AJ, Brittliffe K (2006). Online randomized controlled trial of brief and full cognitive behaviour therapy for depression. Psychological Medicine 36: 1737–1746.

Connelly M, Rapoff MA, Thompson N, Connelly W (2006). Headstrong: a pilot study of a CD-ROM intervention for recurrent pediatric headache. Journal of Pediatric Psychology 31: 737–747.

Craske MG, Stein MB, Sullivan G, et al (2011). Disorder-specific impact of coordinated anxiety learning and management treatment for anxiety disorders in primary care. Archives of General Psychiatry 68: 378–388.

Cuijpers P, Donker T, Johansson R, et al (2011). Self-guided psychological treatment for depressive symptoms: a meta-analysis. PLoS ONE 6: e21274.

Cuijpers P, Donker T, van Straten A, Li J, Andersson G (2010). Is guided self-help as effective as face-to-face psychotherapy for depression and anxiety disorders? A systematic review and meta-analysis of comparative outcome studies. Psychological Medicine 40: 1943–1957.

Cuijpers P, Marks I, van Straten A, Cavanagh K, Gega L, Andersson G (2009). Computer-aided psychotherapy for anxiety disorders: a meta-analytic review. Cognitive Behaviour Therapy 38: 66–82.

Cuijpers P, van Straten A, Andersson G (2008). Internet-administered cognitive behavior therapy for health problems: a systematic review. Journal of Behavioral Medicine 31: 169–177.

Donker T, Bennett K, Bennett A, et al (2013). Internet-delivered interpersonal psychotherapy versus internet-delivered cognitive behavioral therapy for adults with depressive symptoms: randomized controlled noninferiority trial. Journal of Medical Internet Research 15: e82.

Donkin L, Christensen H, Naismith SL, Neal B, Hickie IB, Glozier N (2011). A systematic review of the impact of adherence on the effectiveness of e-therapies. Journal of Medical Internet Research 13: e52.

Farrer L, Christensen H, Griffiths KM, Mackinnon A (2011). Internet-based CBT for depression with and without telephone tracking in a national helpline: randomised controlled trial. PLoS ONE 6: e28099.

Farrer L, Gulliver A, Chan JKY, et al (2013). Technology-based interventions for mental health in tertiary students: systematic review. Journal of Medical Internet Research 15: e101.

Ferriter M (1993). Computer aided interviewing and the psychiatric social history. Social Work and Social Sciences Review 4: 255–263.

Foroushani PS, Schneider J, Assareh N (2011). Meta-review of the effectiveness of computerised CBT in treating depression. BMC Psychiatry 11: 131.

Furmark T, Carlbring P, Hedman E, et al (2009). Guided and unguided self-help for social anxiety disorder: randomised controlled trial. British Journal of Psychiatry 195: 440–447.

Garcia-Lizana F, Munoz-Mayorga I (2010). Telemedicine for depression: a systematic review. Perspectives in Psychiatric Care 46: 119–126.

Gega L, Kenwright M, Mataix-Cols D, Cameron R, Marks IM (2005). Screening people with anxiety/depression for suitability for guided self-help. Cognitive Behaviour Therapy 34: 16–21.

Gega L, Norman I, Marks I (2007). Computer-aided vs. tutor-delivered teaching of exposure therapy for phobia/panic: a randomised controlled trial with pre-registration nursing students. International Journal of Nursing Studies 44: 147–157.

Gega L, Smith J, Reynolds S (2013). Cognitive behaviour therapy (CBT) for depression by computer vs. therapist: patient experiences & therapeutic processes. Psychotherapy Research 23: 218–231.

Gerhards SAH, Abmac TA, Arntz A, et al (2011). Improving adherence and effectiveness of computerised cognitive behavioural therapy without support for depression: a qualitative study on patient experiences. Journal of Affective Disorders 129: 117–125.

Gerhards SAH, de Graaf LE, Jacobs LE, et al (2010). Economic evaluation of online computerised cognitive behavioral therapy without support for depression in primary care: randomised trial. British Journal of Psychiatry 196: 310–318.

Greist JH, Klein MH, VanCura LJ (1973). A computer interview by psychiatric patient target symptoms. Archives of General Psychiatry 29: 247–253.

Greist JH, Marks IM, Baer L, et al (2002). Behavior therapy for obsessive-compulsive disorder guided by a computer or by a clinician compared with relaxation as a control. Journal of Clinical Psychiatry 63: 138–145.

Griffiths KM, Calear AL, Banfield M (2009). Systematic review on Internet support groups (ISGs) and depression (1): do ISGs reduce depressive symptoms? Journal of Medical Internet Research 11: e40.

Griffiths KM, Farrer L, Christensen H (2010). The efficacy of internet interventions for depression and anxiety disorders: a review of randomised controlled trials. Medical Journal of Australia 192: S4–S11.

Grosse S (2008). Assessing cost-effectiveness in healthcare: history of the $50,000 per QALY threshold. Expert Review of Pharmacoeconomics & Outcomes Research 8: 165–178.

Gyani A, Shafran R, Layard R, Clark DM (2013) Enhancing recovery rates: lessons from year one of IAPT. Behaviour Research and Therapy 51: 597–606.

Hawton K, Salkovskis PM., Kirk J, Clark DM, Editors (1989). Cognitive Therapy for Psychiatric Problems: A Practical Guide. Oxford University Press, Oxford, UK.

Hedman E, Andersson E, Lindefors N, Andersson G, Rück C, Ljótsson B. (2013) Cost-effectiveness and long-term effectiveness of internet-based cognitive behaviour therapy for severe health anxiety. Psychological Medicine 43: 363–374.

Hedman E, Andersson E, Ljótsson B, Andersson G, Rück C, Lindefors N (2011). Cost-effectiveness of internet-based cognitive behavior therapy vs. cognitive behavioral group therapy for social anxiety disorder: results from a randomized controlled trial. Behaviour Research and Therapy 49: 729–736.

Hedman E, Ljótsson B, Lindefors N (2012). Cognitive behavior therapy via the Internet: a systematic review of applications, clinical efficacy and cost-effectiveness. Expert Review of Pharmacoeconomics & Outcomes Research 12: 745–764.

Hilvert-Bruce Z, Rossouw PJ, Wong N, Sunderland M, Andrews G (2012). Adherence as a determinant of effectiveness of internet cognitive behavioural therapy for anxiety and depressive disorders. Behaviour Research and Therapy 50: 463–468.

Hind D, O'Cathain A, Cooper CL, et al (2010). The acceptability of computerised cognitive behavioural therapy for the treatment of depression in people with chronic physical disease: a qualitative study of people with multiple sclerosis. Psychology and Health 25: 699–712.

Holländare F, Anthony SA, Randestad M, et al (2013). Two-year outcome of internet-based relapse prevention for partially remitted depression. Behavior Research and Therapy 51: 719–722.

Johansson R, Ekbladh S, Hebert A, et al (2012). Psychodynamic guided self-help for adult depression through the internet: a randomised controlled trial. PLoS ONE 7: e38021.

Johansson R, Nyblom A, Carlbring P, Cuijpers P, Andersson G (2013). Choosing between Internet-based psychodynamic versus cognitive behavioral therapy for depression: a pilot preference study. BMC Psychiatry 13: 268.

Kaltenthaler E, Brazier J, De Nigris E, et al (2006). Computerized cognitive behavior therapy for depression and anxiety update: a systematic review and economic evaluation. Health Technology Assessment 10: 1–70.

Kaltenthaler E, Sutcliffe P, Parry G, Beverley C, Rees A, Ferriter M (2008). The acceptability to patients of computerized cognitive behavior therapy for depression: a systematic review. Psychological Medicine 38: 1521–1530.

Kazantzis N, L'Abate L, Editors (2007). Handbook of Homework Assignments in Psychotherapy: Research, Practice, and Prevention. Springer, New York, NY.

Kelders SM, Kok RN, Ossebaard HC, Van Gemert-Pijnen JE (2012). Persuasive system design does matter: a systematic review of adherence to web-based interventions. Journal of Medical Internet Research 14: e152.

Kenardy J, McCafferty K, Rosa V (2003). Internet-delivered indicated prevention for anxiety disorders: a RCT. Behavioural and Cognitive Psychotherapy 31: 279–289.

Kenter R, Warmerdam L, Brouwer-Dudokdewit C, Cuijpers P, Van Straten A (2013). Guided online treatment in routine mental health care: an observational study on uptake, drop-out and effects. BMC Psychiatry 13: 43.

Kessler D, Lewis G, Kaur S, et al (2009). Therapist-delivered internet psychotherapy for depression in primary care: a randomised controlled trial. Lancet 374: 628–634.

Klein B, Austin D, Pier C, et al (2009). Internet-based treatment for panic disorder: does frequency of therapist contact make a difference? Cognitive Behaviour Therapy 38: 100–113.

Knowles SE, Toms G, Sanders C, et al (2014). Qualitative meta-synthesis of user experience of computerised therapy for depression and anxiety. PLoS ONE 9: e84323.

Kohl LF, Crutzen R, de Vries NK (2013). Online prevention aimed at lifestyle behaviors: a systematic review of reviews. Journal of Medical Internet Research 15: e146.

Learmonth D, Rai S (2008). Taking computerized CBT beyond primary care. British Journal of Clinical Psychology 47: 111–118.

Lillevoll KR, Wilhelmsen M, Kolstrup N, et al (2013). Patients' experiences of helpfulness in guided Internet-based treatment for depression: qualitative study of integrated therapeutic dimensions. Journal of Medical Internet Research 15: e126.

Lintvedt OK, Griffiths KM, Sørensen K, et al (2013). Evaluating the effectiveness and efficacy of unguided internet-based self-help intervention for the prevention of depression: a randomized controlled trial. Clinical Psychology and Psychotherapy 20: 10–27.

Ljótsson B, Andersson G, Andersson E, et al (2011). Acceptability, effectiveness, and cost-effectiveness of internet-based exposure treatment for irritable bowel syndrome in a clinical sample: a randomized controlled trial. BMC Gastroenterology 11: 110.

MacGregor AD, Hayward L, Peck DF, Wilkes P (2009). Empirically grounded clinical interventions: clients and referrers' perceptions of computer-guided CBT (FearFighter). Behavioural and Cognitive Psychotherapy 37: 1–9.

Marks IM, Kavanagh K, Gega L (2007). Hands-on Help: Computer-aided Psychotherapy. Maudsley Monograph—No. 49. Psychology Press, Hove, UK.

Marks IM, Kenwright M, McDonough M, Whittaker M, Mataix-Cols D (2004). Saving clinicians' time by delegating routine aspects of therapy to a computer: a randomized controlled trial in phobia/panic disorder. Psychological Medicine 34: 9–18.

Mayo-Wilson E, Montgomery P (2013). Media-delivered cognitive behavioral therapy and behavioral therapy (self-help) for anxiety disorders in adults. Cochrane Database of Systematic Reviews 9: CD005330.

McCrone P, Knapp M, Proudfoot J, et al (2004). Cost-effectiveness of computerised CBT for anxiety and depression in primary care. British Journal of Psychiatry 185: 55–62.

McCrone P, Marks IM, Greist JH, et al (2007). Cost-effectiveness of computer-aided behavior therapy for obsessive-compulsive disorder. Psychotherapy and Psychosomatics 76: 249–250.

Melville KM, Casey LM, Kavanagh DJ (2010). Dropout from Internet-based treatment for psychological disorders. British Journal of Clinical Psychology 49: 455–471.

Mihalopoulos C, Kiropoulos L, Shih ST, Gunn J, Blashki G, Meadows G (2005). Exploratory economic analyses of two primary care mental health projects: implications for sustainability. Medical Journal of Australia 183(Suppl 10): S73–S76.

Mohr DC, Burns MN, Schueller SM, Clarke G, Klinkman M (2013). Behavioral intervention technologies: evidence review and recommendations for future research in mental health. General Hospital Psychiatry 35: 332–338.

Mohr DC, Siddique J, Ho J, Duffecy J, Jin L, Fokuo JK (2010). Interest in behavioral and psychological treatments delivered face-to-face, by telephone, and by internet. Annals of Behavioural Medicine 40: 89–98.

Mora L, Nevid J, Chaplin W (2008). Psychologist treatment recommendations for Internet-based therapeutic interventions. Computers in Human Behavior 24: 3052–3062.

Murray K, Pombo-Carril MG, Bara-Carril N, et al (2003). Factors determining uptake of a CD-ROM-based CBT self-help treatment for bulimia: patient characteristics and subjective appraisals of self-help treatment. European Eating Disorders Review 11: 243–260.

Murray K, Schmidt U, Pombo-Carril M-G, et al (2007). Does therapist guidance improve uptake, adherence and outcome from a CD-ROM based cognitive-behavioral intervention for the treatment of bulimia nervosa? Computers in Human Behavior 23: 850–859.

National Institute for Health and Care Excellence (NICE) (2009). Quick Reference Guide. Depression: treatment and management of depression in adults, including adults with a chronic physical health problem. NICE Clinical Guidelines 90 and 91. NICE, London, UK.

National Institute for Health and Care Excellence (NICE) (2013a). Guide to the methods of technology appraisal. NICE, London, UK.

National Institute for Health and Care Excellence (NICE) (2013b). Social anxiety disorder: recognition, assessment and treatment. NICE Clinical Guideline 159. NICE, London, UK.

Neil AL, Batterham P, Christensen H, Bennett K, Griffiths KM (2009). Predictors of adherence by adolescents to a cognitive behavior therapy website in school and community-based settings. Journal of Medical Internet Research 11: e6.

Neil AL, Christensen H (2009). Efficacy and effectiveness of school-based prevention and early intervention programs for anxiety. Clinical Psychology Review 29: 208–215.

Neve M, Morgan PJ, Jones PR, Collins CE (2010). Effectiveness of web-based interventions in achieving weight loss and weight loss maintenance in overweight and obese adults: a systematic review with meta-analysis. Obesity Reviews 11: 306–321.

Olmstead TA, Ostrow CD, Carroll, KM (2010). Cost-effectiveness of computer-assisted training in cognitive-behavioral therapy as an adjunct to standard care for addiction. Drug and Alcohol Dependence 110: 200–207.

Palmqvist B, Carlbring P, Andersson G (2007). Internet-delivered treatments with or without therapist input: does the therapist factor have implications for efficacy and cost? Expert Review of Pharmacoeconomics & Outcomes Research 7: 291–297.

Paul CL, Carey ML, Sanson-Fisher RW, Houlcroft LE, Turon HE (2013). The impact of web-based approaches on psychosocial health in chronic physical and mental health conditions. Health Education Research 28: 450–471.

Postel MG, de Haan HA, De Jong CAJ (2008). E-Therapy for mental health problems: a systematic review. Telemedicine and E-Health 14: 707–714.

Postel MG, de Haan HA, ter Huurne ED, Becker ES, de Jong CA (2010). Effectiveness of a web-based intervention for problem drinkers and reasons for dropout: randomized controlled trial. Journal of Medical Internet Research 12: e68.

Powell J, Hamborg T, Stallard N, et al (2012). Effectiveness of a web-based cognitive-behavioral tool to improve mental well-being in the general population: randomized controlled trial. Journal of Medical Internet Research 15: e2.

Proudfoot J, Ryden C, Everitt B, et al (2004). Clinical effectiveness of computerized cognitive behavioral therapy for anxiety and depression in primary care. British Journal of Psychiatry 185: 46–54.

Reger MA, Gahm GA (2009). A meta-analysis of the effects of Internet- and computer-based cognitive-behavioral treatments for anxiety. Journal of Clinical Psychology 65: 53–75.

Richardson T, Stallard P, Velleman S (2010). Computerised cognitive behavioural therapy for the prevention and treatment of depression and anxiety in children and adolescents: a systematic review. Clinical Child and Family Psychology Review 13: 275–290.

Robinson R, West R (1992). A comparison of computer and questionnaire methods of history-taking in a genitourinary clinic. Psychology and Health 6: 77–84.

Roth A, Fonagy P, Editors (2008). What Works for Whom? A Critical Review of Psychotherapy Research. 2nd Edition. Guilford, New York, NY.

Ruwaard J, Lange A, Schrieken B, Emmelkamp P (2011). Efficacy and effectiveness of online cognitive behavioral treatment: a decade of interapy research. Studies in Health Technology & Informatics 167: 9–14.

Schulz KF, Grimes DA (2002). Sample size slippages in randomised trials: exclusions and the lost and wayward. Lancet 359: 781–785.

So M, Yamaguchi S, Hashimoto S, Sado M, Furukawa TA, McCrone P (2013). Is computerised CBT really helpful for adult depression? A meta-analytic re-evaluation of CCBT for adult depression in terms of clinical implementation and methodological validity. BMC Psychiatry 13: 113.

Spek V, Cuijpers P, Nyklíček I, Riper H, Keyzer J, Pop V (2007). Internet-based cognitive behavior therapy for symptoms of depression and anxiety: a meta-analysis Psychological Medicine 37: 319–328.

Spence SH, Holmes JM, March S, Lipp OV (2006). The feasibility and outcome of clinic plus Internet delivery of cognitive-behavior therapy for childhood anxiety. Journal of Consulting and Clinical Psychology 74: 614–621.

Stallard P, Richardson T, Velleman S (2010). Clinician's attitudes towards the use of computerised cognitive behaviour therapy (cCBT) with children and adolescents. Behavioural and Cognitive Psychotherapy 38: 545–560.

Titov N, Andrews G, Choi I, Schwencke G, Mahoney A (2008). Shyness 3: randomized controlled trial of guided versus unguided Internet-based CBT for social phobia. Australian and New Zealand Journal of Psychiatry 42: 1030–1040.

Titov N, Andrews G, Schwencke G, et al (2010). Randomized controlled trial of Internet cognitive behavioural treatment for social phobia with and without motivational enhancement strategies. Australian and New Zealand Journal of Psychiatry 44: 938–945.

Trusheim MR, Berndt ER, Douglas FL (2007). Stratified medicine: strategic and economic implications of combining drugs and clinical biomarkers. Nature Reviews Drug Discovery 6: 287–293.

van Beugen S, Ferwerda M, Hoeve D, et al (2014). Internet-based cognitive behavioral therapy for patients with chronic somatic conditions: a meta-analytic review. Journal of Medical Internet Research 16: e88.

van Gemert-Pijnen JE, Nijland N, van Limburg M, et al (2011). A holistic framework to improve the uptake and impact of eHealth technologies. Journal of Medical Internet Research 13: e111.

van Spijker BAJ, Majo C, Smit F, van Straten A, Kerkhof AJFM (2012). Reducing suicidal ideation: cost-effectiveness analysis of a randomized controlled trial of unguided web-based self-help. Journal of Medical Internet Research 14: e141.

Vangberg HCB, Lillevoll KR, Waterloo K, Eisemann M (2012). Does personality predict depression and use of an Internet-based intervention for depression among adolescents? Depression Research and Treatment, Article ID 593068.

Vernmark K, Lenndin J, Bjärehed J, et al (2011). Internet administered guided self-help versus individualized e-mail therapy: a randomized trial of two versions of CBT for major depression. Behaviour Research and Therapy 48: 368–376.

Waller R, Gilbody S (2009). Barriers to the uptake of computerized cognitive behavioral therapy: a systematic review of the quantitative and qualitative evidence. Psychological Medicine 39: 705–712.

Walters ST, Wright JA, Shegog R (2006). A review of computer and Internet-based interventions for smoking behavior. Addictive Behaviors 31: 264–277.

Wangberg SC, Gammon D, Spitznogle K (2007). In the eyes of the beholder: exploring psychologists' attitudes towards and use of e-therapy in Norway. Cyberpsychology and Behavior 10: 418–423.

Wantland DJ, Portillo CJ, Holzemer WL, Slaughter R, McGhee EM (2004). The effectiveness of Web-based vs. non-Web-based interventions: a meta-analysis of behavioral change outcomes. Journal of Medical Internet Research 6: e40.

Warmerdam L, Smit F, van Straten A, Riper H, Cuijpers P (2010). Cost-utility and cost-effectiveness of internet-based treatment for adults with depressive symptoms: randomized trial. Journal of Medical Internet Research 12: e53.

White A, Kavanagh D, Stallman H, et al (2010). Online alcohol interventions: a systematic review. Journal of Medical Internet Research 12: e62.

Whitfield G, Williams C (2004). If the evidence is so good—why doesn't anyone use them? A national survey of the use of computerized cognitive behaviour therapy. Behavioural and Cognitive Psychotherapy 32: 57–65.

Wood SK, Eckley L, Hughes K, et al (2014). Computer-based programmes for the prevention and management of illicit recreational drug use: a systematic review. Addictive Behaviors 39: 30–38.

Wright JH, Turkington D, Sudak DM, Thase ME (2010). High-Yield Cognitive-Behavior Therapy for Brief Sessions: An Illustrated Guide. American Psychiatric Publishing, Arlington, VA.

Wylie-Rosett J, Swencionis C, Ginsberg M, et al (2001). Computerized weight loss intervention optimizes staff time: the clinical and cost results of a controlled clinical trial conducted in a managed care setting. Journal of the American Dietetic Association 101: 1155–1162.

12 Virtual Reality in Exposure Therapy

The Next Frontier

Eric Malbos

INTRODUCTION

"The engineers of the future will be poets. This is what virtual reality holds out to us—the possibility of walking in to the constructs of the imagination" (McKenna, 1995). This quote from the American philosopher Terence McKenna highlights the boundless potential of a new medium in the postmodern world: virtual reality (VR). The aim of this chapter is to examine the therapeutic use of VR in mental disorders.

VR is made possible by a collection of technologies, including computers, head-mounted displays (HMDs), motion trackers, and data gloves, which allow individuals to interact efficiently and intuitively with a three-dimensional (3D) virtual environment using natural senses and skills (Riva et al., 2002b). Thus, VR can be regarded as a novel human-computer interaction paradigm where the user is an active participant in the interaction (Riva and Wiederhold, 2002). This is enabled by two crucial characteristics of this medium: (1) the real-time aspect of interactions with objects or virtual humans and (2) the possibility of a new sense of presence or existing in computer-generated environments (the feeling of "being there") (Heeter, 1992). Such immersion into synthesized worlds can be achieved via specific equipment, most commonly a HMD that is embedded in a helmet and connected to a head motion tracker (Figure 12.1A) and a computer. Another apparatus consists of several large screens arranged in the shape of a "curve" that wraps around the person (Figure 12.1B). Less often, a cave automatic virtual environment (CAVE) is used, consisting of a room where each wall is a screen in itself displaying 3D images produced by several video

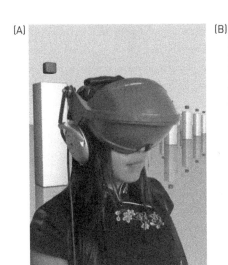
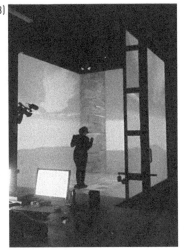
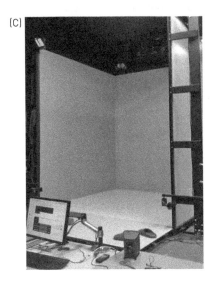

FIGURE 12.1

Virtual reality apparatus: head mounted display with embedded motion tracker (A) and cave automatic virtual environment (B and C). (B and C courtesy of Center for Virtual Reality of the Mediterranean.)

projectors (Figure 12.1C). Other equipment for analyzing and integrating the human body representation and its digital model include steering wheels, joysticks or other navigation controls, spatial motion trackers, and sound production systems.

The early prototype for a VR platform dates back to the late 1960s, when Ivan Sutherland attempted to create an avant-garde display system that reacted to viewers' actions. Given the name "Ultimate Display," this magnum opus integrated several key features of VR: computer-generated images, stereoscopic vision, and synchronization of the view with movements of the head (Sutherland, 1965). This milestone was followed by the systematic introduction by the National Aeronautics and Space Administration and the US Army in the 1980s of reality simulation in training activities, such as the Visually Coupled Airborne System Simulator. Currently, VR has multiple applications in the military domain (piloting, telerobotics), medicine (modeling superior brain functions, spatial learning, pain control), science (inaccessible matter manipulation), communications (teleconferencing), art (architecture visualization, design demonstration), engineering (testing design properties), and video gaming (in-depth immersion with virtual characters) (Gobbetti and Scateni, 1998).

VR has also demonstrated value in mental health, specifically as a tool for the administration of psychotherapy. The initial attempt took place in 1992 at Clark Atlanta University's Virtual Reality Technology Laboratory. The objective was to exploit the immersive properties of VR to treat one subject suffering from aviophobia (fear of flying). Through eight 30-minute sessions of exposure to a virtual environment representing an aircraft cabin, the subject was able to achieve symptom control (North and North, 1994).

Exposure is a central tenet of cognitive-behavioral therapy (CBT), widely considered the standard psychotherapeutic treatment for anxiety disorders, including specific phobias (Deacon and Abramowitz, 2004; National Institute of Clinical Excellence, 2007; National Institute of Mental Health, 2010). Typically, CBT for phobias includes in vivo exposure, which requires the patient to be gradually and repeatedly confronted with feared objects or spaces (e.g., planes, elevators, spiders). The goal is to achieve habituation and extinction, leading to a decrease in fear and avoidance behavior. Via the use of VR, in vivo exposure to the feared stimulus can be replaced by exposure to artificially created stimuli inside a computerized world. This approach has been called virtual reality exposure therapy (VRET). Like CBT, it uses exposure to attain habituation to feared triggers and anxiety extinction, but it does so in a more flexible and controllable environment than real life (Rothbaum et al., 2001).

Theoretically, VRET could address some shortcomings inherent in CBT. For instance, a relatively high proportion of patients are reluctant to undergo traditional exposure therapy. It is estimated that 60% to 80% of patients with specific phobias never seek professional help, and among those who do, 25% refuse to undergo exposure (Botella et al., 2007). That is typically due to fear of confronting the phobogenic stimulus during therapy. There are also the practical obstacles to facing feared stimuli such as planes, trains, elevators, or crowded places if they are difficult or inconvenient to access (Cottraux, 1995). Indeed, traditional exposure therapy depends on various uncontrollable random events that may disrupt the progress of therapy (e.g., people or crowd behavior, weather and transport conditions, mechanical issues). In addition, the following factors should be considered: cost may hamper treatment; exposure in some environments, such as planes, trains, and buses, may be expensive; and the time needed to conduct the therapy, including transportation to and from the therapist's office, may produce prohibitive expenses (Rothbaum et al., 2006).

VRET can help address some of these limitations. The patient does not need to leave the office and may potentially undergo the entire treatment in camera (i.e., in private), feeling reassured by the controlled environment and by the confidential nature of the intervention (Banos et al., 2002). Also, VR features graded fear-eliciting environments, which can ease the process and prevent the occurrence of sensitization incidents (i.e., accidental exposure to a highly anxiogenic situation; Rothbaum et al., 2000). If required, exposure to a particular event or situation may be repeated relatively easily, as many times as necessary. During the process, patient reactions can be closely monitored by the therapist via objective measures such as vital signs and subjective instruments such as questionnaires (Malbos et al., 2012). VRET still typically involves a face-to-face interaction with the therapist; therefore, the VRET session can be an opportunity to review with the patient previously learned techniques, such as relaxation strategies, mindfulness, and cognitive methods.

The high degree of control over the virtual environment can inspire additional motivation and comfort in the patient. To that effect, some trials have shown a general preference for VRET over standard CBT (Garcia-Palacios et al., 2007). For example, when requested to choose between VRET and traditional exposure in a trial that compared both interventions for diverse phobias, 76% of participants stated that they preferred VRET. Moreover, when given the option to undergo these two exposure programs, the refusal rate for exposure therapy was higher than for the VRET (27% versus 3%).

VRET may also save time and money. There is no need with VRET to take time to reach the outdoor exposure site with the therapist or to spend money on plane tickets or train rides. The notion that VRET may save money can surprise practitioners and patients—the usual assumption is that VRET is prohibitively expensive due to the need to invest in necessary equipment. However, as the technology used by VRET becomes more ubiquitous, accessibility to equipment continues to improve and the associated price tag continues to decrease (Malbos et al., 2008).

TREATMENT USING VIRTUAL REALITY EXPOSURE THERAPY

Positive results from experiments since 1992 suggest that VRET may be effective in the treatment of anxiety disorders such as specific phobias, agoraphobia and post-traumatic stress disorder (PTSD), and eating disorders (Riva et al., 2003; Powers and Emmelkamp, 2008). In addition, more recent studies have begun to test the potential of the VRET in targeting obsessive-compulsive disorder (OCD), substance use disorders, and the social impairment of schizophrenia. Interestingly, data are lacking on using VRET in the treatment of mood disorders.

Anxiety Disorders

VRET has been tested in a number of clinical trials involving various anxiety disorders, and two meta-analyses have demonstrated its clinical efficacy (Powers and Emmelkamp, 2008; Opris et al., 2012). Study protocols tend to be similar in VRET; subjects with an anxiety diagnosis are typically placed in a prolonged and repeated fashion in a virtual representation of the situation they avoid or fear. VRET is administered in 5 to 12 weekly sessions lasting 30 to 60 minutes each, and the effect is measured via subjective methods (questionnaires administered before and after the exposure) and objective methods (physiological parameters such as heart rate, body temperature, and skin conductance) (Malbos et al., 2008, 2013).

Aviophobia (fear of flying)

Since the aforementioned 1992 experiment, several studies of aviophobia, including trials that compared VRET to a wait list control and to traditional CBT, have been conducted. High interest in this particular phobia may be partially explained by economic factors; annual losses by airlines in the United States caused by aviophobia exceed $1 billion (Rothbaum et al., 2000), creating a strong financial impetus for the airline industry to support research in this field.

Controlled trials of VRET for aviophobia were conducted by Rothbaum and others in 2000 (N = 45) and 2006 (N = 73). Both compared the intervention to a wait list control and to standard in vivo exposure. In both studies, subjects undergoing active treatment (whether VRET or in vivo exposure) received four sessions, with superior therapeutic efficacy demonstrated for VRET compared to the wait list control and an equivalent effect when compared to in vivo exposure (Rothbaum et al., 2000, 2002, 2006). The positive change was maintained at the 6- and 12-month follow-up assessments, and participants were able to make real flights thereafter. This supports de facto the possibility of a generalization of the VRET benefits to real-life fearful situations. Of note, the same virtual spaces, aircraft cabins, and 3D models (Figure 12.2) can also be used in the treatment of other phobias, including agoraphobia and claustrophobia (Malbos et al., 2013).

Acrophobia (fear of heights)

The first test of VRET in the treatment of acrophobia (fear of heights) was conducted in a 19-year-old subject in 1995 (Rothbaum et al., 1995). The observed reduction in the severity of acrophobia propelled the same team to conduct a trial in 17 acrophobic subjects. Similar symptom improvement was noted on all scales for the VRET group (Rothbaum and Hodges, 1999). Another study compared 10 subjects receiving VRET to 33 receiving in vivo exposure (Emmelkamp et al., 2002), and similar results were observed in both groups. In addition, the researchers used a low-cost commercially available personal computer with a HMD attached, suggesting that access to VRET in standard practice settings should not require large investments in technology or infrastructure. One subsequent study compared HMD and CAVE and reported similar therapeutic effects for the two delivery systems (Krijn et al., 2004).

Arachnophobia (fear of spiders)

The first test of VRET in the treatment of arachnophobia (fear of spiders) was conducted in 1996 in a 37-year-old subject. After 12 sessions, the symptoms improved

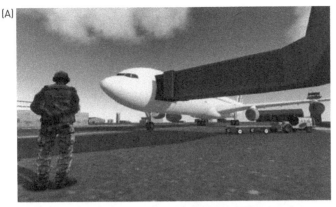

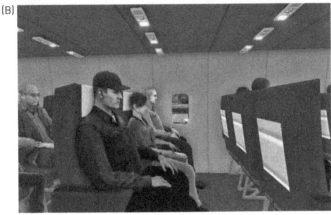

FIGURE 12.2
Virtual environment for aviophobia with boarding platform and Airbus 340 airplane (A). The plane features a virtual cabin with avatars waiting for takeoff (B).

enough for the patient to be able to camp outdoors. A peculiar aspect of this experiment was the incorporation of a fake hairy spider into the VRET procedure, introducing a tactile element and a sense of physicality (Carlin et al., 1997). The first controlled study to compare VRET to a wait list control in arachnophobia was conducted in 2002 in 23 subjects (Garcia-Palacios et al., 2002). Eighty three percent of those assigned to VRET showed significant clinical improvement compared to none in the wait list control group.

Claustrophobia

The first published case report of VRET in the treatment of claustrophobia described a 43-year-old woman whose phobia prevented her from undergoing a tomography scan necessary for the assessment of a suspected spinal cord lesion (Botella et al., 1998). VRET yielded a significant reduction in her anxiety. Subsequently, Malbos et al. (2008) conducted a study in six claustrophobic subjects using affordable VR equipment and virtual environments constructed with an inexpensive game level editor (Figure 12.3). Game level editors are developed by video game companies for the mainstream gaming market and often possess powerful 3D engines that are

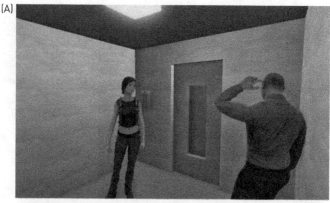

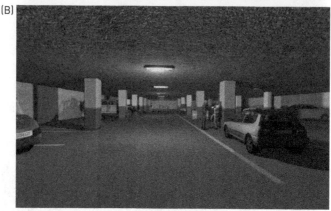

FIGURE 12.3

Virtual reality exposure therapy for claustrophobia: virtual environment simulating an elevator (A) and a dark underground parking lot (B).

compatible with a large array of personal computer hardware and are meant to be used by the average gamer. Although rather low-cost ($10–$60), the graphic, animation, and realistic features of game level editors can often match professional software; their aim is to immerse the player into a realistic 3D environment. In this specific study, VRET yielded significant clinical improvement in all subjects, with generalization noted to feared real life situations (e.g., elevators, planes) (Malbos et al., 2008).

Driving Phobia

VRET for driving phobia typically consists of driving a virtual car (Figure 12.4). A significant clinical improvement was reported in a single case study (Wald and Taylor, 2000) and a study of 10 subjects (Walshe et al., 2003). In both studies, the virtual environment was derived from a driving video game.

Social Phobia

The use of VR to create a flexible and controllable virtual audience was introduced in 1998 in a controlled study of VRET in 16 subjects with fear of public speaking

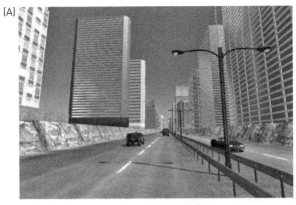

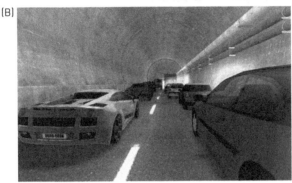

FIGURE 12.4

Virtual reality exposure therapy for agoraphobia and driving phobia: virtual highway without traffic (A) and traffic jam in a 3-km tunnel (B).

(North et al., 1998). Study results suggested that VRET might be effective for this disorder. Similar outcomes were observed in a subsequent uncontrolled study in 10 subjects (Anderson et al., 2005) and a controlled trial that compared VRET to conventional CBT in 58 subjects (Safir et al., 2012). To test VRET in broader social situations that may produce anxiety, Klinger et al. (2005) compared it to conventional CBT in 36 subjects with a wide range of socially induced distress (e.g., occurring in public forums, bars, meeting rooms, elevators). The study showed similar efficacy between VRET and treatment in vivo.

Agoraphobia with or without Panic Disorder

Agoraphobia involves a fear and avoidance of a wide range of distinct places from which escape might be difficult or embarrassing (e.g., planes, subways, cinemas, crowded places, highways, standing in lines). The first study of VRET in agoraphobia dates back to 1996 (North et al., 1996). Subsequently, a controlled trial in 12 agoraphobic subjects compared "experiential cognitive therapy" (a therapy that integrates the use of VR with traditional multicomponent CBT strategy) with standard CBT and a wait list control. Experiential cognitive therapy was as efficacious as CBT and required fewer sessions for analogous outcomes (Vincelli et al., 2003). This finding was corroborated by a subsequent, larger, controlled trial in 40 subjects (Botella et al., 2004). More recently, a study used a contextually graded virtual environment design, which presented 18 subjects with a hierarchy of anxiogenic cues. These cues included virtual road tunnels of increasing length, virtual flights with progressively worsening weather, virtual subway rides of gradually increasing duration, and virtual supermarkets with progressively longer customer queues (Figures 12.5 and 12.6; Malbos et al., 2013). In addition to demonstrating that virtual environments can be created by a therapist at a reasonable cost, this study showed a significant therapeutic efficacy for VRET in all domains (behavioral, physiological, and subjective).

Obsessive-Compulsive Disorder

The diverse nature of the anxiogenic triggers that lead to compulsions such as washing or checking in patients with OCD makes it difficult to create a virtual environment that would address the needs of a broad range of patients. The high level of customization required may explain the limited number of VRET studies in OCD. However, a pilot study showed that VR exposure induced a detectable level of anxiety in 33 subjects with OCD (Kim et al., 2009); this suggested a possibility of using VRET

(A)

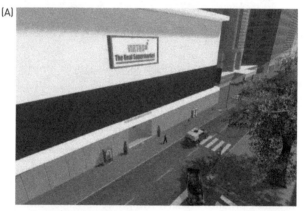

(B)

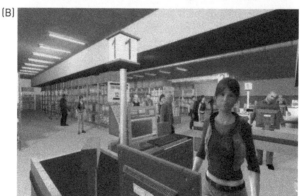

FIGURE 12.5

Virtual mall (A) and supermarket (B). Note three-dimensional objects, dynamic shadows, cashiers, and virtual queue.

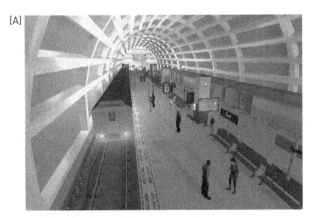

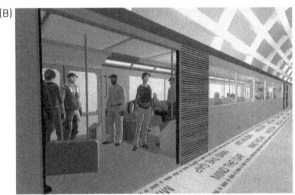

FIGURE 12.6

Virtual underground train station (A and B). The number of three-dimensional passengers can vary depending on desired exercise difficulty. This is used in virtual reality exposure therapy for diverse phobias, including agoraphobia and claustrophobia.

for OCD because emotional arousal is required to obtain a therapeutic effect from exposure (Foa and Kozak, 1986). Researchers then created virtual environments for a sample of 24 OCD subjects with cleaning compulsions, and results showed a decreasing level of anxiety over the course of the VRET sessions (Kim et al., 2011). Further studies are needed to assess the use of VRET in the treatment of OCD.

Posttraumatic Stress Disorder

The high prevalence of PTSD among war veterans and the impossibility of simulating war situations in conventional CBT have prompted the search for alternate treatments. The first test of VRET in PTSD was conducted in 1999 in a single case (Rothbaum et al., 1999) and was followed by an uncontrolled trial that used a combination of VRET, relaxation tools, and imagery techniques in nine combat veterans (Rothbaum et al., 2001). Both studies focused on the Vietnam War and therefore included a virtual environment resembling the landscape of Southeast Asia (i.e., with tropical jungle, rice fields). Although the first study showed a decrease in the scores on PTSD rating scales, the second study found a significant reduction in anxiety and avoidance, along with a shift from severely to moderately intense PTSD symptoms. In the second study, follow-up assessments at 3 months (N = 5) and 6 months (N = 8) showed stable benefit.

Regarding nonwar traumas involving civilians, one case report described improvement with VRET in a survivor of the September 11, 2001 terrorist attacks (Difede and Hoffman, 2002). This was followed by a controlled trial in 13 survivors, with results showing a significant improvement compared to the wait list control group (Difede et al., 2007). More recently, a controlled trial of VRET versus conventional CBT in 10 subjects with PTSD of diverse etiologies (physical abuse, automobile accident, assault) suggested efficacy of both CBT and VRET, with a statistical difference in favor of the latter (Banos et al., 2011). Finally, the use of VRET for the treatment of survivors of motor vehicle accidents with PTSD was examined in an uncontrolled clinical experiment. The outcome indicated significant reductions in post-trauma symptoms involving reexperiencing, avoidance, and emotional numbing (Beck et al., 2007).

Eating Disorders

Conventional CBT in the treatment of eating disorders incorporates body image modification, cognitive tools, behavioral procedures (e.g., exposure to objects of temptation to extinguish a pathological response), visuomotor techniques (e.g., visualization of the body schema), and nutrition and dietary education. Studies of VRET in eating disorders were initiated in 1997 by Riva's team in Italy (Riva and Mellis, 1997). In addition to cognitive methods, these studies used virtual environments constructed to resemble anxiogenic situations, such as a room with a virtual scale, feared social settings (e.g., restaurants, public swimming pools), and objects and activities of temptation (e.g., cooking, food, refrigerator). To alter the misconception regarding body image, subjects were shown pictures of virtual humans of different body height, weight, and age, and asked to choose the best fit for their current and ideal body (Riva et al., 2002a). A comparison of scores in 20 subjects with binge-eating disorder before and after this VR exercise revealed a significant reduction in body dissatisfaction and social avoidance. These findings were supported by a more recent study in a similar population (Marco et al., 2013). A controlled study in 120 subjects who were either obese or had an eating disorder (binge-eating disorder or bulimia nervosa) demonstrated a superior therapeutic effect for VRET compared with a traditional CBT psychonutrition program (Riva and Molinari, 2009). Similar outcomes were reported in a controlled study involving 90 obese patients with binge-eating disorder (Cesa et al., 2013).

Substance Use Disorders

Many psychotherapeutic approaches to drug dependence center on the concept of cue reactivity. Cues trigger the desire, or "craving," to use drugs. This craving can then induce drug consumption or relapse. Conventional CBT for substance dependence includes repeated exposure to cues while resisting drug consumption. This aims at reducing reactivity to drug cues through extinction. However, in traditional therapy, sessions are run so that relevant situations are shown on slides, photographs, or film; also, therapists seldom accompany patients to the real locations that activate their craving. Therefore, researchers have investigated the simulation of these cues inside a computerized environment composed of bar like settings, 3D bartenders, virtual humans, and virtual customers (Figure 12.7).

An early study exposed five heroin addicts to a virtual scene consisting of a bar with a heroin-like substance and injection paraphernalia on the counter (Kuntze et al., 2001). The study reported a significant activation of the autonomic nervous system during exposure (with changes in heart rate, respiratory rate, oxygen saturation, and blood pressure), along with subjective discomfort and a strong desire to use the substance. Similar effects were detected in a sample of 47 smokers with tobacco dependence (Garcia-Rodriguez et al., 2012). Also, a study in 15 subjects with alcohol dependence tracked cravings when they were exposed to virtual environments that evoked alcohol consumption (e.g., going out, bars, kitchen). A unique aspect of this study was the incorporation of olfactory stimuli consisting of a variety of odors—whiskey, beer, cigarette, pizza—emanating from a scent palette or scent beads (Ryan et al., 2010). During exposure, binge drinkers reported significantly more cravings than nonbinge drinkers. Across these studies among

(A)

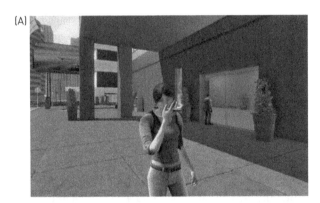

(B)

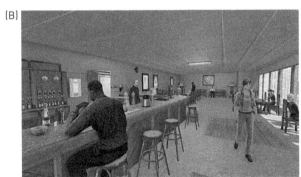

FIGURE 12.7
Virtual environment for social phobia, substance use disorders, and schizophrenia. An avatar smoking (A) and a bar (B). Social context can be used for rehabilitation and to induce cues for individuals with substance use disorders.

heroin, tobacco, and alcohol users, the induction of craving while in a virtual space demonstrates the potential therapeutic use of VR exposure.

A study of 46 nicotine-dependent subjects who crushed virtual cigarettes as a way of modifying their response to virtual smoking cues showed a significant reduction in relapse rates (Girard et al., 2009). Also, exposure to virtual alcohol cues (e.g., a bar, bottles of alcohol) in eight abstinent subjects with a history of alcohol dependence revealed reduced craving associated with these cues (Lee et al., 2007). Although these preliminary studies suggest potential benefits of VRET in the treatment of substance use disorders, studies comparing VRET with other treatments remain to be conducted.

Schizophrenia

Because reality confusion and hallucinations are among the core features of schizophrenia, VRET may seem contraindicated in this disorder. However, a small trial in four subjects who agreed to work with computers and HMDs to complete cognitive tasks (e.g., freehand drawing with a mouse and 3D visualization) showed that they tolerated the procedure well and that they were very interested in this technology (da Costa and de Carvalho, 2004). Additionally, there was good acceptance by subjects of virtual cognitive and social rehabilitation tasks (e.g., involving temporospatial orientation, combining auditory and visual information on a virtual piano, solving 3D puzzles, use of a virtual telephone). Subsequently, a study tested VR for cognitive and social rehabilitation in 91 subjects with schizophrenia, randomized to either a VR treatment group or traditional role playing (Park et al., 2011). Motivation measures documented a higher interest in VR compared to conventional treatment. There was a significant improvement in social competence from both interventions and, in the VR group, a greater effect on conversational skills and assertiveness.

Despite these preliminary results, it is important to be cautious, especially given the heterogeneity within schizophrenia. There is an insufficiently examined and real risk that the virtual aspect of VRET might strengthen delusions, cause new symptoms, or exacerbate deficits in reality testing. Clinicians and researchers should therefore proceed with caution when considering use of VRET in psychotic individuals.

CONCLUSION

VR, a modern space built out of a new human-machine relationship, is a medium that allows individuals to create and interact with nonexisting worlds without the constraints of concrete environments and materials. Synthesized worlds may then be exploited for an infinite number of applications. VRET is one such application. It adapts VR to well-established CBT methods, offering a new treatment that has accumulated some promising preliminary data. Indeed, studies of several psychological disturbances, including phobias, eating disorders, PTSD, OCD, substance use disorders, and schizophrenia, suggest efficacy on subjective and objective (behavioral and physiological) measures. Assuming lack of contraindications, such as severe myopia or photosensitive epilepsy that might be triggered by certain visual patterns such as flashing lights, government-funded controlled trials suggest that VRET, like traditional CBT, may be attempted as a first-line intervention in the treatment of some anxiety disorders. However, because of the effort and expertise needed to construct virtual environments, VRET is currently utilized more for treating conditions with common triggers (e.g., transportation phobia, animal phobia, situational phobia, PTSD following automobile accidents) than in the treatment of disorders with very unique or idiosyncratic cues (e.g., certain forms of OCD, PTSD, or phobias). The latter group would require the creation of customized virtual environments for every case—a time-consuming and expensive requirement given present technology and resources.

One can envision how VRET, through added convenience, enhanced practicality, and lower costs, can eventually address some limitations inherent to traditional CBT. Its resemblance to highly popular video games or 3D cinema may also add to its attractiveness and help its dissemination (Garcia-Palacios et al., 2002, 2007), as may the greater degree of control it offers the patient (Malbos et al., 2013). Still, several limitations of the current research need to be addressed before VRET can be widely recommended and used. First, the studies mostly involved a small number of subjects (generally less than 50), and larger, more representative studies are crucial. Second, better designed controlled trials against standard treatments are needed. Third, only a few studies involved long-term follow-up assessments, seriously limiting knowledge of long-term efficacy. Finally, there is great variability in, and lack of consensus on the equipment used, making comparisons among studies difficult.

Technological obstacles also remain, both at the level of savoir faire and availability. Although currently limited, HMDs and wireless models are likely to become more widely available in the future, which will decrease costs and make VRET more practical and affordable for small mental health clinics, individual therapists, and patients undertaking virtual exposure at home. Indeed, generalization of VR technology for computer and game consoles, as well as mass production, have already allowed a significant reduction in the price of VR equipment; although a ready-to-use HMD for personal computer can be purchased for about $1500, several very immersive prototype models intended for the general market (e.g., Oculus Rift, Gameface) can be expected to be available for less. Regarding software for researchers or clinicians wishing to use or even create therapeutic virtual environments, Riva has suggested free downloadable software for those with limited computer knowledge (NeuroVR 2.0, www.neurovr.org) (Riva et al., 2007). Other researchers advocate use of certain video game level editors to produce realistic immersive virtual environments at reduced cost ($10–$60); these have demonstrated therapeutic effects (Walshe et al., 2003; Bouchard et al., 2006; Malbos et al., 2008, 2013).

In conclusion, VRET is part of the fast-moving field of VR, which can be utilized as an experimental or therapeutic tool. However, its application is not limited to these fields. VR is not a substitute for human imagination; on the contrary, it allows individuals to create, visualize, and explore their own ideas. With the advent of new interfaces in the coming decades, such as omnidirectional treadmills, immersive suits, and computer-brain interfaces (Clausen, 2009), individuals in the future may see today's VR similarly to how people now regard the first nuclear reactor by Fermi, the discovery of other galaxies by Hubble, or the first flight into space by Gagarin—an early step into a domain that transcends them and prompts them to go forward.

DISCLOSURE STATEMENT

The author discloses no relationships with commercial entities and professional activities that may bias his views.

REFERENCES

Anderson PL, Rothbaum BO, Hodges LF (2005). Cognitive behavioral therapy for public-speaking anxiety using virtual reality for exposure. Depression and Anxiety 22: 156–158.

Banos RM, Botella C, Perpina C (2002). Virtual reality treatment of flying phobia. IEEE Transactions on Information Technology in Biomedicine 6: 206–212.

Banos RM, Guillen V, Quero S, Garcia-Palacios A, Alcaniz M, Botella C (2011). A virtual reality system for the treatment of stress-related disorders: a preliminary analysis of efficacy compared to a standard cognitive behavioral program. Human-Computer Studies 69: 602–613.

Beck JG, Palyo SA, Winer EH, Schwagler BE, Ang EJ (2007). Virtual reality exposure therapy for PTSD symptoms after a road accident: an uncontrolled case series. Behavior Therapy 38: 39–48.

Botella C, Banos RM, Perpina C (1998). Virtual reality treatment of claustrophobia: a case report. Behaviour Research and Therapy 36: 239–246.

Botella C, Garcia-Palacios A, Villa H (2007). Virtual reality exposure in the treatment of panic disorder and agoraphobia: a controlled study. Clinical Psychology and Psychotherapy 14: 164–175.

Botella C, Villa H, Garcia-Palacios A, Banos R (2004). Clinically significant virtual environments for the treatment of panic disorder and agoraphobia. Cyberpsychology and Behavior 7: 527–535.

Bouchard S, Cote S, St-Jacques J (2006). Effectiveness of virtual reality exposure in the treatment of arachnophobia using 3D games. Technology and Health Care 14: 19–27.

Carlin A, Hoffman H, Werghorst S (1997). Virtual reality and tactile augmentation in the treatment of spider phobia: a case report. Behaviour Research and Therapy 35: 153–158.

Cesa GL, Manzoni GM, Bacchetta M, et al (2013). Virtual reality for enhancing the cognitive behavioral treatment of obesity with binge eating disorder: randomized controlled study with one-year follow-up. Journal of Medical Internet Research 15: e113.

Clausen J (2009). Man, machine and in between. Nature 457: 1080–1081.

Cottraux J (1995). Les Thérapies Cognitivo-Comportementales [in French]. Masson, Paris, France.

da Costa RMEM, de Carvalho LAV (2004). The acceptance of virtual reality devices for cognitive rehabilitation: a report of positive results with schizophrenia. Computer Methods and Program in Biomedicine 73: 173–182.

Deacon B, Abramowitz J (2004). Cognitive and behavioral treatments for anxiety disorders: a review of meta-analytic findings. Journal of Clinical Psychology 60: 429–441.

Difede J, Cukor J, Jayasinghe N, et al (2007). Virtual reality exposure therapy for the treatment of posttraumatic stress disorder following September 11, 2001. Journal of Clinical Psychiatry 68: 1639–1647.

Difede J, Hoffman H (2002). Virtual reality exposure therapy for World Trade Center post-traumatic stress disorder: a case report. Cyberpsychology and Behavior 5: 529–535.

Emmelkamp PMG, Krijn M, Hulsbosch AM (2002). Virtual reality treatment versus exposure in vivo: a comparative evaluation in acrophobia. Behaviour Research and Therapy 40: 509–516.

Foa EB, Kozak MJ (1986). Emotional processing of fear: exposure to corrective information. Psychological Bulletin 99: 20–35.

Garcia-Palacios A, Botella C, Hoffman H (2007). Comparing acceptance and refusal rates of virtual reality exposure vs. in vivo exposure by patients with specific phobias. Cyberpsychology and Behavior 10: 722–724.

Garcia-Palacios A, Hoffman H, Carlin A (2002). Virtual reality in the treatment of spider phobia: a controlled study. Behaviour Research and Therapy 40: 983–993.

Garcia-Rodriguez O, Pericot-Valverde I, Gutierrez J, Ferrer-Garcia M, Secades-Villa R (2012). Validation of smoking-related virtual environments for cue exposure therapy. Addictive Behaviors 37: 703–708.

Girard B, Turcotte V, Bouchard S, Girard B (2009). Crushing virtual cigarettes reduces tobacco addiction and treatment discontinuation. Cyberpsychology and Behavior 12: 477–483.

Gobbetti E, Scateni R (1998). Virtual Reality: Past, Present and Future. Ios Press, Amsterdam, the Netherlands.

Heeter C (1992). Being there: the subjective experience of presence. Presence: Teleoperators and Virtual Environments 1: 262–271.

Kim K, Kim CH, Kim SY, Roh D, Kim SI (2009). Virtual reality for obsessive compulsive disorders: past and future. Psychiatry Investigation 6: 115–121.

Kim K, Roh D, Kim SI, Kim CH (2011). Provoked arrangement symptoms in obsessive-compulsive disorder using a virtual environment: a preliminary report. Computers in Biology and Medicine 42: 422–427.

Klinger E, Bouchard S, Légeron P (2005). Virtual reality therapy versus cognitive behavior therapy for social phobia: a preliminary controlled study. Cyberpsychology and Behavior 8: 76–88.

Krijn M, Emmelkamp PMG, Biemond R (2004). Treatment of acrophobia in virtual reality: the role of immersion and presence. Behavior Research and Therapy 42: 229–239.

Kuntze M, Stoemer R, Mager R, Roessler A, Mueller-Spahn F, Bullinger AH (2001). Immersive virtual environments in cue exposure. Cyberpsychology and Behavior 4: 497–501.

Lee JH, Kwon H, Choi J, Yang BH (2007). Cue-exposure therapy to decrease alcohol craving in virtual environment. Cyberpsychology and Behavior 10: 617–623.

Malbos E, Mestre DR, Note ID, Gellato C (2008). Virtual reality and claustrophobia: multiple components therapy involving game editor virtual environments exposure. Cyberpsychology and Behavior 11: 695–697.

Malbos E, Rapee RM, Kavakli M (2012). A behavioral presence test in threatening virtual environments. Presence: Teleoperators and Virtual Environments 21: 268–280.

Malbos E, Rapee RM, Kavakli M (2013). A controlled study of agoraphobia and the independent effect of virtual reality exposure therapy. Australian and New Zealand Journal of Psychiatry 47: 160–168.

Marco JH, Perpiña C, Botella C (2013). Effectiveness of cognitive behavioral therapy supported by virtual reality in the treatment of body image in eating disorders: one year follow-up. Psychiatry Research 209: 619–625.

McKenna T (1995). The deoxyribonucleic hyperdimension. Available at http://deoxy.org/deoxy.htm. Retrieved on April 15, 2009.

National Institute of Clinical Excellence (2007). Anxiety: Management of Anxiety in Adults in Primary and Community Care. National Institute for Health and Clinical Excellence. Retrieved on November 10, 2009 from www.nice.org.uk/CG022NICEguideline.

National Institute of Mental Health (2010). Treatment of Anxiety Disorders. National Institute of Mental Health. Retrieved on July 25, 2011 from http://www.nimh.nih.gov/health/publications/anxiety-disorders/treatment-of-anxiety-disorders.shtml.

North MM, North SM (1994). Virtual environment and psychological disorders. Electronic Journal of Virtual Culture 2: 37–42.

North MM, North SM, Coble JR (1996). Effectiveness of virtual environments desensitization in the treatment of agoraphobia. Presence: Teleoperators and Virtual Environments 5: 346–352.

North MM, North SM, Coble JR (1998). Virtual reality therapy: an effective treatment for the fear of public speaking. International Journal of Virtual Reality 3: 1–6.

Opris D, Pintea S, Garcia-Palacios A, Botella C, Szamosközi S, David D (2012). Virtual reality exposure therapy in anxiety disorders: a quantitative meta-analysis. Depression and Anxiety 29: 85–93.

Park KM, Ku J, Choi SH, Jang HJ, Park JY, Kim SI (2011). A virtual reality application in role-plays of social skills training for schizophrenia: a randomized, controlled trial. Psychiatry Research 189: 166–172.

Powers MB, Emmelkamp PMG (2008). Virtual reality exposure therapy for anxiety disorders: a meta-analysis. Journal of Anxiety Disorders 22: 561–569.

Riva G, Alcaniz M, Anolli L (2003). The VEPSY UPDATED project: clinical rationale and technical approach. Cyberpsychology and Behavior 6: 433–439.

Riva G, Bachetta M, Baruffi M (2002a). Virtual reality based multidimensional therapy for the treatment of body image disturbances in binge eating disorders: a preliminary controlled study. IEEE Transactions on Information Technology in Biomedicine 6: 224–234.

Riva G, Gaggiolo A, Villani D, et al (2007). NeuroVR: an open source virtual reality platform for clinical psychology and behavioral neurosciences. Studies in Health Technologies and Informatics 125: 394–399.

Riva G, Mellis L (1997). Virtual reality for the treatment of body image disturbances. Studies in Health Technologies and Informatics 44: 95–111.

Riva G, Molinari E (2009). Virtual reality in the treatment of eating disorders and obesity. Cybertherapy and Rehabilitation 2: 16–19.

Riva G, Molinari E, Vincelli F (2002b). Interaction and presence in the clinical relationship: virtual reality, a communicative medium between patient and therapist. IEEE Transactions on Information Technology in Biomedicine 6: 198–205.

Riva G, Wiederhold BK (2002). Introduction to the special issue on virtual reality environments in behavioral sciences. IEEE Transactions on Information Technology in Biomedicine 6: 193–197.

Rothbaum BO, Hodges L (1999). The use of virtual reality exposure in the treatment of anxiety disorders. Behavior Modification 23: 507–525.

Rothbaum BO, Hodges L, Alarcon R (1999). Virtual reality exposure therapy for PTSD Vietnam veterans: a case study. Journal of Traumatic Stress 12: 263–271.

Rothbaum BO, Hodges L, Anderson PL (2002). Twelve-month follow-up of virtual reality and standard exposure therapies for the fear of flying. Journal of Consulting and Clinical Psychology 70: 428–432.

Rothbaum BO, Hodges L, Kooper R (1995). Effectiveness of computer generated (virtual reality) graded exposure in the treatment of acrophobia. American Journal of Psychiatry 152: 626–628.

Rothbaum BO, Hodges L, Ready D (2001). Virtual reality exposure therapy for Vietnam veterans with post-traumatic stress disorder. Journal of Clinical Psychiatry 62: 617–622.

Rothbaum B, Hodges L, Smith S (2000). A controlled study of virtual reality exposure therapy for fear of flying. Journal of Consulting and Clinical Psychology 68: 1020–1026.

Rothbaum BO, Page A, Zimand E, Hodges L, Lang D, Wilson J (2006). Virtual reality exposure therapy and standard therapy in the treatment of fear of flying. Behavior Therapy 37: 80–90.

Ryan J, Kreiner D, Chapman MD, Stark-Wroblewski K (2010). Virtual reality cues for binge drinking in college students. Cyberpsychology, Behavior and Social Networking 13: 159–162.

Safir MP, Wallach HS, Bar-Zvi M (2012). Virtual reality cognitive-behavior therapy for public speaking anxiety: one-year follow-up. Behavior Modification 36: 235–246.

Sutherland IE (1965). The ultimate display. Proceedings of International Federation for Information Processing (IFIP) 65: 506–508.

Vincelli F, Anolli L, Bouchard S (2003). Experiential cognitive therapy in the treatment of panic disorders with agoraphobia: a controlled study. Cyberpsychology and Behavior 6: 321–328.

Wald J, Taylor S (2000). Efficacy of virtual reality exposure therapy to treat driving phobia: a case report. Journal of Behavior Therapy and Experimental Psychiatry 31: 249–257.

Walshe DG, Lewis EJ, Kim SI (2003). Exploring the use of computer games and virtual reality in exposure therapy for fear of driving following a motor vehicle accident. Cyberpsychology and Behavior 6: 329–334.

13 Mobile Therapy

An Overview of Mobile Device–Assisted Psychological Therapy and Prevention of Mental Health Problems

Sylvia Kauer and Sophie C. Reid

INTRODUCTION

The Internet is a common source of health information and support, with Internet-enabled smartphones increasingly becoming the device of choice to access this material (Fox and Duggan, 2012). For example, it is estimated that 31% of Americans use their cell phones to look for health-related information (Fox and Duggan, 2012). Also, more than 45,000 health, medical, and fitness apps are available in the Apple App store alone (James, 2013). Within that category are a plethora of mental health–related apps, too. Indeed, mobile therapy (mTherapy) is an increasingly common resource for accessing information and support for mental health problems (Harrison et al., 2011).

This mTherapy, which refers to any therapeutic mobile intervention or app for mental health, is a burgeoning area of development in health technology. It can take many forms, including text messaging, voice calls, and apps. Apps that track mood, sleep, diet, exercise, and various symptoms in real time are gaining in popularity and have been shown to increase awareness of the tracked behavior or symptom and to lead to measurable improvement (Kauer et al., 2012). As well as tracking, mTherapy can include appointment or medication reminders, self-motivating messages, and homework between therapy sessions. As such, it may be beneficial across a broad range of psychiatric disorders (Depp et al., 2010).

Mobile telephones have taken on a practical and emotional significance in people's lives (Morris and Aguilera, 2012). Young people have been shown to readily engage with mTherapy and comply with self-monitoring using mobile devices (Silk et al., 2003; Reid et al., 2009). Mobile phones may be beneficial as therapeutic devices; they are affordable, especially in Western countries; they are familiar; and they have vast functionality (Morris and Aguilera, 2012). Also, the penetration of mobile phone ownership gives users an alternative to carrying a separate device purposely built for mTherapy (Ben-Zeev et al., 2013). As the vast majority of people carry mobile phones, they can access therapeutic apps and text messages discreetly anytime and anywhere. Therefore, people with psychiatric disorders can use their mobile phones for treatment at almost any time without attracting attention, thereby avoiding stigma.

Many individuals affected by anxiety, depression, or other psychiatric disorders often do not require intensive treatment; they may suffer from only mild symptoms. In such cases, mTherapy has the potential to engage these people in low-intensity treatment, initiating a stepped care approach that can increase in intensity as needed (van Straten et al., 2010). Individuals with serious mental illness have also demonstrated a willingness to use mobile apps for self-management (Ben-Zeev et al., 2013). Their treatment may benefit from mTherapy as well; it may facilitate mood monitoring between therapeutic sessions and offer reminders for appointments or medication administration times.

DOES MOBILE THERAPY WORK?

Despite the large array of apps and tools available and regularly used, few studies have evaluated whether they result in improvements in mental health and well-being. In 2011, a systematic review identified only three randomized controlled trials (RCTs) that investigated the efficacy of mTherapy in the treatment of any mental health problem (Ehrenreich et al., 2011). Of the three RCTs identified, only one showed a significant improvement in anxiety. Clinicians and researchers are inundated with papers describing programs, examining user experience and satisfaction, and outlining the feasibility of mTherapy, yet there are still few data on mental health outcomes, the very reason these apps were designed. Although it is critical that mTherapies are "user friendly" and feasible, it is imperative that investigators also focus on whether these apps actually improve the lives of mentally ill people. The remainder of this chapter addresses this question by examining the scientific literature to investigate the effectiveness of mTherapy in the prevention and treatment of psychiatric disorders.

A Medline and PsycInfo literature search was conducted in November 2013 using PRISMA guidelines (Liberati et al., 2009). The search terms used (Figure 13.1) were based on four themes: mental disorders, mobile devices, prevention and

---

Search terms

PsycInfo:

(depress* OR anxiety OR mental disorder OR mental il*)

AND (*therapy OR counselling OR intervention OR prevention)

AND (benefits OR engagement OR trust OR satisfaction OR improvement OR prevent)

AND (mobile phone OR cellular phone OR PDA OR mobile device)—*resulted in 76 publications*

Medline:

(depress* OR anxiety OR mental disorder OR mental il*)

AND (therapy OR counseling OR intervention OR prevention)

AND (mobile phone OR cellular phone OR PDA OR mobile device)

AND (benefits OR engagement OR trust OR satisfaction OR improvement OR prevent)—*resulted in 41 publications*

Inclusion and exclusion criteria

Includes:

- A mobile device
- Prevention, early intervention, and treatment programs
- A focus on improving mental health

Excludes:

- Unrelated technology: apps that were developed for entertainment without a therapeutic aim (e.g., the impact popular mobile games have on mental health)
- Methodological or development paper without evaluation
- Mobile devices used for data collection, not for therapeutic reasons

---

FIGURE 13.1

Search terms for the literature search and the inclusion and exclusion criteria.

therapy, and mental health outcomes. Articles were selected on the basis of the inclusion criteria listed in Figure 13.1.

The literature search uncovered a total of 121 publications (Figure 13.2), of which 27 were duplicates. After applying the exclusion criteria (Figure 13.1), based on abstracts and titles, 54 publications were excluded, leaving a total of 40 full texts to screen. A further 15 were excluded after reading the full texts, resulting in 25 studies for inclusion in this review.

The following psychiatric disorders and mental health problems were investigated by these studies: schizophrenia (Spaniel et al., 2008; Depp et al., 2010; Granholm et al., 2012; Ben-Zeev et al., 2013); bipolar disorder (Depp et al., 2010; Miklowitz et al., 2012); major depressive disorder (Aguilera and Muñoz, 2011; Burns et al., 2011; Wichers et al., 2011; Agyapong et al., 2012; Whittaker et al., 2012; Watts et al., 2013); "mild mental health problems" (Morris et al., 2010; Reid et al., 2011; Lappalainen et al., 2013; Proudfoot et al., 2013; Villani et al., 2013); anxiety disorders (Grassi et al., 2007; Pallavicini et al., 2009; Preziosa et al., 2009; Ehrenreich et al., 2011); eating disorders (Shapiro et al., 2010; Cardi et al., 2013); phobias (Botella et al., 2007; Flynn et al., 2013); and suicidal behaviors (Marasinghe et al., 2012).

The interventions investigated include symptom tracking apps (Depp et al., 2010; Morris et al., 2010; Burns et al., 2011; Reid et al., 2011; Wichers et al.,

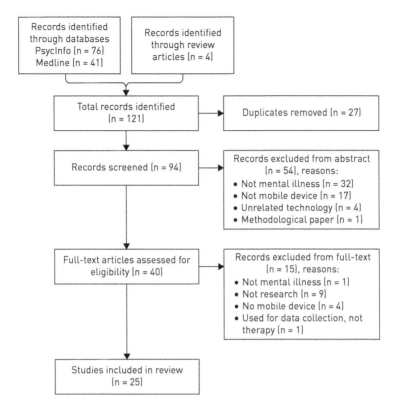

FIGURE 13.2

Preferred Reporting Items for Systematic Reviews and Meta-Analyses (PRISMA) flow diagram.

2011; Ben-Zeev et al., 2013; Proudfoot et al., 2013); mobile apps with a narrative recording to facilitate exposure or relaxation therapy (Grassi et al., 2007; Pallavicini et al., 2009; Preziosa et al., 2009; Cardi et al., 2013; Villani et al., 2013); cognitive-behavioral therapy (CBT)-based apps (Depp et al., 2010; Ehrenreich et al., 2011; Whittaker et al., 2012; Lappalainen et al., 2013; Watts et al., 2013); text messaging (Spaniel et al., 2008; Depp et al., 2010; Shapiro et al., 2010; Aguilera and Muñoz, 2011; Agyapong et al., 2012; Granholm et al., 2012; Miklowitz et al., 2012); phone calls (Marasinghe et al., 2012; Flynn et al., 2013); and a therapeutic game (Botella et al., 2007). The following sections describe the various forms of mTherapy used and the available data on their efficacy in prevention and treatment.

Tracking Apps

Seven studies investigated self-monitoring, or tracking apps, in which a patient tracks mood or other variables of interest multiple times over several days (Table 13.1). Two of these studies focused on severe mental illness (Depp et al., 2010; Ben-Zeev et al., 2013); four on depression (Burns et al., 2011; Reid et al., 2011; Wichers et al., 2011; Proudfoot et al., 2013); and one on mild mental health problems (Morris et al., 2010). Two studies did not involve face-to-face support in conjunction with mTherapy (Morris et al., 2010; Proudfoot et al., 2013).

Table 13.1 Studies Using Tracking Apps

Study	N	Disorder	Study Design	Intervention	Findings
Depp et al. (2010)	10	Bipolar disorder	Longitudinal study	PRISM: a tracking intervention consisting of automated experience sampling and psychoeducation	Reduction in depressive symptoms but no change in manic symptoms
	8	Schizophrenia	Longitudinal study	MATS: a tracking app consisting of computer-initiated text messages	25% reduction in text responses to MATS in the second half of the trial compared to the first half
	9	Schizophrenia	Longitudinal study	STEP: two phone calls between face-to-face cognitive-behavioral therapy sessions; phone calls used to check in, provide an overview, and remind about next session and homework	86% reported increase in skills utilization Participants found the program acceptable, and 57% enjoyed their homework assignments
Morris et al. (2010)	5 adults	Mild symptoms ("stress")	Case series	MyExperience: a mobile phone mood tracking app (includes mood scales and therapies) Mood Map and Mind Scan (encourages cognitive appraisal)	Anger, anxiety, and sadness ratings were lower postintervention
Burns et al. (2011)	8	Major depressive disorder	Case series	Mobilyze!: a tracking app Uses mobile phones to gather data about subjects and their environment Subjects self-report their mood Data also accessible through a web interface	Participants less likely to meet the criteria for major depressive disorder, depressive symptoms decreased, and anxiety decreased
Reid et al. (2011)	114 adolescents	"Mild mental health problems"	Randomized controlled trial	mobiletype: a mobile phone–based self-monitoring program (mood, stress, coping, exercise, sleep, diet, and drug and alcohol use) completed up to three times a day for 2–4 weeks Subjects received feedback reports from their monitoring that they reviewed with their physicians	No significant differences between the intervention group and attention-control group in depressive symptoms over time Emotional self-awareness significantly increased in the intervention group over time compared to the attention-control group

Study	N	Diagnosis	Study design	Intervention	Results
Wichers et al. (2011)	22	Major depressive disorder	Longitudinal study	PsyMate: three to four beeps per day for self-monitoring positive emotions and activities for 6 weeks with feedback offered in graphic form	Participants rated the app highly, liked the graphic feedback, and tried to implement the suggestions from the feedback 60% would like to continue using PsyMate.
Ben-Zeev et al. (2013)	12	Schizophrenia	Qualitative study	FOCUS: a tracking app Addresses medication adherence, mood regulation, sleep, social functioning, and coping with auditory hallucinations Contains self-assessment and flagging if self-assessment reveals areas that could benefit from self-management Once-daily reminders	All participants felt confident that they would be able to use the program Eight satisfied with ease of use and helpfulness Seven used coping strategies during testing
Proudfoot et al. (2013)	720	Mild depression, anxiety, or stress	Randomized controlled trial	MyCompass: a web-based mobile phone self-help tool offering symptom and behavior tracking, text message reminders, graphic feedback, tips and strategies, and self-help modules based on cognitive-behavioral therapy	MyCompass group showed decrease in depression, anxiety, and stress compared to an attention-control intervention group and a wait list control group

Most commonly, mobile phones were used as the tracking device (Depp et al., 2010; Morris et al., 2010; Burns et al., 2011; Reid et al., 2011; Proudfoot et al., 2013). A study by Reid et al. (2011) provides an illustration of self-monitoring of young people with early signs of depression seen in general practice settings. This study was the first RCT investigating the effects of self-monitoring in young people and using mobile phones rather than personal digital assistants. One hundred and fourteen young people completed the app, mobiletype, four times a day over 2 to 4 weeks between appointments with their general practitioners. Each entry took approximately 2 minutes to complete and consisted of questions about mood, stress level, daily activities, coping strategies, alcohol use, sleep, and diet. Participants in the control group completed a similar protocol matched to the intervention for duration and attention from the general practitioner; they also monitored their daily activities, sleep, and diet. Feedback was presented to the participants and their general practitioners for review via a secure website. Both groups had a significant decrease in depressive symptoms, and there were no differences between them. Secondary analyses, however, demonstrated that the intervention group had a significant increase in emotional self-awareness compared to the control group (Kauer et al., 2012). Also, general practitioners reported that mobiletype was superior in terms of improving communication with young people about mental health issues and understanding of their needs compared to participants in the control group. Furthermore, significant advantages for mobiletype were reported for making decisions about medication and referrals and helping to diagnose mental health problems (Reid et al., 2013).

Following this inaugural study, Proudfoot et al. (2013) conducted an RCT with adults experiencing mild depressive symptoms (N = 720) and found that tracking led to a significant reduction in these symptoms compared to controls. The app, MyCompass, also contained a CBT component that participants could complete online. Another useful feature was users' option to choose when and how often they wanted to receive reminders to complete the app and what symptoms and mood states to track (Harrison et al., 2011).

Other research investigating tracking has been less rigorous. Depp et al. (2010) tracked both the depressive and manic symptoms of 10 patients with bipolar affective disorder using an app that not only tracked symptoms but also provided self-management strategies when symptoms were present. Interestingly, a significant reduction in depressive, but not manic, symptoms was found. A case series (N = 5; Morris et al., 2010) using the MyExperience tracking app reported an increase in participants' self-awareness and improvement in coping with stress. MyExperience was programmed for touchscreen mobile phones, with participants rating their mood on a graph and on Likert scales throughout the day.

Two further studies investigated tracking in depressed subjects and found that participants were highly satisfied with PsyMate (N = 22; Wichers et al., 2011) and Mobilyze! (N = 8; Burns et al., 2011). Although these studies did not provide information on outcomes, both apps were innovative; PsyMate provided users with daily feedback about their mood and Mobilyze! used sensors to predict mood based on environmental context. Further evaluation of these apps is needed.

Tracking apps have also been used to track medication adherence in schizophrenia patients. Ben-Zeev et al. (2013) tested an app designed to increase adherence to a medication regimen in 12 patients with schizophrenia. All participants felt confident that they would be able to use the system (8 strongly agreed and 4 agreed).

Taken as a whole, these seven studies suggest that tracking one's mood and behavior can lead to users' increased awareness. In the case of mobiletype (Kauer et al., 2012), tracking one's mood led to an increase in emotional self-awareness, which in turn seemed to decrease depressive symptoms. Tracking medication adherence functioned to increase the salience of medication regimens and serve as a reminder to take therapeutic actions. The extent to which this may have a direct impact on mental health outcomes, however, is still to be extensively examined.

Text Messaging

Text messaging, also referred to as Short Message Service or SMS, has been used therapeutically in two distinct ways: to track mood and symptoms (similar to tracking apps) and to send supportive messages to participants (Table 13.2). Studies have investigated the use of text messaging as a tracking device in subjects with bipolar affective disorder (N = 19; Miklowitz et al., 2012), female subjects with bulimia nervosa (N = 38; Shapiro et al., 2010), subjects with schizophrenia and other psychotic disorders (N = 45; Spaniel et al., 2008), and female subjects with major depressive disorder (N = 10; Aguilera and Muñoz, 2011). All four studies were conducted in conjunction with face-to-face therapy. In these studies, patients were sent a text message at least once a day and asked to respond via text messaging in the form of numbers on a Likert scale (i.e., 1, 2, 3, 4, and 5 corresponding to five items on a 5-point Likert scale).

Results suggested that tracking via text messaging might be beneficial. Subjects with bipolar affective disorder reported stable mood during the study (Miklowitz et al., 2012); subjects with bulimia nervosa were shown to have fewer binge-eating and purging episodes (Shapiro et al., 2010); and subjects with psychotic disorders had fewer hospitalizations. No mental health outcomes were evaluated by Aguilera and Muñoz (2011), although participants found tracking via text messaging a positive experience. Adherence was moderate to high in these studies—65% (Aguilera and Muñoz, 2011), 81% (Miklowitz et al., 2012), and 87% (Shapiro et al., 2010).

Text messaging was also used to provide supportive messages to patients between therapeutic sessions in three studies. These involved patients enrolled in a dual depression and alcohol abuse treatment program (N = 26; Agyapong et al., 2012); a community sample of adults with schizophrenia who were also receiving treatment (N = 42; Depp et al., 2010; Granholm et al., 2012); and a sample of disadvantaged young people of various cultural backgrounds who were not experiencing symptoms of depression or self-harm (Whittaker et al., 2012). All three studies yielded promising results. Compared to the control group, a significant improvement in depression scores was seen in patients with a dual diagnosis of

Table 13.2 Studies Using Text Messaging

Study	N	Disorder	Study Design	Intervention	Findings
Spaniel et al. (2008)	45	Schizophrenia	Longitudinal study	ITAREPS program: subjects completed an early warning signs questionnaire by SMS weekly; if the questionnaire indicated a high risk, the clinician was alerted and tracking continued for three more weeks	Significant reduction in the number of psychiatric hospitalizations of the similar length
Shapiro et al. (2010)	31 adult women	Bulimia nervosa	Longitudinal study	In addition to group cognitive-behavioral therapy for 12 weeks, participants completed a paper-based diary to record food intake and purging and sent one SMS daily indicating binge eating, purging, and peak urges	Binge eating decreased Number of purges decreased
Aguilera and Muñoz (2011)	10	Major depressive disorder (participants enrolled in group cognitive-behavioral therapy)	Longitudinal study	Participants were sent two to three text messages daily over 2 months asking about mood, number of positive thoughts, and number of pleasant activities	65% response Overall, positive experiences reported by participants
Agyapong et al. (2012)	50	Major depressive disorder and alcohol use disorder (participants enrolled in an inpatient dual diagnosis program)	Randomized controlled trial	Supportive text messages were sent twice daily for 3 months 180 text messages were sent covering stress, well-being, abstinence, cravings, medication adherence, and general support Control group subjects were sent text messages once fortnightly thanking them for participation	Significant decrease in 3-month depression scores, compared to control group subjects
Granholm et al. (2012)	42	Schizophrenia or schizoaffective disorder	Longitudinal study	Computer-initiated text messages Three sets of four text messages were sent daily targeting medication adherence, socialization, or auditory hallucinations in random order	Among independent individuals, medication adherence improved, number of social interactions increased, and auditory hallucinations decreased
Miklowitz et al. (2012)	19 adults	Bipolar affective disorder	Longitudinal study	FIMM: Daily monitoring via text messaging or email	Stable moods reported throughout the study Knowledge of mood management strategies significantly increased
Whittaker et al. (2012)	835 adolescents	Depression (participants from a low socioeconomic status in a multicultural high school)	Randomized controlled trial	MEMO program: key messages based on cognitive-behavioral therapy were sent two times a day for 9 weeks	Intervention helped participants to be more positive and to get rid of negative thoughts, which was significantly different from the control groups

depression and alcohol abuse (Agyapong et al., 2012). Although the findings were preliminary, subjects with schizophrenia who completed the program showed a significant reduction in severity of hallucinations, a significant increase in social interactions, and a significant improvement in medication adherence among those living independently (Depp et al., 2010; Granholm et al., 2012). This was likely due either to the cognitive interventions within the program that aimed to reduce the beliefs in the voices or to increased adherence to medication. In the study of young people, a significantly higher proportion receiving the intervention indicated that they became more positive and had fewer negative thoughts compared to the control group (N = 1348; Whittaker et al., 2012).

Text messaging programs are inexpensive, simple, flexible, accessible, and can be automated and tailored to suit the needs of both patient and provider. These qualities render them potentially helpful for prevention and protection against relapse. Unlike apps, text messaging programs work readily on all mobile phones without the need for programming or extensive testing, allowing for ease of design and distribution by researchers and health providers. As with mobile phone apps, text messaging programs are not intrusive and not stigmatizing.

Text messaging programs may not be useful for everyone, however. Individuals who are highly disorganized or have limited cognitive functioning may find responding to a text message using Likert-scale coding systems overly complicated (Ben-Zeev et al., 2013). Also, characters in text messaging programs are limited, and therefore only a few questions can be asked and answered at a time. Furthermore, although programs utilizing text messaging are generally inexpensive in the developed world, users typically still pay for them, and this may affect patients' willingness or ability to use them, as opposed to apps that can share data over wireless networks that tend to be less expensive or free.

Overall, it is difficult to determine the effect of text messaging on treatment. There may be some effect in terms of increased medication adherence, decreased hospitalization, and some improvement in symptoms, but due to small sample sizes and lack of RCTs, this is difficult to discern. Further research using controlled trials where subjects are randomized to text messaging or no-text messaging groups is needed to determine whether text messaging interventions result in improved mental health outcomes.

Telephone Calls

Two studies investigated the effects of phone calls on mental health. Phone calls can be used in innovative ways as part of an mTherapy intervention. Flynn et al. (2013) conducted a study with two patients experiencing a driving phobia. Hands-free mobile phones were installed in their automobiles, allowing them to call their therapist or anyone else when anxious. The participants were encouraged to drive three times each week for 8 weeks, with the number of phone calls slowly reduced until no calls were made during week 8. One participant increased the number of miles driven over the course of the study, whereas there was no improvement in the second participant.

As described in an RCT conducted in suicidal patients (Marasinghe et al., 2012), another important role for phone calls can be with high-risk groups. In this study, young people (N = 68) admitted to a psychiatric hospital for self-harming or suicidal behavior were given face-to-face treatment while in the hospital. After discharge, phone calls were made over 24 weeks to assess the participants' mood and suicidal ideation and provide relaxation, problem solving, and meditation training. Weekly text messages were sent reminding participants to use these strategies. Patients receiving this intervention had a significant decrease in suicidal ideation and depression compared to those receiving usual care.

Advantages of using phone calls as interventions are similar to those of text messages, perhaps with the added scope of telepsychotherapy with a psychologist as in Marasinghe et al. (2012). Nevertheless, interventions using such calls can be time-consuming or costly for the service provider and the user. In addition, recent research suggests that phone calls may no longer be the preferred means for communication, particularly for young people who often prefer to communicate via text messaging (Smith, 2011). Also, phone calls are difficult, if not impossible, to automate, particularly in a therapeutic context. Both aforementioned studies (Marasinghe et al., 2012; Flynn et al., 2013) used these calls in conjunction with therapy. Therefore, a therapist was available on the other end of the phone. The increased burden on providers was not discussed in these studies, but one can imagine that it was substantial. In general, better engagement, rapport, and contact with a therapist correlate with improvements in mental health (Leach, 2005). Consequently, the use of phone calls may be beneficial in conjunction with therapy, but given the limitations discussed, it is perhaps best reserved for high-risk patients.

Mobile Narratives

Mobile narratives refer to narrative recordings, either audio or audiovisual, on mobile devices (Grassi et al., 2007). They may also involve elements of virtual or augmented reality via the representation of digital imagery (such as a tropical island or other relaxing scenery, combined with music or soothing narratives) to facilitate exposure or relaxation for those experiencing stress or anxiety (Pallavicini et al., 2009). Five studies investigated mobile narratives in anxiety (Grassi et al., 2007; Pallavicini et al., 2009; Preziosa et al., 2009), anorexia nervosa (Cardi et al., 2013), and stress among nurses (Villani et al., 2013) (Table 13.3). Different techniques were used. Two studies (Preziosa et al., 2009; Villani et al., 2013) relied on the principles of stress inoculation training to increase awareness of stressful situations, teach skills to deal with the stress, and rehearse these skills. One study used exposure therapy (Cardi et al., 2013), and two used relaxation training (Grassi et al., 2007; Pallavicini et al., 2009). Pallavicini et al. (2009) included sensory glasses and controllers in conjunction with the mobile narrative to create a sense of virtual reality and allow subjects to become immersed in the experience.

All studies were RCTs and demonstrated that use of mobile narratives with visual and audio components was associated with reductions in anxiety and stress

Table 13.3 Studies Using Mobile Narratives

Study	N	Disorder	Study design	Intervention	Findings
Grassi et al. (2007)	120 students	Anxiety	Randomized controlled trial	Four 10-minute sessions over 2 days. Four groups: (1) Mobile narrative during train trip (2) Video of a tropical beach only (3) Relaxation audio only (4) No intervention (control)	Only mobile narrative group had significant decrease in anxiety
Pallavicini et al. (2009)	12 adults	Generalized anxiety disorder	Randomized controlled trial	Eight sessions of virtual reality therapy via phone, including exposure and relaxation, with or without biofeedback	Decrease in anxiety in biofeedback group compared to no biofeedback and wait list control groups
Preziosa et al. (2009)	30 female university students	Examination-related anxiety	Randomized controlled trial	Stress Inoculation Training (SIT) narratives over 6 sessions with five groups: (1) Audio at home (2) Portable audio (3) Audio/visual at home (4) Portable audio/visual (5) Control	Reduction in anxiety for 80% of participants in both audio/visual groups compared to 50% of participants in portable audio group and 0% of participants in audio at home group. No results presented for the control group
	90 commuters to university aged 20–25 years	Mild anxiety	Randomized controlled trial	SIT narratives over 6 sessions with three groups: (1) Mobile narrative trip to beach (2) Music videos (3) Control	Mobile narrative group exhibited a reduction in anxiety and greater relaxation compared to other two groups
Cardi et al. (2013)	20 inpatients and 18 outpatients	Anorexia nervosa	Randomized controlled trial	A mobile narrative consisting of a short video clip to encourage users to reappraise and accept food. The music intervention consisted of modern classical music for 20 minutes	Inpatients ate twice as much food as outpatients. Inpatients ate more in the music intervention group and outpatients ate more in the mobile narrative group
Villani et al. (2013)	30 female nurses	Mild mental health problems ("stress")	Randomized controlled trial	Mobile Stress Inoculation Training (M-SIT; relaxation and skills acquisition and rehearsal) compared to neutral video delivered over mobile phones over 4 weeks	Significant reduction in anxiety over time in the M-SIT group compared to the control group

and an improved ability to relax compared to subjects in mp3 audio groups who listened to music only and those in video groups who watched a relaxing scene only, or wait list groups. Some additional findings are worth highlighting. Biofeedback appeared to increase the effects of the mobile narrative (Preziosa et al., 2009). Also, inpatients with anorexia nervosa seemed to benefit more from music than from mobile narratives, in contrast to outpatients who benefited more from the mobile narratives (Cardi et al., 2013). In addition, two of the mobile narrative studies were stand-alone programs, conducted without a therapist (Pallavicini et al., 2009; Cardi et al., 2013), suggesting that mobile narratives can be utilized with or without therapy.

Sample sizes were small and ranged between 13 and 120 participants, limiting the generalizability of these studies. Further, four of the five studies were conducted by the same research group (Grassi et al., 2007; Pallavicini et al., 2009; Preziosa et al., 2009; Villani et al., 2013).

In summary, mobile narratives show promise as a tool that can help in exposure therapy and relaxation. However, the research investigating the use of mobile narratives in the treatment of psychiatric disorders is still in its infancy, requiring replication in large-scale RCTs conducted in representative samples.

Mobile Cognitive-Behavioral Therapy

Cognitive-behavioral therapy using mobile devices (mCBT) was investigated in two pilot RCTs in depression (Lappalainen et al., 2013; Watts et al., 2013) and in a systematic literature review (Ehrenreich et al., 2011). In the systematic review, three RCTs focused on anxiety disorders and other eight on smoking cessation. Only one of the three studies investigating anxiety disorders showed a reduction in anxiety (Ehrenreich et al., 2011). Of the pilot RCTs, one demonstrated a reduction in depressive symptoms in men (N = 23) with generally mild symptoms; participants also showed an improvement in the symptoms of stress, self-rated health, ability to work, and life satisfaction (Lappalainen et al., 2013). The second pilot RCT found a reduction of depression in adults (N = 35) with major depressive disorder over an 8-week intervention (Watts et al., 2013). Mobile CBT was composed of several modules consistent with traditional CBT (i.e., psychoeducation, thought-emotion monitoring, and cognitive challenging). These studies were conducted in conjunction with other treatment and with a clinician. Results are promising, but as with computerized CBT, problems with adherence can be expected when there is no support provided by a research team or a therapist to motivate users to continue working through the program (Christensen et al., 2006).

Therapeutic Games

In a case study, a puzzle game called "The Cockroach Game" was used to expose a woman who was receiving therapy for cockroach phobia to cockroaches on her mobile phone (Botella et al., 2007). In this game, the patient matched puzzle pieces of an unrelated picture while virtual cockroaches crawled on the phone's screen.

The patient had to interact with the cockroaches by flicking them off the screen or redirecting them off the puzzle pieces. Advancement to the next level was based on achieving clinical goals. This game was based on "augmented reality," where virtual elements are added to increase exposure to the object of the specific phobia. The patient found the game useful and reported a decrease in fear and avoidance of cockroaches.

The use of this game is innovative and demonstrates how games can be used in a serious mTherapy program. This approach may increase engagement for users by combining therapeutic aspects with entertainment. Further research is obviously needed to examine the therapeutic use of games. Nevertheless, we will almost certainly see an increase in therapeutic games with the increasing "gamification" of society.

WITH OR WITHOUT FACE-TO-FACE TREATMENT?

Of the studies examined in this review, eight were stand-alone programs (Grassi et al., 2007; Preziosa et al., 2009; Morris et al., 2010; Whittaker et al., 2012; Lappalainen et al., 2013; Proudfoot et al., 2013; Villani et al., 2013; Watts et al., 2013). As might be expected, stand-alone programs tended to be for those with mild mental health problems. Only one study explored the use of a stand-alone program for a diagnosable disorder (Watts et al., 2013). There were 15 studies using mTherapy in conjunction with other treatment (pharmacological or psychotherapeutic) for depression (Aguilera and Muñoz, 2011; Burns et al., 2011; Reid et al., 2011; Wichers et al., 2011; Agyapong et al., 2012) and other severe psychiatric disorders (Spaniel et al., 2008; Pallavicini et al., 2009; Depp et al., 2010; Shapiro and Bauer, 2010; Ehrenreich et al., 2011; Granholm et al., 2012; Marasinghe et al., 2012; Miklowitz et al., 2012; Ben-Zeev et al., 2013; Flynn et al., 2013).

For some interventions (such as phone calls, text messaging, and some tracking apps), a clinician may be required to examine the data, provide feedback, or make and receive text messages or phone calls. Mobile narratives and mCBT are more likely to be used as a stand-alone program for individuals experiencing mild disorders or as an adjunct to therapy between sessions. Therefore, the way the tool is used and the infrastructure surrounding the tool are important to consider, as is the severity of symptoms. Like face-to-face CBT and other mental health interventions, a single treatment modality may be insufficient on its own. Hence, the chapter authors would recommend that mTherapy be considered as one component of an overall treatment approach, potentially following a stepped care framework that begins with mTherapy and progresses to more intensive treatments as needed. Alternatively, mTherapy can be used as an adjunct, along with other interventions being administered.

BARRIERS AND OTHER CONSIDERATIONS

A major consideration in the use of mobile devices for the treatment of psychiatric disorders is directing the user to the evidence-based mTherapy interventions amidst 45,000 health, medical, and well-being apps (James, 2013). Finding an appropriate mTherapy in the Apple App Store or the Google Play Store is the 21st-century mental health equivalent of searching for a needle in a haystack. Evidence and safety are key principles required in the development of mTherapies. It has been cautioned that "any app that provides medical advice may result in harm to the consumer if the advice is incorrect" (Tegan, 2013, p. 40). Yet these are principles by which commercial companies are not required to abide. Although the medical community is bound to the "do no harm" dictum, the same does not apply to individuals who develop health-related apps, often for profit. Regulatory bodies such as the Food and Drug Administration (United States) and the Therapeutic Goods Administration (Australia) assess only those apps that are submitted to their scrutiny. Long-term financial support, commitment, and oversight are required to conduct the necessary research and embed evidence-based mTherapies within preestablished treatment and service provision frameworks.

Another issue to consider in evaluating mTherapies is the breakneck speed with which the technology is moving. With technology becoming obsolete at increasingly rapid rates, the generalizability of results evaluating apps is limited. Apps require constant updating to run on the latest model of mobile phones or software. Research, in comparison, can be painstakingly slow, with grant review, research ethics committee approval, and subject recruitment sometimes taking years. A paradigm shift is required if the research community is to keep up with the breathtaking pace of technology evolution. Research institutes and universities have the research expertise but often have only limited funds and so tend to develop and evaluate the initial conception of product. Continuing on to develop a state-of-the-art product ready for mainstream adoption can be very challenging in research settings. In contrast, commercial companies focus on developing an app with mass appeal, good functionality, and ease of use but rarely concern themselves with the effectiveness of the product. Government-brokered partnerships between developers and research institutions would likely help develop evidence-based, high-quality products that are also attractive enough to allow for their wide adoption.

Like many interventions, mTherapies work only if correctly implemented and consistently used. Stand-alone, unguided, and unsupported web-based CBT programs such as MoodGYM have been shown to be efficacious in RCTs where participation in the program is supported by research staff. Yet, in a real-world study, 51% of users used the web-based program only once, with less than 7% progressing beyond two of the five modules (Christensen et al., 2006). The same has been found for many mobile apps purchased through the iPhone app store; only 30% of purchased apps and 20% of free apps are used the day after purchase (Tegan, 2013). Embedding mTherapies within preestablished treatment systems and frameworks would allow consumers to be directed to the best evidence-based therapies and would increase the likelihood of the consumer receiving the level of intervention required to produce therapeutic benefits.

CONCLUSION

This chapter has focused on 25 publications that investigated the benefit of mTherapy in the prevention and treatment of mild mental health problems; suicidal behavior; and various psychiatric conditions, including schizophrenia, bipolar disorder, major depressive disorder, anxiety disorders, eating disorders, and phobias. Studies of apps or text messages used to track behavior and mood were most rigorous, suggesting that tracking apps may be beneficial. Mobile narratives used for relaxation or exposure therapy may also assist in decreasing anxiety and phobias. There are inadequate data at this stage to support recommending mCBT apps, phone calls, or therapeutic games for the treatment of patients with psychiatric disorders; however, these innovative approaches are still in their infancy and may improve with time. Overall, more research is needed in this field before we can draw meaningful conclusions about the effects of mTherapy on mental health problems.

There is little evidence that the vast majority of mTherapy apps available to the general public improve mental health, and it is difficult for research to stay up-to-date with the latest trends in technology. Partnership between commercial companies and research institutes is necessary to deliver the best evidence-based care and ensure that no harm is done. Real-world studies are also needed to determine the characteristics of those who are likely to engage with mTherapy, tailoring apps to individuals and using a prescription system with support from general practitioners and therapists. It is essential that mTherapy be considered as one component of treatment, with medication, face-to-face therapy, and other treatments being used in a stepped care approach or in combination. The severity of the disorder as well as the availability of therapists and other infrastructure is an important consideration when implementing mTherapy.

The world is becoming increasingly technical, with more and more services available online and, by extension, on mobile phones. As well as the mTherapies discussed here, there are other mobile monitoring devices that purport to track other aspects of well-being, such as activity, fitness, and sleep. These include Jawbone UP, Fitbit and, more recently, PhyODE W/Me, which correlates autonomic nervous system variables with how a person is feeling. To our knowledge, no studies have been conducted to evaluate the impact of these devices on mental health outcomes. That, of course, will not prevent people from adopting them, perhaps on a massive scale. Rather than fight this process, it is critical that investigators systematically evaluate available tools to assess safety at the very least and, one would hope, establish efficacy.

DISCLOSURE STATEMENT

The authors disclose no relationships with commercial entities and professional activities that may bias their views.

REFERENCES

Aguilera A, Muñoz RF (2011). Text messaging as an adjunct to CBT in low-income populations: a usability and feasibility pilot study. Professional Psychology: Research and Practice 42: 472–478.

Agyapong VIO, Ahern S, McLoughlin DM, Farren CK (2012). Supportive text messaging for depression and comorbid alcohol use disorder: single-blind randomised trial. Journal of Affective Disorders 141: 168–176.

Ben-Zeev D, Kaiser SM, Brenner CJ, et al (2013). Development and usability testing of FOCUS: a smartphone system for self-management of schizophrenia. Psychiatric Rehabilitation Journal 36: 289–297.

Botella C, García-Palacios A, Villa H, et al (2007). Virtual reality exposure in the treatment of panic disorder and agoraphobia: a controlled study. Clinical Psychology and Psychotherapy 14: 164–175.

Burns MN, Begale M, Duffecy J, et al (2011). Harnessing context sensing to develop a mobile intervention for depression. Journal of Medical Internet Research 13: e55.

Cardi V, Lounes N, Kan C, Treasure J (2013). Meal support using mobile technology in anorexia nervosa. Contextual differences between inpatient and outpatient settings. Appetite 60: 33–39.

Christensen H, Griffiths KM, Groves C, Korten A (2006). Free range users and one hit wonders: community users of an Internet-based cognitive behaviour therapy program. Australian and New Zealand Journal of Psychiatry 40: 59–62.

Depp CA, Mausbach B, Granholm E, et al (2010). Mobile interventions for severe mental illness: design and preliminary data from three approaches. Journal of Nervous and Mental Disease 198: 715–721.

Ehrenreich B, Righter B, Rocke DA, Dixon L, Himelhoch S (2011). Are mobile phones and handheld computers being used to enhance delivery of psychiatric treatment? A systematic review. Journal of Nervous and Mental Disease 199: 886–891.

Flynn TM, Taylor P, Pollard CA (2013). Use of mobile phones in the behavioral treatment of driving phobias. Journal of Behavioral Therapy and Experimental Psychiatry 23: 299–302.

Fox S, Duggan M (2012). Mobile health 2012. Pew Internet: Washington, DC. Available at http://www.pewInternet.org/~/media//Files/Reports/2012/PIP_MobileHealth2012_FINAL.pdf. Retrieved on December 23, 2012.

Granholm E, Ben-Zeev D, Link PC, Bradshaw KR, Holden JL (2012). Mobile assessment and treatment for schizophrenia (MATS): a pilot trial of an interactive text-messaging intervention for medication adherence, socialization, and auditory hallucinations. Schizophrenia Bulletin 38: 414–425.

Grassi A, Preziosa A, Villani D, Riva G (2007). A relaxing journey: the use of mobile phones for well-being improvement. Annual Review of CyberTherapy and Telemedicine 5: 1–15.

Harrison V, Proudfoot J, Wee PP, et al (2011). Mobile mental health: review of the emerging field and proof of concept study. Journal of Mental Health 20: 509–524.

James S (2013). Learning from mobile health missteps (editorial). Pulse+IT Magazine, p. 6.

Kauer SD, Reid SC, Crooke AHD, et al (2012). Self-monitoring using mobile phones in the early stages of adolescent depression: randomized controlled trial. Journal of Medical Internet Research 14: e67.

Lappalainen P, Kaipainen K, Lappalainen R, et al (2013). Feasibility of a personal health technology-based psychological intervention for men with stress and mood problems: randomized controlled pilot trial. JMIR Research Protocols 2: e1.

Leach MJ (2005). Rapport: a key to treatment success. Complementary Therapies in Clinical Practice 11: 262–265.

Liberati A, Altman DG, Tetzlaff J, et al (2009). The PRISMA statement for reporting systematic reviews and meta-analyses of studies that evaluate health care interventions: explanation and elaboration. Annals of Internal Medicine 151: 65–94.

Marasinghe RB, Edirippulige S, Kavanagh D, Smith A, Jiffry MTM (2012). Original article of mobile phone-based psychotherapy in Q Effect suicide prevention: a randomized controlled trial in Sri Lanka. Journal of Telemedicine and Telecare 18: 151–155.

Miklowitz DJ, Price J, Holmes EA, et al (2012). Facilitated integrated mood management for adults with bipolar disorder. Bipolar Disorders 14: 185–197.

Morris ME, Aguilera A (2012). Mobile, social, and wearable computing and the evolution of psychological practice. Professional Psychology: Research and Practice 43: 622–626.

Morris ME, Kathawala Q, Leen TK, et al (2010). Mobile therapy: case study evaluations of a cell phone application for emotional self-awareness. Journal of Medical Internet Research 12: e10.

Pallavicini F, Algeri D, Repetto C, Gorini A, Riva G (2009). Biofeedback, virtual reality and mobile phones in the treatment of generalized anxiety disorder (GAD): a phase-2 controlled clinical trial. Journal of CyberTherapy and Rehabilitation 2: 315–327.

Preziosa A, Grassi A, Gaggioli A, Riva G (2009). Therapeutic applications of the mobile phone. British Journal of Guidance and Counselling 37: 313–325.

Proudfoot J, Clarke J, Birch M-R, et al (2013). Impact of a mobile phone and web program on symptom and functional outcomes for people with mild-to-moderate depression, anxiety and stress: a randomised controlled trial. BMC Psychiatry 13: 312.

Reid SC, Kauer SD, Dudgeon P, et al (2009). A mobile phone program to track young people's experiences of mood, stress and coping. Development and testing of the mobiletype program. Social Psychiatry and Psychiatric Epidemiology 44: 501–507.

Reid SC, Kauer SD, Hearps SJC, et al (2011). A mobile phone application for the assessment and management of youth mental health problems in primary care: a randomised controlled trial. BMC Family Practice 12: 131.

Reid SC, Kauer SD, Hearps SJC, et al (2013). A mobile phone application for the assessment and management of youth mental health problems in primary care: health service outcomes from a randomised controlled trial of mobiletype. BMC Family Practice 14: 84.

Shapiro JR, Bauer S (2010). Use of short message service (SMS)-based interventions to enhance low intensity CBT. In Bennett-Levy J, Christensen H, Farrand P, Griffiths K, Klein B, Lau MA, Proudfoot J, Kavanagh D, Editors, Oxford Guide to Low Intensity CBT Interventions. Oxford University Press, New York, NY, pp. 281–286.

Shapiro JR, Bauer S, Andrews E, et al (2010). Mobile therapy: use of text-messaging in the treatment of bulimia nervosa. International Journal of Eating Disorders 43: 513–519.

Silk JS, Steinberg L, Morris AS (2003). Adolescents' emotion regulation in daily life: links to depressive symptoms and problem behavior. Child Development 74: 1869–1880.

Smith A (2011). Americans and text messaging. Pew Internet: Washington, DC. Available at http://pewInternet.org/Reports/2011/Cell-Phone-Texting-2011.aspx. Retrieved on February 18, 2014.

Spaniel F, Vohlídka P, Hrdlicka J, et al (2008). ITAREPS: information technology aided relapse prevention programme in schizophrenia. Schizophrenia Research 98: 312–317.

Tegan S (2013). Medical apps and mobile health regulation. Pulse+IT Magazine, pp. 39–41.

Van Straten A, Seekles W, Beekman ATF, Cuijpers P (2010). Stepped care for depression in primary care: what should be offered and how? Medical Journal of Australia 192: S36–S39.

Villani D, Grassi A, Cognetta C, et al (2013). Self-help stress management training through mobile phones: an experience with oncology nurses. Psychological Services 10: 315–22.

Watts S, Mackenzie A, Thomas C, et al (2013). CBT for depression: a pilot RCT comparing mobile phone vs. computer. BMC Psychiatry 13: 49.

Whittaker R, Merry S, Stasiak K, et al (2012). MEMO—A mobile phone depression prevention intervention for adolescents: development process and postprogram findings on acceptability from a randomized controlled trial. Journal of Medical Internet Research 14: e13.

Wichers M, Hartmann J, Kramer IMA, et al (2011). Translating assessments of the film of daily life into person-tailored feedback interventions in depression. Acta Psychiatrica Scandinavica 123: 402–403.

14 Electronic Mental Health Records in the United States
Promise and Pitfalls

David J. Peterson and Jeffrey G. Miller

INTRODUCTION

It seems that almost everyone in the industrialized world is racing toward the digitalization of the patient's paper medical record. Norway leads with a reported 98% adoption rate (Gregg, 2013). According to the US Department of Health and Human Services, a significant "tipping point" has been reached with more than half of American medical providers "steering away from paper records" (Radnofsky, 2013). This is significant because, compared to other industrialized countries, the United States has been relatively slow to adopt electronic health records (EHRs), ranking only seventh behind Norway, the Netherlands, the United Kingdom, New Zealand, Australia, and Germany in a recent survey (Gregg, 2013).

In the United States, there is a long list of incentives and benefits for patients, physicians, and group practices to adopt EHRs. Some are financial and are directed toward the provider. Others can be described as "just better health care" and include "a reduction in the incidence of medical errors, readily available health information, reduction of duplicate tests, reductions in treatment delays and better informed patients making better decisions" (Centers for Medicare and Medicaid Services, 2009, p. 1). A 2013 survey of 3700 primary and specialty care physicians from eight countries demonstrates the growing acceptance of EHRs. It concludes that physicians in the United States believed they "achieved . . . improved decision-making and the reduction of medical errors" through use of EHRs (Accenture, 2013, p. 7).

Government policy has also helped accelerate the adoption of EHRs. The 2009 Health Information Technology for Economic and Clinical Health (HITECH) Act offered financial incentives for physicians who incorporate electronic records into their practices and introduced penalties for those who fail to do so (Porter, 2013). The penalties are set to start in 2015 and will be realized through reduced reimbursement for treating patients (Radnofsky, 2013). As a result, EHR adoption has significantly increased. But in the mental health profession, the interest has lagged. If Google search results can be considered a surrogate for measuring interest in a topic, a general search under the term "electronic health record" yields more than 88 million results. When the search is narrowed down to "mental health and electronic health record," the yield is reduced by more than half. Further refining the search to "mental health and electronic health record and confidentiality" returns 2 million results. Thus, as the topic moves from an electronic health record to an electronic mental health record, the visibility in the ether clearly declines.

One could point to the stigma attached to mental illness to partially explain these results. The stigma seems widely prevalent across patients, cultures, and even health care professionals. A 2006 Australian study found that nearly one in four people thought depression was a sign of personal weakness (Government of Western Australia Mental Health Commission, 2014). Such sentiment has led health care organizations such as the Mayo Clinic to offer specific coping strategies to address the shame still associated with mental illness (Mayo Clinic, 2014). This is hardly only a lay person's problem; a 2013 report by the Mental Health Commission of Canada showed that "some of the most deeply felt stigma" came from health care professionals themselves (Pellegrini, 2014, p. 1). As an example, the report describes the physician's "failure to investigate a patient's pain symptoms because. . . [of a] history of mental illness" (Pellegrini, 2014, p. 1).

It follows that a potentially stigmatizing record should be heavily guarded. Linked to stigma is the issue of privacy and the need to maintain confidentiality. Although those are crucial to the maintenance of any medical record, they take on particular significance when it comes to mental health records. In an article on electronic mental health records, Bresnick (2013, p. 1) argues that there is a "myth in the healthcare industry that mental health is somehow a world apart from antibiotics, physicals and x-rays. Most of the time, mental health records are collected separately, stored separately, and treated as an issue of secondary importance." "Privacy," Bresnick continues, "is most often cited as the reason why it's too difficult to integrate mental health records with the rest of the patient's electronic record" (Bresnick, 2013, p. 2). Indeed, there are legitimate legal (in the form of legislation protecting privacy) and ethical issues regarding patient privacy. This focus on privacy and the mandated protections it has spawned represent the principal challenges to the integration of mental health information into the EHR. The aim of this chapter is to review advantages and disadvantages of electronic mental health records and discuss their implications for patient care in the United States.

Understanding the challenge of integrating mental health information into the EHR requires an understanding of the legislation protecting the confidentiality of mental health information and the mental health profession's obligations to confidentiality.

In the United States, the first formal attempt to protect the confidentiality of patient health information dates back to the passage of the Drug Abuse Prevention, Treatment and Rehabilitation Act of 1972. Unless a patient's consent was obtained, this regulation prohibited the disclosure of any information about patients in federally assisted alcohol and drug abuse programs. It was described as one of the "strongest federal and state patient confidentiality laws" and required compliance from any provider in alcohol or drug abuse treatment programs (Peterson and Wickeham, 2011, p. 77).

The Health Insurance Portability and Accountability Act (HIPAA) was passed in 1996. In addition to ensuring some portability of health insurance, the HIPAA also contained more rules regarding the privacy and security of patient health information. With regard to safeguarding mental health information, HIPAA specifically addressed protections around "psychotherapy note(s)," defining them as notes written by a mental health professional "documenting or analyzing the contents of conversations during a private or a group, joint, or family counseling session and that are separated from the rest of the individual's medical record" (US Department of Health and Human Services, 2003, p. 21). To capture the additional protections afforded the psychotherapy note, the note had to be maintained and housed separately from the general medical record. The psychotherapy note definition, however, expressly excludes medication prescriptions and monitoring, counseling session start and stop times, the modalities and frequencies of treatment furnished, results of clinical tests, and any summary of the diagnosis, functional status, treatment plan, symptoms, prognosis, and progress to date, whereas it allows for this information to be included in the progress note (US Department of Health and Human Services, 2003, p. 21). Naturally, this affects the type and amount of mental health information that can be maintained and integrated with the general medical EHR (Peterson and Wickeham, 2011). In fact, Smolyansky et al. (2013) argue that once providers fully understood the definition of true psychotherapy notes and that their notes were progress notes as opposed to psychotherapy notes, integrating mental health records into the main medical record would be deemed appropriate and in accordance with HIPAA. They also report that when implementing an HIPAA-compliant EHR system at Cincinnati Children's Hospital Medical Center, a consensus was reached that all of the medical record is to be considered confidential and that denying access to portions of the record to other members of the health care team can jeopardize patient safety.

Although EHRs offer providers a more complete view of a patient's medical history, most of them contain features with additional levels of confidentiality for the mental health portion. These protections vary by product, but they are similar in intent. One such protection is often referred to as "break the glass." This allows providers to access mental health notes within the EHR but requires them to electronically acknowledge that they are accessing confidential information. This creates a "digital trail" that can be reviewed to determine the legitimacy of the need for access. But this is not universal. Some EHRs do not require primary care or emergency department care providers to take such additional "break the glass" steps, because it is deemed that their access to the entirety of the medical record is necessary for the safety and quality of patient care delivery.

Moreover, 2009 saw the adoption of federal legislation that introduced financial incentives and penalties to stimulate the adoption of EHRs. Known as the HITECH Act, it encouraged health care providers to adopt EHRs and added penalties and fines for breaches of protected data and inappropriate disclosures by providers. Overall, the HITECH Act aimed to assist with the development of "meaningful use" of the EHR. The goals of meaningful use are to improve quality, safety, and efficiency of health care; reduce health care disparities; engage patients and families; improve care coordination; ensure adequate privacy and security protections; and promote the exchange of electronic data (Ancker et al., 2012).

Finally, the next few years will most likely witness new policies that stem from the 2010 United States Patient Protection and Affordable Care Act and the 2008 Paul Wellstone Mental Health and Addiction Equity Act (Tai et al., 2012). These policies will expand health care coverage to previously uninsured individuals and provide parity in insurance coverage for mental health and substance use problems. For this to be realized relatively smoothly, there will be increased demand to integrate mental health services into primary care and to standardize behavioral and psychosocial data, which should be facilitated by using an integrated EHR. This will be especially important for the many patients with coexisting psychiatric and physical health conditions (Tai et al., 2012).

Sometimes the mental health profession itself complicates the integration of mental health information into the EHR. For many mental health professionals, the compact between patient and provider to protect privacy is sacrosanct and inviolable, and this often translates into resistance to participation in any development of an integrated record. But although the development of integrated EHRs can raise confidentiality concerns, one questions how integrated the care really can be if only a few members of the health care team have all the information. Indeed, a 2011 meeting of the National Institutes of Health and the Society for Behavioral Medicine concluded that the integration of health data could enhance care quality, patient-centeredness, and the efficiency of patient-provider encounters (Institute of Medicine, 2011).

Navigating federal law (not to mention state laws) and the profession's long-held conventions on patient privacy are real challenges. However, data from interviews with providers suggest that after implementing and utilizing an EHR, most of those challenges seem to dissipate. According to Smolyansky et al. (2013), 4 years after implementing EPIC, one of the most popular integrated EHRs in the United States, "the hesitations initially voiced about an integrated electronic medical record are gone" (p. 21). Furthermore, Clemens (2012) argues that as the interaction of physical and psychiatric disorders becomes better understood, and as the somewhat artificial barriers between them fall, there will be a trend toward assuming that psychiatric treatments "no longer carry the stigma traditionally ascribed to them and they can be integrated with general medical care" (p. 46). To that end, mental health providers can do more to help eliminate stigma. Many providers seem more concerned about having a diagnosis of depression than human immunodeficiency virus on a patient's "problem list," begging the question of which carries more stigma.

PROMISES

Despite the controversy surrounding the implementation of electronic health and mental health records, legislative, economic and industry forces will continue to push for their adoption. The potential benefits of this move cannot be ignored. These benefits include increased efficiency, improved access to medical information and medical records, remote access in critical situations, avoidance of medication errors and drug interactions, availability of aggregated data for analysis and research, reduction in medical errors and costs, prevention of loss of records, and patient empowerment through greater engagement in health care provision. Blumenthal (2009) identified that the goals of transitioning to electronic records were to improve patient care through use of quality measures, care coordination, widespread data exchange, enhanced patient access to health records, and implementation of the required standards of care to ensure health record privacy and security. Reitz et al. (2012) described benefits that included increased long-term efficiency, improved organization, and a more complete record. In their study, most respondents believed that EHRs brought added value to interdisciplinary communication, made them aware of other providers' treatment plans, and enabled them to better support those treatment plans. For Takian et al. (2012), who reported on implementing an integrated EHR in England, the benefits also included greater safety because some mentally ill individuals may not be able to provide adequate history. By providing context and background, EHRs can be a valuable tool in diagnosis and treatment.

A major advantage of an integrated EHR is access to the patient information by the interdisciplinary team. This allows integration of services and helps coordinate care. Such access will be particularly essential as mental health services become increasingly embedded in primary care and other specialty clinics. Consequently, an "unintegrated" EHR might be counterproductive in that it would defeat the purpose of integrated care. For example, a mental health intervention is often requested to help patients cope better with a medical diagnosis and increase their adherence to medication regimens. If the medical team is unable to review the mental health provider's notes and has to rely on face-to-face or other forms of communication, how would the team members know in a reliable and timely manner when to move forward with medications or other treatment goals?

Another major benefit of the EHR is increased efficiency. Building and incorporating "charting templates" in the record has resulted in more consistency in documenting the patient encounter while enabling pertinent data to be imported into the encounter note. An undeniable added advantage is improved legibility; one only has to review old paper charts to recall the poor quality of documentation and the frequent difficulty with reading notes. Completeness is another benefit of the EHR. For example, an integrated record will contain a comprehensive current and past medication list. The list will include medications and their doses as prescribed by all providers involved in the patient's care and will automatically alert the prescriber to potentially harmful interactions. No longer would the provider have to wonder about the identity and strength of "blue blood pressure pill" the patient takes in the morning. Furthermore, the ability to electronically prescribe simplifies the traditionally time-consuming process of writing each prescription by hand. Like electronic notes, electronic prescriptions are also legible, decreasing guesswork and follow-up phone calls between pharmacy and prescriber.

Finally, many proponents point to "patient empowerment" as an advantage of EHRs. This can occur by electronically allowing patients to access predetermined portions of their medical record, such as laboratory results, and by facilitating communication with their provider (Tennessee Office of eHealth Initiatives, 2012, p. 1). Similar to an e-mail system, this communication is protected within the EHR and becomes part of the medical record. It allows patients to ask questions, provide health updates, request refills, and schedule appointments. The provider, in turn, can respond. All this is accomplished within the security of the EHR and with increased time savings for both provider and patient. Patient access to EHRs and communication with providers are, in fact, measures of "meaningful use."

Two case illustrations inspired by real patients suggest the advantages of a properly integrated EHR.

The first case describes a patient before the implementation of an EHR. This patient had been treated in an outpatient mental health clinic for major depressive disorder and had made several suicide attempts. Following an exacerbation in his mood, he was dropped off by family members at the emergency department of the hospital associated with his outpatient clinic. The patient requested hospitalization for depression but denied having a history of psychiatric treatment or any previous suicidal thinking or attempts. Although his outpatient treatment had occurred at the same facility, his psychiatric records were separate and inaccessible. He was therefore admitted to the inpatient unit on standard observation precautions. Within 24 hours of admission, he had hung himself on the ward. One wonders whether the outcome might have been different if the admitting physician had had access to the patient's outpatient record and, as a result, had ordered closer monitoring and more frequent safety checks.

A second case depicts a patient after the implementation of an EHR. Although the mental health record was integrated into the electronic chart, it was "hidden" from other providers with no "break the glass" feature available. The patient had a tendency to seek out multiple providers for opiate medications. The psychiatrist had clearly identified this in his note and strongly discouraged other providers from prescribing those medications to the patient. However, because his note was not visible to the primary care physician, the patient obtained more medication from this provider only 2 days after the psychiatrist had made his recommendation. Two days after the patient was given the additional prescription, she was admitted to the medical unit in a delirious state from an unintentional overdose on opiate medications. Again, the outcome might have been different if the primary care provider had been able to see the psychiatrist's note.

PITFALLS

Although the advantages of EHRs are many, there are a few pitfalls. A recent issue of *Medical Economics* (2013) ranks 100 companies that produce an EHR in the United States. To be sure, a handful of them dominate the market, but when one assesses, as the journal did, many versions of EHRs available for sale, one realizes the truth of the adage, "if you've seen one EHR, you've seen one EHR." With so many systems on the market, standardization is almost nonexistent, communication between them is spotty, and the features and capabilities of each range from minimal to robust. Such inconsistencies contribute to provider dissatisfaction with EHRs, can slow their adoption rate, and are often cited as reasons not to use EHRs because patients using multiple health care systems will not have their complete medical chart in one EHR (Verdon, 2014).

Also, considerable staff, capital, and ongoing financial resources are required to launch and maintain EHRs. Providers and other clinic staff need to be trained on systems, which can be costly and requires that staff take time away from other responsibilities to attend training sessions. In addition, there are difficulties during the initial implementation. This has forced many clinics to decrease the number of patients scheduled for several weeks after the launch of EHRs, as staff become more familiar with it (Takian et al., 2012; Smolyansky et al., 2013). Beyond that, remaining current is crucial and requires regular retraining and the installation of system upgrades; this represents an ongoing commitment in time and money.

Furthermore, providers have stated that the EHR terminal and keyboard become "the third person" in the room, which can have a negative impact on the provider-patient relationship (Cerrato, 2013). Because mental health interventions are built around a solid rapport with patients, this can pose particular challenges. Indeed, mental health providers have lagged behind other medical professionals in adopting EHRs (Clemens, 2012). Part of their hesitation can be explained by loss of eye contact with patients while entering data, which could weaken the therapeutic bond and the communication of empathy and lead to reticence and withholding on the part of patients. Still, others have found that an EHR can actually facilitate conversation by serving as an "ice breaker" and have successfully incorporated it into the patient encounter and used it as an information tool. Regarding patients' perspectives, Smolyansky et al. (2013) reported that the use of EHRs by mental health providers was viewed as neutral to positive in anecdotal patient feedback. Patients familiar with EHRs typically had no concerns with the inclusion of their mental health records in the EHR.

The biggest pitfall surrounding EHR adoption, however, is the fear of potential abuse or loss of confidential health information. These issues account for the penalties embedded in the HITECH Act and HIPAA legislation, their emphasis on data protection, and their careful identification and definition of what data are protected. But, conversely, one could also argue that confidentiality is actually enhanced with an EHR, because it is possible to digitally track any access to protected information. Prior to EHRs, there were rooms and storage units full of filing cabinets with paper charts, and unauthorized staff members could view any record without being caught. Now there is the possibility of an audit trail to track whether a chart has been accessed, by whom, and when, all in an effort to protect patient confidentiality.

CONCLUSION

In an age where digital technology permeates every aspect of life, the movement to digitalize the medical record is hardly surprising, and incorporating a patient's mental health information into it seems like a natural corollary. But it is also unsurprising that a record so intensely personal should, in its digital incarnation, continue to require careful protections guaranteed in traditional charting. These protections have made their way into regulations and legislation to ensure that confidentiality is respected and that compliance is maintained, while simultaneously allowing the delivery of integrated health care. On balance, most would probably argue that there are more advantages than disadvantages to the integration of mental health information into the EHR. Legislative efforts seem to support this integration, financial incentives (and penalties) are being built to encourage it, and there seems to be growing awareness from providers and patients alike that better health care can result from it. Properly coordinated, integrated medical and mental health care can result in more efficient and less error-prone care. All this arguably translates into improved wellbeing for individuals and populations.

However, the integration of information that by nature is deeply personal and potentially damaging cannot unfold recklessly. It requires material and human resources, a well-trained staff, financial and operational sustainability, knowledge of the regulatory and legal environments, and familiarity with policies and protocols developed to protect the confidentiality and integrity of both the medical and mental health records. Ensuring that all this is in place represents a challenge. In addition, there is a question of an unknown and potentially negative impact of the use of digital technology on the relationship between patients and mental health professionals.

The physicians Robin Cook and Eric Topol may have summed it up best in an opinion piece for the *Wall Street Journal*; "digital medicine is coming over the next few years with the force of a hurricane whether we doctors—and we patients—are ready or not" (Cook and Topol, 2014). "This is huge," and a "large benefit from this new world of digital medicine will come in lower costs... but we'll also have to deal with problems and unanticipated consequences, *mostly related to privacy* [emphasis added]" (Cook and Topol, 2014). Mental health information will be in the eye of this hurricane, providing a powerful example of the promise of digitalized medicine, so long as the pitfalls—primarily relating to compromised privacy—can be avoided.

DISCLOSURE STATEMENT

The authors disclose no relationships with commercial entities and professional activities that may bias their views.

REFERENCES

Accenture (2013). Doctors survey: US country profile. Available at http://www.accenture.com/SiteCollectionDocuments/PDF/Accenture-Doctors-Survey-US-Country-Profile-Report.pdf Retrieved on March 21, 2013.

Ancker JS, Edwards AM, Miller MC, Kaushal R (2012). Consumer perceptions of electronic health information exchange. American Journal of Preventive Medicine 43: 76–80.

Blumenthal D (2009). Stimulating the adoption of health information technology. New England Journal of Medicine 360: 1477–1479.

Bresnick J (2013). The missing link: making the case for EHRs in behavioral health. Available at http://ehrintelligence.com/2013/05/17/the-missing-link-making-the-case-for-ehrs-in-behavioral-health/ Retrieved on March 21, 2014.

Centers for Medicare and Medicaid Services (2009). Medicare and Medicaid health information technology. Title IV of the American Recovery and Reinvestment Act. Available at http://www.cms.gov/apps/media/press/factsheet.asp?Counter=3466 Retrieved on May 10, 2014.

Cerrato P (2013). Do your EHR manners turn patients off? Available at http://medscape.com/viewarticle/809237 Retrieved on May 23, 2014.

Clemens NA (2012). Privacy, consent, and the electronic mental health record: the person vs. the system. Journal of Psychiatric Practice 18: 46–50.

Cook R, Topol E (2014). How digital medicine will soon save your life. Available at http://online.wsj.com/news/articles/SB10001424052702303973704579351080028045594 Retrieved on March 21, 2014.

Government of Western Australia Mental Health Commission (2014). What is stigma? Available at http://www.mentalhealth.wa.gov.au/mental_illness_and_health/mh_stigma.aspx Retrieved on March 21, 2014.

Gregg H (2013). Top 10 countries for EHR adoption. Available at http://www.beckershospitalreview.com/healthcare-information-technology/top-10-countries-for-ehr-adoption.html Retrieved on March 21, 2014.

Institute of Medicine (2011). Engineering a Learning Healthcare System: A Look at the Future-Workshop Summary. National Academies Press, Washington, DC.

Mayo Clinic (2014). Mental health: overcoming the stigma of mental illness. Available at http://www.mayoclinic.org/diseases-conditions/mental-illness/in-depth/mental-health/art-20046477 Retrieved on March 21, 2014.

Medical Economics (2013). The top 100 EHR companies. Available at http://medicaleconomics.modernmedicine.com/medical-economics/news/top-100-ehr-companies-part-4-4 Retrieved on March 21, 2014.

Pellegrini C (2014). Mental illness stigma in health care settings a barrier to care. Canadian Medical Association Journal 186: E17.

Peterson D, Wickeham D (2011). New challenge for academic psychiatry: the electronic health record. Academic Psychiatry 35: 76–79.

Porter M (2013). Adoption of electronic health records in the United States. Available at https://xnet.kp.org/kpinternational/other/otherUS/html Retrieved on March 21, 2014.

Radnofsky L (2013). Electronic health data gaining favor. Available at http://online.wsj.com/news/articles/SB10001424127887323463704584 Retrieved on March 21, 2014.

Reitz R, Common K, Fifield P, Stiasny E (2012). Collaboration in the presence of an electronic health record. Families, Systems & Health 30: 72–80.

Smolyansky BH, Stark LJ, Pendley J, Robins PM, Price K (2013). Confidentiality and electronic medical records for behavioral health records: the experience of pediatric psychologists at four children's hospitals. Clinical Practice in Pediatric Psychology 1: 18–27.

Tai B, Boyle M, Ghitza U, Kaplan RM, Clark HW, Gersing K (2012). Meaningful use of electronic behavioral health data in primary health care. Science Translational Medicine 4: 119mr3.

Takian A, Sheikh A, Barber N (2012). We are bitter, but we are better off: case study of the implementation of an electronic health record system into a mental health hospital in England. BMC Health Services Research 12: 484.

Tennessee Office of eHealth Initiatives (2012). Electronic health records. Available at http://www.tn.gov/ehealth/ehr.shtml Retrieved on May 23, 2014.

United States Department of Health and Human Services (2003). Summary of the HIPAA privacy rule. Available at http://hhs.gov/ocr/privacy/hipaa/understanding/summary/privacysummary.pdf Retrieved on March 28, 2013.

Verdon D (2014). Physician outcry on EHR functionality, cost will shake the health information technology sector. Available at http://medicaleconomics.modernmedicine.com/medcidal-econcomics//news/physician-outcry-ehr-functionality-cost-will-shake-health-information-technol Retrieved on March 21, 2014.

Index

Page numbers followed by "f" and "t" indicate figures and tables.